BREAST CANCER:
TRENDS IN RESEARCH AND TREATMENT

MONOGRAPH SERIES OF THE EUROPEAN ORGANIZATION FOR RESEARCH ON TREATMENT OF CANCER

The Monograph Series of the EORTC deals with selected topics related to cancer treatment. Volumes are usually, but not necessarily, based on the proceedings of an EORTC symposium. The responsibility of the Editorial Advisory Board is to approve the subject of each monograph; the Board does not review individual manuscripts.

Breast Cancer:
Trends in Research and Treatment

A Monograph of the
European Organization for Research on
Treatment of Cancer

Editors

Jean-Claude Heuson, M.D.

Associate Professor
Associate Attending Physician
Department of Medicine
Institut Jules Bordet
Tumor Center of the Free University
  of Brussels
Brussels, Belgium

Wolrad H. Mattheiem, M.D.

Associate Professor
Head, Breast and Pelvic Service
Department of Surgery
Institut Jules Bordet
Tumor Center of the Free University
  of Brussels
Brussels, Belgium

Marcel Rozencweig, M.D.

Department of Medicine
Institut Jules Bordet
Tumor Center of the Free University
  of Brussels
Brussels, Belgium

Raven Press ■ New York

Raven Press, 1140 Avenue of the Americas, New York, New York 10036

Made in the United States of America

International Standard Book Number 0-89004-096-6
Library of Congress Catalog Card Number 76-22910

Preface

The First EORTC Breast Cancer Working Conference, on which this volume is based, was held in September 1975. The conference was a logical outcome of many years of work by the EORTC Breast Cancer Cooperative Group[1], and a necessary starting point for expanding its activities and implementing new projects.

The methodology of multi-institutional clinical trials had been well established and was ready for testing new ideas. Elaboration of new projects implied full participation of all specialists in the various disciplines involved in breast cancer research. The first goal of the conference was to exchange mutual information among these researchers and particularly among basic researchers, clinicians, and epidemiologists. The presentations and especially the roundtable discussions following each session indicate that this goal was fully achieved.

Eminent specialists from Europe and the United States described the current status of knowledge in virology, immunology, and endocrinology in relation to breast cancer in both humans and experimental models. The results of palliative treatments and of the recently introduced use of postoperative chemotherapy aiming at the definitive cure of poor-prognosis cases were reported and assessed. The concept and usefulness of early detection and mass screening were debated.

This volume, based on the proceedings of the conference, includes chapters on virology, immunology, experimental models, endocrine aspects, palliative treatment, curative treatment, epidemiology, and screening, as well as section introductions and roundtable discussions. It should appeal to the breast cancer specialist interested in an updating of the subject and to the physician confronted with breast cancer in his daily practice.

The conference pursued a second objective and indeed a more ambitious one: to bring together experimentalists and clinicians in order to carry out well-defined projects directed toward the common target—a better understanding of and the appropriate means of prevention, detection, and cure of breast cancer. The EORTC Breast Cancer Task Force was created to fulfill this second objective as reported in the last section of this volume. It assigned to itself the task of defining key research projects, encouraging teams to implement them, and finding the necessary funds.

---

[1] The EORTC Breast Cancer Cooperative Group was created by Professor H. J. Tagnon in 1958. It is composed of 15 active members from various European countries. Chairman: J. C. Heuson. Secretary: W. H. Mattheiem.

We believe we have succeeded in achieving our first objective, as evidenced by this volume. It is our strong hope that within a year or two a second publication will demonstrate the validity of our efforts and the success of the EORTC Breast Cancer Task Force.

The Editors

Acknowledgments

I wish to acknowledge the many people who helped organize the symposium on which this volume is based. The Programme Committee formulated the framework and selected and invited the speakers, chairmen of the sessions, and members of the Roundtables. We are especially indebted to the participants. Dr. Mattheiem, Secretary of the Breast Cancer Group, is to be thanked, as is Dr. Staquet, coordinator of the EORTC, who was a very helpful adviser and who obtained the participation of Raven Press for the rapid publication of the proceedings. Dr. Staquet's secretary, Miss Dominique Eeckhoudt, was of invaluable help. Dr. Rozencweig, Secretary of the symposium, has undoubtedly been the major instrument in the success of the symposium. He mastered the organizational problems, which proved unexpectedly numerous, with remarkable efficiency. We are all indebted to him. The enthusiastic drive of Dr. Tagnon, Chairman of the EORTC, is gratefully acknowledged.

Finally, I wish to acknowledge the very generous technical and financial support of Imperial Chemical Industries.

J. C. Heuson

Contents

Virology

Immunology

Experimental Models

Endocrine Aspects

Palliative Treatment

Contributors

Etienne-Emile Baulieu

Unité de Recherches sur le Métabolisme Moléculaire et la Physio-Pathologie des Stéroides de l'Institut National de la Santé et de la Recherche Médicale Département de Chimie Biologique Faculté de Médecine Paris-Sud 94270 Bicêtre, France

P. Bentvelzen

Radiobiological Institute TNO Rijswijk, The Netherlands

Arthur E. Bogden

Department of Immunobiology Mason Research Institute Worcester, Massachusetts 01608

Gianni Bonadonna

Istituto Nazionale Tumori Milan 20133, Italy

R. D. Bulbrook

Department of Clinical Endocrinology Imperial Cancer Research Fund Laboratories Lincoln's Inn Fields London WC2A 3PX, England

Paul P. Carbone

Eastern Cooperative Oncology Group 850 Sligo Avenue, Suite 601 Silver Springs, Maryland 20910

Stephen K. Carter

Northern California Cancer Program 770 Welch Road Palo Alto, California 94010

D. Colcher

Meloy Laboratories Springfield, Virginia 22150

M. De La Garza

University of Texas Health Science Center San Antonio, Texas 78284

W. Drohan

Meloy Laboratories Springfield, Virginia 22150

E. Engelsman

Antoni van Leeuwenhoek Ziekenhuis The Netherlands Cancer Institute Amsterdam, The Netherlands

J. C. Heuson

Department of Medicine Institut Jules Bordet Tumor Center of the Free University of Brussels 1000 Brussels, Belgium

J. A. Heuson-Stiennon

Laboratoire d'Histologie Faculté de Médecine Université Libre de Bruxelles Brussels, Belgium

J. Hilgers

Department of Biology The Netherlands Cancer Institute Amsterdam, The Netherlands

K. B. Horwitz

University of Texas Health Science Center San Antonio, Texas 78284

P. Kimball

Meloy Laboratories Springfield, Virginia 22150

R. J. B. King

Hormone Biochemistry Department Imperial Cancer Research Fund

Lincoln's Inn Fields
London WC2A 3PX, England

G. Leclercq

Service de Médecine et Laboratoire
    d'Investigation Clinique
Institut Jules Bordet
1000 Brussels, Belgium

N. Legros

Service de Médecine et Laboratoire
    d'Investigation Clinique
Institut Jules Bordet
1000 Brussels, Belgium

Marc Lippman

Medicine Branch
National Cancer Institute
National Institutes of Health
Bethesda, Maryland 20014

Zoltan J. Lucas

Department of Surgery
Stanford University
Stanford, California 94305

Wolrad H. Mattheiem

Department of Surgery
Institut Jules Bordet
Tumor Center of the Free University
    of Brussels
1000 Brussels, Belgium

W. L. McGuire

University of Texas Health
    Science Center
San Antonio, Texas 78284

R. Michalides

The Netherlands Cancer Institute
Amsterdam, The Netherlands

J. L. Pasteels

Laboratoire d'Histologie
Faculté de Médecine
Université Libre de Bruxelles
Brussels, Belgium

J. Schlom

National Cancer Institute
National Institutes of Health
Bethesda, Maryland 20014

G. Schochetman

Meloy Laboratories
Springfield, Virginia 22150

J. A. Smith

Hormone Biochemistry Department
Imperial Cancer Research Fund
Lincoln's Inn Fields
London WC2A 3PX, England

Agnes M. Stark

Women's Cancer Detection Society
Department of Gynaecological Oncology
Queen Elizabeth Hospital
Gateshead
Tyne & Wear, England

Henri J. Tagnon

Service de Médecine Interne et
    Laboratoires d'Investigation Clinique
Institut Jules Bordet
1000 Brussels, Belgium

D. Jane Taylor

Breast Cancer Program Coordinating
    Branch
Division of Cancer Biology and
    Diagnosis
National Cancer Institute
National Institutes of Health
Bethesda, Maryland 20014

Pinuccia Valagussa

Istituto Nazionale Tumori
Milan 20133, Italy

Umberto Veronesi

Istituto Nazionale Tumori
Milan 20133, Italy

Marvin Zelen

State University of New York at Buffalo
Buffalo, New York 14226

Discussants

P. Alberto
P. Band
E. E. Baulieu
P. Bentvelzen
A. Billiau
J. Blonk-Van Der Wijst
A. E. Bogden
G. Bonadonna
R. D. Bulbrook
A. Burny
P. P. Carbone
S. K. Carter
A. Clarysse
F. J. Cleton
J. L. Daehnfeldt
E. Engelsman
H. Hansen
J. L. Hayward
J. C. Heuson
J. Hildebrand
J. Hilgers
W. F. Jungi
P. Juret
Y. Kenis
R. J. B. King
I. Konyves

F. Labrie
G. Leclerq
F. J. Lejeune
M. Lippman
Z. L. Lucas
H. Maass
W. H. Mattheiem
W. L. McGuire
H. Mouridsen
T. Palshof
T. Powles
L. M. van Putten
M. A. Rich
C. Robyn
S. Saez
J. Schlom
M. Spittle
A. M. Stark
J. S. Stjernsward
H. J. Tagnon
L. Thiry
M. Tubiana
D. Vakil
J. Wybran
M. Zelen

Breast Cancer: Trends in Research and Treatment, edited by J. C. Heuson,
W. H. Mattheiem, and M. Rozencweig. Raven Press, New York © 1976.

Introduction: Virology

A. Billiau

This volume was organized to evaluate the present status in combating human
mammary cancer. The motive for starting with mammary tumor virus is, to my
understanding at least, an irrational one. For although clinicians and epidemiologists—and many experimental workers as well—are aware of the possibility that
mammary cancer in man may ultimately be found to be caused by a virus, little
role is played by this awareness in the current daily strategy to combat cancer. So
the virus believed to be at the origin of cancer is like a transcendent principle, a
god in whom they believe but over whom they have no power—a god whom they
venerate every now and then (at meetings such as this for example) but who has
little significance to the daily routine. So in starting with virology, I think the
organizers have tried to placate the transcendent—the virus that is perhaps at the
root of the worries which bring us here. Therefore they have invited several of the
high priests of the virus to tell us about mammary tumor virus.

At present it is established that cancer results from delicate changes in the
genetic makeup of the cell, that viruses DNA as well as RNA can change the
genetic makeup of the cell by incorporating some or all of their viral genome in
that of the cell. In this way the viruses can replicate and transmit themselves,
either by going from cell to cell in repeating infectious cycles or by replicating in
conjunction with the cellular genome. Some of the material presented here pertains to this aspect. The viral genetic information in cells can be detected by
comparing nucleic acids of cells with those of the viruses that are incriminated,
and secondly by looking for proteins which correspond not to the cellular genes
but to some of the genes of the incriminated viruses. Similarly, *in vivo,* viruses
and especially cancer viruses can be transmitted horizontally, as occurs for most
common virus diseases, or vertically, from parents to offspring, as is most often
the case for oncogenic viruses. Virologists therefore believe that cancer is caused
by viruses which we inherit from our parents, rather than by viruses which infect
us during our lifetime, and mammary tumor virus in mice has been shown to be
transmitted from parent to offspring in several ways, including the secretion of
virus particles in the milk. The next chapters will therefore discuss the following
concepts:

(1) the vertical transmission of mammary tumor virus, including the presence of
   virus in milk;

1

(2) the presence of viral nucleic acid sequences in mammary tumors of animals and man; and

(3) the presence of virus-coded proteins in mammary tumors.

Breast Cancer: Trends in Research and Treatment, edited by J. C. Heuson, W. H. Mattheiem, and M. Rozencweig. Raven Press, New York © 1976.

Interaction Between Viral and Genetic Factors in Murine Mammary Cancer: Possible Implications for Human Disease

J. Hilgers and P. Bentvelzen

Department of Biology, The Netherlands Cancer Institute, Sarphatistraat 108, Amsterdam; and Radiobiological Institute, TNO, Rijswijk, The Netherlands

The concept of breast cancer as a hereditary disease finds its origin in the familiar occurrence in man (1). The existence of mouse families with either a high or a low incidence of mammary cancer leads to the same hypothesis, which was substantiated by the development of genetically homogenous mouse strains (for review, see ref. 2). However, the use of these inbred strains permitted discovery of an extrachromosomal factor that has been proved to be a virus (3).

This virus, exhibiting milk transmission, prompted intensive research for a maternal effect in man. Failure in this respect has been interpreted as evidence against the viral nature of the human disease. However, there seem to be some molecular biological indications for the implication of viral genetic material in human breast cancer (4). This apparent contradiction compels us to "revisit the mouse world" for an analysis of the biology of mouse mammary tumor viruses, particularly in regard to transmission and virus-host genetic interactions.

Since discovery of the milk factor by Bittner, the finding of genetic transmission by Mühlbock and Bentvelzen (5) has changed the outlook on the necessity of milk transmission as proof for a viral etiology completely. The various modes of transmission of mammary tumor virus (MTV) known today are presented in Table 1. After the initial discovery of milk transmission (3), confirmed by Andervont and McEleney (6) and Van Gulik and Korteweg (7), Fekete and Little (8) noted some indications for transplacental transmission. As far as we can evaluate, this is a rather erratic event. More important seems to be the extrachromosomal male transmission discovered by Andervont (9) and confirmed by Foulds (10), Mühlbock (11), and Bittner (12). In most cases the infection is transmitted by the mother, who transfers the virus via the milk after infection during mating. In a few instances there is direct infection of the zygotes *in utero* (13). A still unconfirmed mode of transmission was described by Peacock (14), where the newborns could be infected by drops of semen of the infected male, which starts to copulate directly after the partus.

3

TABLE 1. *Discoveries of the various modes of transmission of mammary tumor virus*

Mode of transmission/discoverer	Year	Reference
Extrachromosomal vertical		
Staff, Jackson Laboratories	1933	*Science*, 78:465
Korteweg	1934	*Ned. Tijdschr. Geneeskund.*, 78:240
Milk		
Bittner	1936	*Science*, 84:162
Andervont and McEleney	1938	*Public Health Rep.*, 53:777
Van Gulik and Korteweg	1940	*Proc. Kon. Ned. Akad. Wetensch.*, C43:58
Transplacental[a]		
Fekete and Little	1942	*Cancer Res.*, 2:525
Male (indirect) via mother		
Andervont	1945	*J. Natl. Cancer Inst.*, 5:391
Foulds	1949	*Br. J. Cancer*, 3:230
Mühlbock	1952	*J. Natl. Cancer Inst.*, 12:819
Bittner	1952	*Cancer Res.*, 12:387
Male (direct) *in utero*		
Andervont	1963	*J. Natl. Cancer Inst.*, 31:261
Male (direct) postnatally[a]		
Peacock	1953	*Br. J. Cancer*, 7:352
Chromosomal vertical		
Male		
Bentvelzen	1968	Thesis, Hollandia, Amsterdam
Mühlbock and Bentvelzen	1968	*Perspect. Virol.*, 6:75
Female		
Zeilmaker	1969	*Int. J. Cancer*, 4:261
Horizontal		
Arthropod-borne[a]		
Pogossiantz	1956	*Acta Un. Int. Cancr.*, 12:690
Cage[a]		
Stutman	1975	*Unpublished observations*

[a]Not confirmed.

Besides "extrachromosomal vertical transmission," there are some indications for horizontal transmission, i.e., transmission of one individual to another irrespective of relationship. Pogossiantz (15) reported transmission of the virus from a high-cancer strain to a susceptible low-cancer strain by means of fleas. In general, experiments on horizontal transmission in "insect-free" environments yielded negative results, although there is a recent claim that inside the cage such transmission might take place with low efficiency, resulting in some late-appearing tumors (Stutman, *personal communication*).

Mühlbock (16) described a new mouse strain of European origin, the GR strain, which has a high incidence of mammary tumors at an early age, and of which either sex can transmit the virus very effectively. When introduced into other mouse strains the virus did not show any capacity for male transmission, indicating that this property was controlled for by the GR host genome (17). Subsequent analysis demonstrated this property to depend on a single mendelian factor. It was hypothesized that this gene represents a DNA provirus (i.e., a DNA copy of the viral genome in the host genome), and thus the virus would be transmitted as a genetic factor of the host (17). Zeilmaker (18) found that the virus in GR females was transmitted not only by the milk but also by the ovum, a finding in line with the genetic transmission concept.

In mouse strains liberated from the milk factor by foster nursing on low-cancer-strain females, mammary tumors can appear at a late age. It was thought that these tumors were induced by the interaction of hormones and an appropriate genetic constitution only (19). However, Bernard et al. (20) found virus particles in these tumors that had the same morphology as those thought to be the classic milk factor. Recently it was demonstrated by inoculation of these purified particles that they represent another, considerably less oncogenic virus strain (21). In crosses between such an artificially established low-cancer strain (C3Hf) and a "true" low-cancer strain (Balb/c), it became apparent that this virus can be transmitted by either parent. Also, in this case it was postulated that the virus was transmitted as a genetic factor (22). Verstraeten and Van Nie (23) found (by means of radioim-munoassay for MTV antigens in milk of segregating populations between C3Hf and Balb/c) that here also one dominant gene controls the transmission and mammary carcinogenesis. Surprisingly this gene is not allelic to the GR gene for male transmission. It is situated on the first linkage group of the mouse and is now called Mtv-1. The GR gene (Mtv-2) has not been mapped as yet.

By means of molecular hybridization it has been found that normal cellular DNA of all mouse strains tested so far contains multiple copies of the MTV genome (24,25). The GR strain has more copies than all other strains tested (26), indicating that the ancestors of this strain acquired a new viral gene, possibly by infection of the germ line with an "exogenous" virus, leading to subsequent genetic fixation and transmission of a now "endogenous" virus or mendelian factor. A curious note is that this "creation" of a new gene has not been accomplished by selection for the appearance of mammary tumors, an indication that this might not be such a rare event after all. The high leukemic mouse strain AKR, which carries several proviruses of murine leukemia viruses (27), was intentionally selected for a high leukemia incidence (28).

Although it has been thought for almost half a century that the "true" low-cancer strains are completely virus-free, the molecular biological findings indicate otherwise, and in fact earlier evidence suggested erratic expression of virus in at least some of such strains (21).

Several reported cases of *de novo* appearance of virulent mammary tumor virus in low-cancer strains (29–33) can now be interpreted as the emergence of a virulent variant of endogenous MTV, which then is transmitted independently of the host genome. The existence of MTV proviruses in all mouse strains tested might imply the "all-viral" etiology of this tumor type in mice. The evidence for this was rather scanty, but the recent finding of MTV expression in late-appearing mammary tumors of the Balb/c strain by radioimmunoassay (Verstraeten and Van Nie, *personal communication*), which was not detectable by electron microscopy or conventional immunological techniques of lower sensitivity (34), now supports this idea. It is therefore important to investigate many other low-cancer strains that do not release virus or viral antigens in the milk for the presence of MTV genome activity or expression in tumors induced by extreme hormonal stimulation. Even then it would be very difficult to deliver real proof that such expression is causally related to the malignant process.

After discovery of the milk factor, it was thought that chromosomal factors were immaterial in determining susceptibility to mammary carcinogenesis (35). However, Korteweg (36) realized that the combination of chromosomal and extrachromosomal factors controls the risk for development of a tumor. Andervont (37) noted a great variation among four different low-cancer strains in their response to the milk-borne virus from the high-cancer strain C3H. Andervont (9) subsequently observed that low-cancer strains resistant to the virus lose the agent very rapidly, indicating that host factors can interfere with replication of the virus and thereby cause resistance to its carcinogenic action. The occasional disappearance of the milk factor from high-cancer strains might in fact be due to fixation of gene mutations which cause interference with virus replication (38).

Resistance to mammary cancer induced by MTV need not necessarily be due to interference with replication. For instance, inadequate hormonal receptiveness of the target organ for this cancer might cause resistance of virgins to the viral action (39).

A specific gene system controlling viral carcinogenesis is the major histocompatibility locus of the mouse (40). Foster nursing of B10 congenic mouse lines for H-2 on C3H females leads to great differences in tumor incidence. For example, whereas the $H-2^b$ and $H-2^m$ haplotypes are resistant, the $H-2^{pa}$, $H-2^r$, and $H-2^k$ are susceptible and the $H-2^a$, $H-2^d$, $H-2^e$, and $H-2^f$ are highly susceptible. Within this complex locus, the H-2D end controls the dominant susceptibility. The action of the H-2 locus on viral mammary carcinogenesis has not yet been elucidated. We hypothesize either a strong immunological response against virus-coded cell surface antigens or an interference of certain membrane configurations coded for by H-2 haplotypes with virus-induced cell surface alterations, leading to neoplastic conversion.

An interesting phenomenon noted by several investigators (37,41) is that F_1 hybrids of two different resistant mouse strains can be fully susceptible to MTV, indicating that different recessive genes can cause considerable resistance to the agent. This might reflect different physiological mechanisms involved in the neoplastic process, but it is also possible that more than one gene controls the same pathway.

Most of the studies on host factors for resistance to mammary cancer in mice were concerned with exogenous virus, but there are already some examples of resistance factors to endogenous mammary tumor virus. Hybrids between C3Hf and some low-cancer strains such as C57BL and O20 have a delayed appearance of mammary tumors associated with a lower amount of the endogenous virus in either milk or tumors (42–44). A noteworthy exception was found in the hybrid (TSI×C3Hf)F$_1$, which had a very much delayed tumor appearance but good virus expression (Hilgers and Boot, *unpublished observations*). It still remains to be established if the factors which inhibit the expression of endogenous virus also cause resistance to exogenous virus.

The implications of these studies in mice to the human situation are that: (a) putative human breast cancer viruses may be transmitted as a genetic factor of the host; and (b) they may be expressed at a low level owing to interfering host genes and are therefore not detectable by conventional means but nevertheless may contribute to mammary carcinogenesis.

ACKNOWLEDGMENT

This work was supported in part by contracts with the National Cancer Institute (United States), contract numbers NO1-CP-33368 (J.H.) and NO1-CP-43328 (P.B.).

REFERENCES

1. Mühlbock, O. (1972): The Fourth Wassink Lecture: The value of experimental cancer research for the understanding of the human disease. In: *RNA Viruses and Host Genome in Oncogenesis,* edited by P. Emmelot and P. Bentvelzen, pp. 339–349. North-Holland Publishing, Amsterdam.
2. Heston, W. E., and Vlahakis, G. (1967): Genetic factors in mammary tumorigenesis. In: *Cancerogenesis: A Broad Critique.* Proceedings of the 12th Annual Symposium on Fundamental Cancer Research. Williams & Wilkens, Baltimore.
3. Bittner, J. J. (1936): Tumor incidence in recriprocal F^1 hybrid mice—A×D high tumor stocks. *Proc. Soc. Exp. Biol. Med.,* 34:42–48.
4. Axel, R., Schlom, J., and Spiegelman, S. (1972): Presence in human breast cancer of RNA homologous to mouse mammary tumour virus RNA. *Nature (Lond.),* 235:32–36.
5. Mühlbock, O., and Bentvelzen, P. (1968): The transmission of the mammary tumor viruses. *Perspect. Virol.,* 6:75–87.
6. Andervont, H. B., and McEleney, W. J. (1938): The influence of nonbreeding and foster nursing upon the occurrence of spontaneous breast tumors in strain C3H mice. *Public Health Rep.,* 53:777–783.
7. Van Gulik, P. J., and Korteweg, R. (1940): The anatomy of the mammary gland in mice with regard to the degree of its disposition for cancer. *Koninkl. Ned. Akad. Wetenschap. Proc. Ser. C.,* 43:891–900.
8. Fekete, E., and Little, C. C. (1942): Observations on the mammary tumor incidence of mice born from transferred ova. *Cancer Res.,* 2:525–530.
9. Andervont, H. (1945): Relation of milk influence to mammary tumors of hybrid mice. *J. Natl. Cancer Inst.,* 5:391–395.
10. Foulds, L. (1949): Mammary tumours in hybrid mice: The presence and transmission of the mammary tumour agent. *Br. J. Cancer,* 3:230–239.
11. Mühlbock, O. (1952): Studies on the transmission of the mouse mammary tumor agent by the male parent. *J. Natl. Cancer Inst.,* 12:819–837.
12. Bittner, J. J. (1952): Transfer of the agent for mammary cancer in mice by the male. *Cancer Res.,* 12:387–398.
13. Andervont, H. B. (1963): In utero transmission of the mouse mammary tumor agent. *J. Natl. Cancer Inst.,* 31:261–272.
14. Peacock, A. (1953): A possible mode of transmission of the mouse mammary tumour agent by the male parent. *Br. J. Cancer,* 7:352–357.

15. Pogossiantz, H. (1956): Some data on the experimental studies of the nature of mammary cancer in mice carried out in the Soviet Union. *Acta Un. Int. Cancr.*, 12:690–700.
16. Mühlbock, O. (1965): Note on a new inbred mouse strain GR/A. *Eur. J. Cancer*, 1:123–124.
17. Bentvelzen, P. (1968): Genetical Control of the Vertical Transmission of the Mühlbock Mammary Tumor Virus in the GR Mouse Strain. *Thesis*, Hollandia, Amsterdam.
18. Zeilmaker, G. H. (1969): Transmission of mammary tumor virus by female GR mice: Results of egg transplantation. *Int. J. Cancer*, 4:261–266.
19. Heston, W. E. (1958): Mammary tumors in agent-free mice. *Ann. N.Y. Acad. Sci.*, 71:931–942.
20. Bernard, W., Guérin, M., and Oberling, Ch. (1956): Mise en évidence de corpuscules d'aspect virusal dans différent souches de cancers mammaires de la souris: Etude au microscope électronique. *Acta Un. Int. Cancr.*, 12:545–554.
21. Hageman, P., Calafat, J., and Daams, J. H. (1972): The mouse mammary tumor viruses. In: *RNA Viruses and Host Genome in Oncogenesis*, edited by P. Emmelot and P. Bentvelzen, pp. 283–300. North-Holland Publishing, Amsterdam.
22. Bentvelzen, P., and Daams, J. H. (1969): Hereditary infections with mammary tumor viruses in mice. *J. Natl. Cancer Inst.*, 43:1025–1035.
23. Verstraeten, A. A., and Van Nie, R. (1974): Radioimmunologic evidence for a linkage relationship between the gene controlling MTV-L expression in milk and the albino (c) locus. In: *Proceedings of the IXth Meeting on Mammary Cancer in Experimental Animals and Man*, Pisa, Italy, p. 34, abstract 19.
24. Varmus, H. E., Bishop, J. M., Nowinski, R. C., and Sarkar, N. H. (1972): Mammary tumor virus specific nucleotide sequences in DNA of high and low incidence mouse strains. *Nature [New Biol.]*, 238:189–190.
25. Parks, W. P., and Scolnick, E. M. (1973): Murine mammary tumor cell clones with varying degrees of virus expression. *Virology*, 55:163–173.
26. Varmus, H. E., Ringold, G., Medeiros, E., Morris, V., and Bishop, J. M. (1974): Characterization of mouse mammary tumor virus genes and their expression in vivo and in tissue culture. In: *Proceedings of the IXth Meeting on Mammary Cancer in Experimental Animals and Man*, Pisa, Italy, abstract 41.
27. Chattopadhyay, S. K., Rowe, W. P., Teich, N. M., and Lowy, D. R. (1975): Definitive evidence that the murine C-type virus inducing locus Akv-1 is viral genetic material. *Proc. Natl. Acad. Sci. U.S.A.*, 72:910–960.
28. Cole, R. K., and Furth, J. (1941): Experimental studies on the genetics of spontaneous leukemia in mice. *Cancer Res.*, 1:957–961.
29. Bittner, J. J. (1941): Changes in the incidence of mammary carcinoma in mice of the "A" stock. *Cancer Res.*, 1:113–114.
30. Bittner, J. J. (1956): Mammary cancer in C3H mice of different sublines and their hybrids. *J. Natl. Cancer Inst.*, 16:1263–1286.
31. Dmochowski, L. (1956): A biology and biophysical approach to the study of the development of mammary cancer in mice. *Acta Un. Int. Cancr.*, 12:582–618.
32. Rudali, G., Yourkovski, N., Juliard, N., and Fautrel, M. (1956): Sur quelques caractères des souris appartenant a la nouvelle lignée cancéreuse. *Bull. Cancer*, 43:364–383.
33. Gardner, W. U., Pfeiffer, C. A., and Trentin, J. J. (1959): Hormonal factors in experimental carcinogenesis. In: *Physiopathology of Cancer*, edited by F. Homburger, pp. 152–237. Hoeber, New York.
34. Hilgers, J. H. M., Theuns, G. J., and Van Nie, R. (1973): Mammary tumor virus (MTV) antigens in normal and mammary tumor-bearing mice. *Int. J. Cancer*, 12:568–576.
35. Murray, W. S., and Little, C. C. (1935): The genetics of mammary tumor incidence in mice. *Genetics*, 20:466–496.
36. Korteweg, R. (1935): Der extrachromosomale Faktor bei der Vererbung der Krebsdisposition bei der Maus. *Verh. 4ᵉ Conf. Leeuwenhoek Ver.*, pp. 57–63.
37. Andervont, H. B. (1940): The influence of foster nursing upon the incidence of spontaneous mammary cancer in resistant and susceptible mice. *J. Natl. Cancer Inst.*, 1:147–153.
38. Andervont, H. B., and Dunn, T. B. (1962): Studies of the mammary tumor agent of strain RIII mice. *J. Natl. Cancer Inst.*, 28:159–185.
39. Bittner, J. J. (1944): Observations on the inherited susceptibility to spontaneous mammary cancer in mice. *Cancer Res.*, 4:159–167.
40. Mühlbock, O., and Dux, A. (1974): Histocompatibility genes (the H-2 complex) and susceptibility to mammary tumor virus in mice. *J. Natl. Cancer Inst.*, 53:993–996.

41. Mühlbock, O. (1956): Biological studies on the mammary tumor agent in different strains of mice. *Acta Un. Int. Cancr.,* 12:665–681.
42. Boot, L. M. (1969): Induction by Prolactin of Mammary Tumors in Mice. Thesis, Noord-Hollandse Uitgevers Maatschappij, N. V., Amsterdam.
43. Röpcke, G. (1975): Interaction of Hypophyseal Isografts and Ovarian Hormones in Mammary Tumour Development in Mice. Thesis, Mondeel, Amsterdam.
44. Verstraeten, A. A., Van Nie, R., Kwa, H. G., and Hageman, Ph. C. (1975): Quantitative estimation of mouse mammary tumor virus (MTV) antigens by radioimmunoassay. *Int. J. Cancer,* 15:270–281.

Breast Cancer: Trends in Research and Treatment, edited by J. C. Heuson,
W. H. Mattheiem, and M. Rozencweig. Raven Press, New York © 1976.

Biochemical Characterization of Mouse Mammary Tumor Viruses and Related Isolates: Mason-Pfizer Virus and the BUdR-Induced Guinea Pig Virus

J. Schlom, D. Colcher, W. Drohan, P. Kimball,
R. Michalides, and G. Schochetman

*National Cancer Institute, Bethesda, Maryland 20014;
and Meloy Laboratories, Springfield, Virginia 22150*

Oncogenic RNA viruses (oncornaviruses) have been traditionally classified on the basis of morphology (1). C-type viruses have been demonstrated to be etiological factors in leukemias, lymphomas, and sarcomas of a variety of avian and mammalian species (2). Intracisternal A-particles have also been associated with some of these diseases (3). The mouse mammary tumor virus (MMTV) is the prototype B-type particle and has been shown to be involved etiologically in mammary carcinoma of a variety of mouse strains (4,5). The intracytoplasmic A-particle is observed with regularity in cells producing MMTV and is believed to be a precursor of the mature B-type particle (6).

Recently two viruses were isolated that have several morphological features in common with the mouse mammary tumor viruses. These agents are the Mason-Pfizer virus (MPV), isolated from a carcinoma of the breast of a rhesus monkey (7), and the bromodeoxyuridine (BUdR)-induced guinea pig virus (B-GPV), which can be isolated by induction with BUdR or iododeoxyuridine (IUdR) from a variety of guinea pig tissues (8–11). Table 1 denotes the structures present at various stages of morphogenesis of the MMTVs, B-GPV, MPV, and avian and mammalian C-type viruses. It can be seen from this table that the MMTVs, B-GPV, and MPV share three features that distinguish them from the avian or mammalian C-type viruses: (a) the presence of intracytoplasmic A-particles; (b) a complete nucleoid formed at the time of budding; and (c) a nucleoid in the mature particle that is eccentric.

Following is a review of our recent biochemical and immunological studies of the MMTVs, MPV, and B-GPV; these studies concern the relationships of these viruses to each other, to other oncornaviruses, and to their species of origin.

MOUSE MAMMARY TUMOR VIRUSES

Characterization of MMTVs Propagated In Vitro from Various Mouse Strains

Various strains of mice have been shown to harbor viral agents capable of

11

TABLE 1. *Comparative morphological properties of MMTVs,
MPV, B-GPV, and C-type viruses*

Property	MMTVs	B-GPV	MPV	C-type
Presence of intracytoplasmic A-particles	+	+	+	–
Nucleoid at budding	Complete	Complete	Complete	Incomplete
Nature of nucleoid in mature particle	Eccentric	Eccentric	Eccentric and cylindrical	Centric
Nature of spikes in mature particle	Long	Long	Short	Short

The data were compiled from references 1, 2, 6, 7, 11, and 57.

causing mammary carcinoma; these agents may differ, however, in a variety of biological parameters (5,12) (Table 2). Until recently the primary sources of mouse mammary tumor viruses have been milk and tumor homogenates, both of which are biochemically complex media. Cell cultures producing MMTV would eliminate major problems of cellular contamination and allow more precise comparative studies of MMTVs from various mouse strains.

Studies on the replication of MMTVs in organ or cell cultures (13–21) provided partial characterization of each of the viruses produced in the culture medium. Recently MMTV has been well characterized from primary cultures of mammary tumors of BALB/cfC3H mice (22–25). We used this technique of culturing mammary tumors and found it useful for producing MMTV from any mouse strain tested that exhibits mammary tumors. Cultures of primary mammary tumors have been successfully cultivated from RIII, GR, DD, C3H, C3Hf, BALB/c, and BALB/cfC3H mice, and MMTVs are produced by all of these cultures (26,27). Furthermore, production of type C virus is sufficiently low that

TABLE 2. *Biological properties of MMTV variants*

Variant	Reference mouse strain	Mode of transmission	Virulence	Tumor type
S	C3H-A^{vy}	Horizontally	+ + + +	Hormone-independent, fast-growing carcinomas
	A	Horizontally	+ + + + +	Fast-growing carcinomas
P	GR	Horizontally and vertically	+ + +	Hormone-dependent P (plaque)-type
PS	RIII	Horizontally	+ + + +	Hormone-independent, fast-growing carcinomas
L	C3H-A^{vy}fB	Vertically	+	Hormone-independent, slow-growing carcinomas

Data are from references 5, 12, and 54.

these tumor cell cultures can serve as a source of viral antigens, enzymes, and nucleic acids for use in answering questions concerning the relatedness among MMTVs from different mouse strains.

Establishment and Maintenance of Tumor Cell Cultures

Mammary tumors from RIII, GR, DD, BALB/c, and BALB/cfC3H mice were minced, and the cells were dissociated and seeded at concentration of $10^6/cm^2$ culture surface area in medium containing insulin and hydrocortisone (26). A typical tumor, 2.5 cm in diameter, yielded $6-25 \times 10^7$ viable cells, depending on the mouse strain. The medium on all mammary tumor cultures was harvested daily. By 3–5 days in culture, confluent monolayers highlighted by acinar-like "domes" (23) characterized the cultures from all strains of mice tested. In general, primary cultures were successfully maintained for 5–8 weeks. Electron microscopic examination of cultures revealed typical intracytoplasmic A-particles, and budding and mature B-type particles.

Assays for MMTV Antigens in Virus from Tumor Cell Cultures

Radioimmunoassays provide sensitive quantitative assays for antigens of murine type-C viruses and MMTV (25,28,29). Therefore we utilized such assays to quantitate and characterize the MMTVs being produced from RIII, GR, DD, BALB/cfC3H, and BALB/c mammary tumor cell cultures. The primary antisera for MMTV antigens used in these studies was prepared against undisrupted BALB/cfC3H MMTV. Precipitation of MMTV by this antiserum has been shown (25) not to be inhibited by MuLV (murine leukemia virus), homogenates of BALB/c lactating mammary glands, defatted BALB/c milk, and fetal calf serum, and to be inhibited by at least 70% with purified gp52 of MMTV from RIII mouse milk. To see if the virus produced by RIII tumor cell cultures reacted with this MMTV-specific antiserum, virus was purified in two successive isopycnic sucrose gradients followed by a single isokinetic gradient. The resulting virus peak was concentrated, and virions were radiolabeled without prior disruption using ^{125}I and lactoperoxidase. After repurification by a single isopycnic sucrose gradient, up to 85% of the label could be precipitated with excess anti-MMTV antiserum. As expected from the specificity of the antiserum, binding of the labeled RIII culture virus could be inhibited substantially (up to 90%) by MMTV purified from RIII milk (Fig. 1, open circles). Samples of purified virus from primary tumor cell cultures of RIII, GR, DD, BALB/cfC3H, and BALB/c mice all inhibited precipitation of the labeled RIII MMTV with similar efficiencies within the range of protein tested (0.1–10.0 μg). The inhibition curves shown in Fig. 1 were plotted in logit form (30), which is used to linearize inhibition curves so that slopes may be compared accurately. It should be noted that the slopes of the inhibition curves for all five MMTVs are essentially the same, thus indicating that in this radioimmunoprecipitation (RIP) inhibition assay, the surface antigens

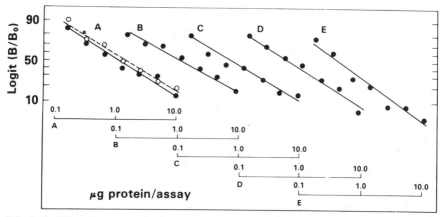

FIG. 1. Radioimmunoprecipitation assay for MMTV antigens in purified virus preparations. All viruses were purified on two successive isopycnic sucrose gradients. The open circles in curve A represent MMTV from RIII milk; all curves of closed circles are for viruses from mammary tumor cell cultures, as follows: A, RIII; B, GR; C, BALB/cfC3H; D, DD; and E, BALB/c. In the ratio (B/B_0), B is the amount of labeled antigen bound in the presence of competing antigen, and B_0 is the amount bound with no competing antigen added. These ratios, expressed as percentages, are plotted in logit form for comparison of slopes. Each point represents average values for several experiments with different samples of each virus (26).

of the MMTVs from these five different mouse strains are immunologically indistinguishable (26).

The MMTV RIA was also used to quantitate the amount of MMTV being produced by the various cultures. As seen in Table 3, 0.8–2.1 μg of density gradient purified MMTV protein is being produced per milliliter of supernatant fluid per 24 hr in cultures from all five mouse strains. Much more MMTV-specif-

TABLE 3. *Production of MMTV in primary mammary tumor cultures*

Mouse strain	MMTV protein μg/ml supernatant[a]	% MuLV protein
RIII	2.1	<0.2
GR	0.8	0.2
DD	0.8	<0.4
BALB/cfC3H	1.0	0.3
BALB/c	0.8	1.3–3.0

[a]Supernates of three to six replicate cultures from each tumor pool were combined in each measurement for the different tumor pools. Samples of 4.0 ml, each harvested on day 14 after culture initiation, were pelleted through 1.0 ml 20% glycerol in TNE in the SW50.1 rotor at 50,000 rpm and 4°C for 30 min. Pellets were resuspended in TNE and assayed by MMTV and MuLV RIP inhibition assays (26, 27).

ic antigen was found in soluble form in the supernatant fluids of tumor cell cultures, however, than was found associated with purified virions from these fluids. An average of 4.9 μg MMTV immunoreactive protein was detected per milliliter of clarified RIII culture supernatant fluid. After high-speed pelleting of the virus, 73.8% of the total antigen remained in the supernate. Moreover, only 13.6% of the total supernatant fluid MMTV antigen was found associated with virus (density range 1.16–1.19 g/ml) after purification in two successive isopycnic sucrose gradients. In contrast to the results for MMTV antigens, the majority of DNA polymerase activity (as measured with oligo $dT_{(12-18)}$:poly rA exogenous template) was virus-associated, and very little activity was detected in high-speed supernates. The conclusion from these experiments is that, unlike viral DNA polymerase, the majority of MMTV surface antigen is found in soluble form in supernatant fluids from primary mammary tumor cell cultures.

The viruses purified from supernatant fluids of primary cell cultures of mammary tumors contained only limited amounts of MuLV. This was measured by a radioimmune precipitation assay for the p30 protein of Friend murine leukemia virus (31,32). The percentage of particles determined to be MuLV by this method was less than 0.4% of the total virus produced by the various mammary tumor cell cultures (Table 3). Only the BALB/c cultures produced virus that contained as much as 1–3% MuLV particles. Virus purified from RIII mouse milk contained approximately 0.2% MuLV particles. Similar results were obtained (courtesy of Dr. C. Sherr, NCI) with an analogous RIP inhibition assay for a murine type C group-specific antigen, using the p30 of an endogenous virus from BALB/c mice (33). Therefore the immunological evidence suggests that primary cell cultures of mouse mammary tumors from several strains of mice produce virus and antigens which are sufficiently low in, or free of, MuLV to be used in comparative biochemical and immunological investigations of MMTV.

Polypeptide Composition of MMTVs from Different Mouse Strains

The polypeptides of the MMTVs of different mouse strains were compared. Cultures were given a mixture of ^{3}H-amino acids, and labeled viruses were purified by isopycnic and isokinetic sucrose gradient centrifugation (26). Polypeptides were solubilized by heating with SDS and urea, and analyzed by polyacrylamide gel electrophoresis. The results of such experiments with MMTVs from RIII, BALB/cfC3H, and DD cultures are presented in Fig. 2. It is apparent that the numbers and sizes of polypeptides in each virus are highly similar, although the relative proportions of the different peaks vary from one strain to another. Eight distinct peaks were observed for all viruses. The four most prominent polypeptides were those with estimated molecular weights of 52,000, 36,000, 28,000, and 10,000 daltons. Four other less prominent but distinct peaks were observed for all viruses, with estimated molecular weights of 46,000, 30,000, 18,000, and 14,000 daltons. Five other polypeptides appeared as distinct peaks or shoulders on major peaks in gels of the viruses, at estimated molecular weights of

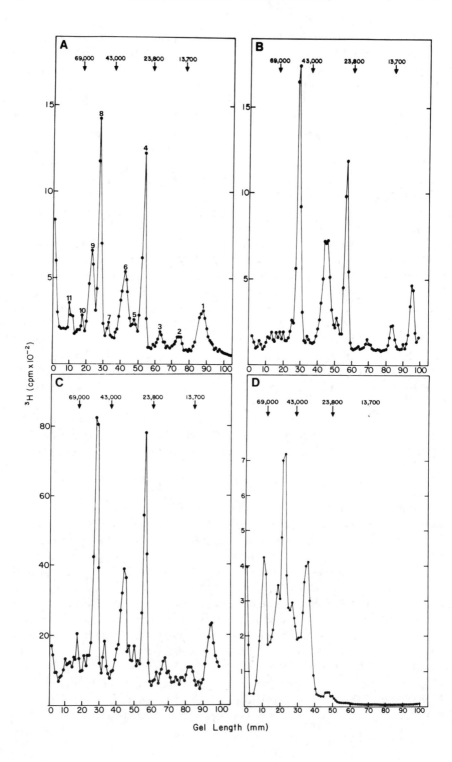

22,000, 38,000, and approximately 60,000, 70,000, and 80,000 daltons.

Primary tumor cell cultures can also be used to identify glycoproteins of MMTVs. Incorporation of ^{3}H-glucosamine in RIII virus was mainly into the polypeptides with apparent molecular weights of 36,000, 52,000, and 70,000 daltons (Fig. 2D). Lesser amounts occurred in those of 38,000, 46,000, and 60,000 daltons. It appears that all the MMTVs examined contain at least eight polypeptides in common.

Biophysical Characterization of Virions and Viral RNA

To detect and characterize the MMTV produced by RIII mouse mammary tumor cell cultures, cells were labeled with a mixture of ^{3}H-uridine, cytidine, and adenosine. Virus was concentrated and purified, and then mixed with purified ^{32}P-labeled MuLV (Rauscher). Comparative densities were determined by analyzing the virus mixture on both CsCl and sucrose equilibrium density gradients. The results of these experiments are summaried in Table 4, where it is seen that MMTV has a higher density than MuLV in both sucrose and CsCl gradients.

Another means of distinguishing murine B-type and C-type particles is by velocity gradient centrifugation. When a mixture of ^{3}H-RNA-labeled virus from RIII cell cultures and ^{32}P-labeled Rauscher leukemia virus was analyzed on an isokinetic sucrose gradient, the majority of the RIII cell culture virus was found to sediment faster (at approximately 800–1,000S) than the MuLV, for which a sedimentation coefficient of 640S was determined previously (34).

To characterize further the MMTV from primary mouse mammary tumor cultures, radioactively labeled RNA was extracted from concentrated virions and analyzed by velocity sedimentation. A distinct peak of TCA-precipitable radioactivity with a sedimentation coefficient of 60–70S was readily observed. The molecular weight of the 60–70S ^{3}H-RNA was estimated to be 8×10^6 as analyzed by electrophoresis on polyacrylamide gels (Fig. 3A). The highest yield of intact 60–70S RNA came from three successive 3-hr collections of unlabeled medium after a 12-hr labeling period (27). The yield of ^{3}H-labeled 60–70S viral RNA varied in several experiments from 25,000 to 100,000 cpm per T75 flask per three 3-hr collection periods; the specific activity of the RNA was approximated at 1.1×10^6 cpm/μg. This ^{3}H-MMTV 60–70S RNA was extremely useful in the molecular hybridization experiments described below.

FIG. 2. Polyacrylamide gel electrophoresis of polypeptides of MMTVs from mammary tumor cell cultures. Viruses were labeled with a mixture of ^{3}H-amino acids (**A, B, C**) or ^{3}H-glucosamine (**D**), and were concentrated, purified, and pelleted as described (26). The virus pellets were solubilized with SDS and applied to gels for electrophoresis. **A:** RIII. **B:** BALB/cfC3H. **C:** DD. **D:** ^{3}H-glucosamine-labeled RIII MMTV. Migration is from left to right. Marker proteins run on parallel gels were, from left to right: BSA, ovalbumin, trypsin, and ribonuclease A.

TABLE 4. *Comparative biochemical properties of MMTV, MPV, B-GPV, and MuLV*

Property	MMTV	B-GPV	MPV	MuLV
Buoyant density in sucrose (g/ml)	1.18	1.18	1.16	1.16
Buoyant density in CsCl (g/ml)	1.21	1.21	1.21	1.17
DNA polymerase [a]				
Active at 20 mM $MgCl_2$	+	+	+	−
Active at 0.4 mM $mnCl_2$	−	−	−	+
Molecular weight of RNA (d)	8×10^6	8×10^6	8×10^6	8×10^6
RNA subunits (d)	$2–3 \times 10^6$	$2–3 \times 10^6$	$2–3 \times 10^6$	$2–3 \times 10^6$
Genome copies in DNA of species of origin [b]	8–54	85–275	<1 [c]	5–15 [d]
Nucleic acid sequence homology (%)				
MMTV	100	<5	<5	<5
B-GPV	<5	100	<5	<5
MPV	<5	<5	100	<5

[a] Viral DNA polymerase assays with poly rC:oligo dG $_{(10-12)}$ as template, as described (95).
[b] Copy numbers are approximations and are given per haploid genome using the calculations described (50), assuming the complexity of the viral RNAs to be approximately 2.4×10^6 (52).
[c] Complete MPV proviral sequences are present in only certain organs of some rhesus monkeys (90).
[d] From ref. 103.

Characterization of MMTV DNA Polymerase Activities

To determine if MMTV from mouse mammary tumor cultures would be a suitable source of viral DNA polymerase, concentrated virus was assayed for DNA polymerase activity using either endogenous RNA or added synthetic polymers as templates (27). In the case of RIII tumor culture virus, a direct comparison was made of the activities with endogenous template, or the exogenous primer templates oligo dG:poly rC, oligo dT:poly rA, and oligo dT:poly dA. When results are expressed in picomoles of DNA synthesized, DNA polymerase activity of the RIII virus was 55 times higher with oligo dG:poly rC template than with the endogenous reaction. Comparison of DNA polymerase activities with the templates oligo dT:poly rA and oligo dT:poly dA also were made with high-speed pellets of MMTV from supernatant fluids of RIII, GR, DD, BALB/c, and BALB/cfC3H mammary tumor cultures. In all cases oligo dT:poly rA was preferred at least 10-fold over oligo dT:poly dA (Table 5). Preference for oligo dT:poly rA over oligo dT:poly dA has been shown to be a characteristic of viral reverse transcriptases (35,36). These results suggest that the virus-associated DNA polymerase activities in the medium of all the mammary tumor cell cultures exhibit properties of viral reverse transcriptase.

The relative effectiveness of magnesium and manganese divalent cations in viral DNA polymerase reactions with oligo dT:poly rA template was determined

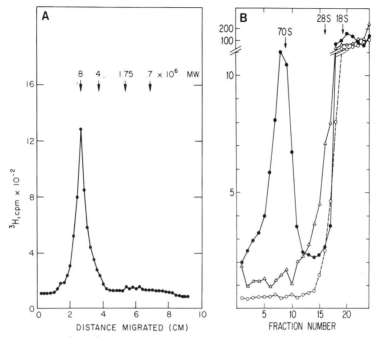

FIG. 3 A: Characterization of ^{3}H-60-70S RNA from RIII tumor cell culture virus. Virus was labeled with a mixture of ^{3}H-ribonucleosides and purified as described (26,27). The RNA was extracted and layered on an isokinetic glycerol gradient for analysis. The RNA in the 60–70S region of the gradient was pooled and precipitated with ethanol. The RNA was then electrophoresed on a gel of 2% acrylamide and 0.5% agarose as described (83). The *arrows* indicate positions in parallel gels of ^{3}H-RNA from VSV (4×10^6), and 28S (1.75×10^6) and 18S (0.7×10^6 daltons) ribosomal ^{3}H-RNA. **B:** Simultaneous detection of ^{3}H-cDNA and viral 60–70S RNA template from DNA polymerase reaction of RIII tumor culture virus. Virus was concentrated (26,27), and the pellet was resuspended in 0.01 M Tris-HCl (pH 8.3) and divided into three aliquots. One was incubated for 1 hr at 37°C in the standard endogenous DNA polymerase reaction (27,29) with all four deoxynucleotide triphosphates present. Another was assayed in the same manner with the exception that pancreatic ribonuclease A was added at 50 μg/ml. The third reaction mixture was incubated without dGTP. All three reactions were stopped by the addition of SLS to 1% and KCl to 0.4 M; the products were analyzed by rate zonal sedimentation on glycerol gradients as described (27,29). *Closed circles* denote complete reaction; *open circles*, ribonuclease treatment; *triangles*, -dGTP.

for the viruses from tumor cultures of each of the five mouse strains (27). In all cases DNA synthesis with magnesium ions was higher than with manganese ions by a factor ranging from 5- to 40-fold (Table 5). A strong preference for magnesium over manganese ions has been shown to be characteristic of reverse transcriptase of MMTV from mouse milk (37,38), whereas the opposite cation preference was demonstrated, using these conditions, for reverse transcriptases from several mammalian C-type viruses (Tables 4 and 5).

The method of simultaneous detection (39) for reverse transcriptase and high-molecular-weight viral RNA template was used to further characterize mammary tumor culture MMTV for DNA synthesis from its endogenous 60–70S RNA

TABLE 5. *DNA polymerase activity of mammary tumor culture viruses*

Virus	Oligo dT:poly rA[a] (cpm $\times$ 10^{-3})'	Ratio of activity (dT:rA/dT:dA)	Mg^{++}/Mn^{++}[b]
MMTV			
RIII	50.3	18.6	33.5
GR	33.4	14.5	18.6
DD	16.6	10.7	41.5
BALB/cfC3H	64.0	11.1	22.0
BALB/c	9.0	27.0	5.6
MuLV			
RLV[c]	1.2	NT[d]	0.015

[a] Cultures were seeded at 10^6 cells/cm^2, and the medium was changed daily. Virus in 4.0 ml medium on day 14 after seeding was concentrated, and DNA polymerase assays using the indicated templates were performed (26,27). Results with oligo dT:poly rA are expressed as counts per minute $\times$ 10^{-3} of ^{3}H-dTMP incorporated per hour per milliliter of supernatant fluid.

[b] DNA polymerase assays utilized oligo dT:poly rA template and either 8 mM MgCl$_2$ or 0.4 mM MnCl$_2$.

[c] Rauscher murine leukemia virus grown in 3T3 cells.

[d] NT, not tested.

template and as a means of preparing ^{3}H-cDNA probe specific for MMTV. The product of a standard DNA polymerase reaction mixture (40) was analyzed by rate zonal sedimentation on isokinetic glycerol gradients. ^{3}H-DNA:RNA complexes routinely appeared in the 60–70S region of the gradient (Fig. 3B). Either treatment of the reaction product with ribonuclease prior to sedimentation or omission of a single nucleotide triphosphate from the reaction eliminated the peak of DNA in the 60–70S region. This indicated that the ^{3}H-cDNA synthesized was: (a) synthesized on a 60–70S RNA; and (b) not the product of a terminal transferase reaction.

Culture Variables and Quantitation of Virus Production

Studies were conducted (27) to determine parameters which might influence MMTV production. Virus yield per milliliter of supernatant fluid was found to be directly proportional to cell density at seeding. This phenomenon was maintained over an eightfold range up to 1.0×10^6 cells/square centimeter of surface. The effect of culture age on virus production was also examined. RIII cultures were seeded at high and low cell densities, and virus was harvested daily for 50 consecutive days without passage of the cells. Assays for viral DNA polymerase activity using oligo dG:poly rC template were made every 5 days up to day 50. The results of these experiments are shown in Fig. 4. In general, it was found that primary cultures from all mouse strains produced MMTV relatively free of MuLV for 30–50 days, after which permanent collapse of the typical dome-like structures occurred concomitantly with a substantial reduction in virus production. Passage of primary cultures led to the production of greater quantities of type C virus.

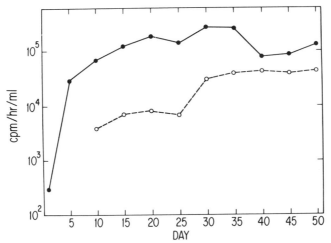

FIG. 4. Assay of MMTV production versus age of primary culture. RIII tumor cultures were seeded at high cell density (1.0 × 10⁶/cm²; *closed circles*) or low cell density (0.12 × 10⁶/cm²; *open circles*), and the medium was changed daily. Samples (4 ml) from indicated days were concentrated by pelleting at 50,000 rpm for 30 min through 20% glycerol and were assayed for DNA polymerase activity using oligo dG:poly rC primer:template as described (26,27).

Several methods were used to estimate the amount of MMTV produced by primary mammary tumor cultures. One method of quantification was particle counts made from low-magnification electron micrographs of concentrated virus. Latex beads of known concentration were added before negative staining to provide an internal counting standard (41). By this means it was determined that an average of 1.1×10^{10} MMTV particles were produced per day per 75 cm² culture. MMTV production by cultures from RIII, GR, DD, BALB/cfC3H, and BALB/c tumors was also quantitated utilizing the MMTV RIP inhibition assay described above. Virus produced in 24 hr was harvested and concentrated by pelleting. The average MMTV production by RIII cultures was 2.1 μg (range 0.9–3.7 μg) protein per milliliter of culture supernate, while MMTV production in GR, DD, BALB/cfC3H, and BALB/c cultures was only slightly lower (Table 3); it can thus be calculated (27) that the average tumor cell culture produces approximately 5×10^{10} particles per day per 75 cm² flask.

General Comments

These studies were undertaken to obtain sources of MMTV and its components from different mouse strains for comparative biochemical and immunological studies. Virions produced in these primary mammary tumor cultures possess the density, sedimentation properties, RNA, and reverse transcriptase activity characteristic of the MMTVs obtained from mouse milk. Furthermore, nucleic acid hybridization studies, cation preferences of the viral DNA polymerases, and the use of radioimmune assays all support the fact that these cell culture-derived MMTVs are relatively free of murine C-type viruses.

Milk and mammary tumors of the RIII, BALB/cfC3H, GR, and DD strains are generally known to contain relatively large amounts of MMTV, but the BABL/c strain has been considered classically to be free of MMTV. Recent studies (40) showed MMTV-related RNA to be present in the relatively rare mammary carcinomas found only in old BALB/c females. There is also recent biological evidence for an MMTV in normal mammary tissue of old BALB/c females (42). It should be noted that the BALB/c tumors used here were generated by transplantation of cells from a spontaneous tumor of an old BALB/c mouse. This is in contrast to the tumors in mice of the other strains, which spontaneously arose in the animal from which the tumor was removed for culture. The significance of this transplantation step for MMTV production in primary cell cultures is not known. However, it is clear that these primary cultures of mammary tumor cells seem to be the first good source of virus for biochemical and immunological studies of the MMTV from BALB/c mice, as well as a good source of MMTVs for comparative biochemical and immunochemical studies of the mouse mammary tumor viruses from a wide variety of mouse strains.

Relationships Among RNA Genomes of MMTVs

Variants of the MMTV have been identified by different biological characteristics such as virulence, host range, mode of transmission, and histological type of tumor induced (Table 2). Variants of the MMTV can be vertically transmitted (i.e., transmitted with cellular genes) or horizontally transmitted by mechanisms such as nursing (4,5,12). The mammary tumor incidence in mouse strains carrying a horizontally transmitted MMTV is usually high (greater than 80%), and tumors arise early in life (6–9 months). The mammary tumor incidence in mouse strains carrying only the vertically transmitted MMTV is usually low (less than 20%), and the tumors usually appear late in life (later than 13 months).

MMTV proviral sequences have been claimed to be uniformly present in the cellular genome of mouse strains with high and low mammary tumor incidence (43), and to be expressed in all tissues of mouse strains irrespective of their mammary tumor history (44). Those studies, however, were conducted using cDNA probes that did not represent the entire viral genome (44) and did not consider a possible difference in nucleic acid sequences between vertically and horizontally transmitted MMTVs. The studies reported here utilized the entire 60–70S RNA genomes of various MMTVs and the technique of competitive molecular hybridization. We found (45) that the nucleic acid sequences of the horizontally transmitted MMTV variants from four mouse strains (RIII, C3H-A^{vy}, GR, and A) are at least 95% homologous to one another and are approximately 25% different from the vertically transmitted MMTV variant from the mouse strain C3H-A^{vy}fB. This C3Hf strain was developed (46) by removing one male and one female C3H-A^{vy} by cesarean section and foster nursing them on a female of strain C57BL, a strain without overt MMTV in its milk. No common nucleic sequences were detected between the RNAs of the MMTVs and those of MuLV (Rauscher), B-GPV, or MPV.

Characterization of MMTV Variants

The RIII, GR, C3H, and C3Hf virus preparations that were the source of viral RNA and were subsequently used in competitive molecular hybridizations did not contain contaminating murine type C virus, as determined by radioimmunoassay for MuLV p30 (Table 3) and cation preference of viral DNA polymerase (Table 5); in competitive molecular hybridization experiments, addition of MuLV RNA to the hybrid formation between radioactively labeled MMTV RNA and mammary tumor DNA had no effect on the final extent of this hybrid formation (Fig. 5). Gel electrophoresis of the radioactively labeled high-molecular-weight RNAs from the MMTVs of RIII, C3H, and GR resulted in a single class of RNA with a molecular weight of 8×10^6 daltons (Fig. 3A) (45). The specific activities of the ^{3}H -labeled 60–70S MMTV RNAs were approximately 1×10^6 cpm/μg.

Competitive Molecular Hybridization

The addition of increasing amounts (0.6–1,200 ng) of unlabeled RNAs from GR, RIII, and C3H MMTVs to the hybridization reaction between the radioactively labeled 60–70S RNA of MMTV(RIII) and the DNA from RIII mammary tumors all resulted in equal displacements of the radioactive MMTV (RIII) 60–70S RNA in the hybrid formations (Fig. 5A). The nucleic acid sequence of MMTV released in the mammary tumor cell cultures of the RIII mouse strain also appears to be identical to that of the MMTV released into RIII milk (Fig. 5A).

The addition of increasing amounts of RNA from GR, RIII, and C3H MMTVs to the hybridization reaction between the radioactively labeled 60–70S RNA from MMTV(GR) and the DNA from GR mammary tumors also resulted in the same equal displacement of the radioactive MMTV(GR) 60–70S RNA in hybrid formations (Fig. 5B). Finally, the addition of increasing amounts of unlabeled RNA from GR, RIII, and C3H MMTVs to the hybridization reaction between radioactive MMTV(C3H) 60–70S RNA and DNA from C3H mammary tumors resulted in a similar equal inhibition of hybrid formations (Fig. 5C). These data indicate that the viral genomes of these three MMTVs from different mouse strains (MMTV-P, PS, and S) (Table 2) are identical in nucleic acid sequences, within the limits of this assay. The fourth MMTV under study, MMTV(A), was obtained from the cell line TA3 (20). The addition of increasing amounts (0.6–1,220 ng) of MMTV(A) RNA to the hybrid formation between radioactive MMTV(C3H) 60–70S RNA and C3H mammary tumor DNA displaced this hybrid formation to the same extent as the addition of MMTV(C3H) RNA. No inhibition of the hybrid formation between radioactive 60–70S MMTV RNAs and mammary tumor DNA was observed after adding increasing amounts of viral

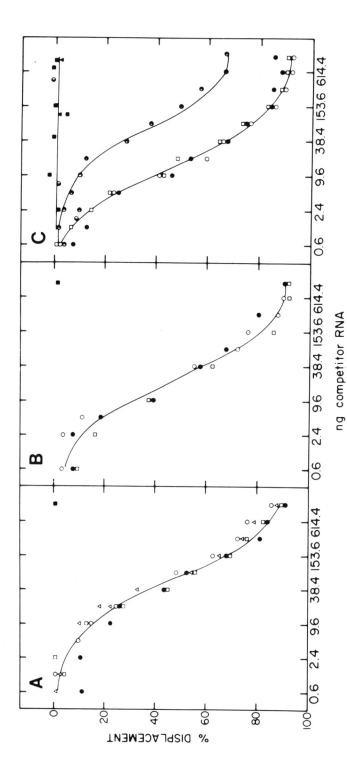

FIG. 5. Displacement of the radioactively labeled MMTV RNAs in a molecular hybridization reaction between radioactive 60–70S MMTV RNAs and DNA from mouse mammary tumors. The following unlabeled viral RNAs were added in the increasing amounts (0.6 ng to 1.2 μg) indicated: ●, MMTV(RIII); ○, MMTV(C3H); □, MMTV(GR); ◑, MMTV(C3Hf); △, MMTV(RIII); ■, RLV; ▲, MPMV; ●, GPV to the hybrid formation between [32]P-60–70S MMTV(RIII) hybridized to RIII mammary tumor DNA (**A**); [3]H-60–70S MMTV(GR) hybridized to GR mammary tumor DNA (**B**); [32]P-60–70S MMTV(C3H) hybridized to C3H-A[vy] mammary tumor DNA (**C**). The hybridization reactions were incubated to a cellular Cot value of 40,000 and assayed for ribonuclease resistance. The results are given as percent inhibition of the labeled MMTV·RNA·DNA hybridization versus amount of unlabeled viral RNA added to the reaction (45).

RNA from MuLV, MPV, or B-GPV to that hybrid formation (Fig. 5), indicating no detectable nucleic acid sequence homology between the horizontally transmitted MMTVs and those viruses.

The relationship in nucleic acid sequences between the C3H milk-transmitted MMTV-S and the vertically transmitted MMTV-L of C3H mice was studied by saturation hybridization and molecular competitive hybridization. In saturation hybridization experiments, a constant amount (2,000 cpm) of ^{32}P 60–70S RNA from C3H MMTV-S (produced by C3H mammary tumors in culture) was hybridized to increasing amounts of cellular DNA fragments from mammary tumors and livers of the same tumor-bearing C3H mice. Liver was chosen because it had been reported negative for MMTV antigens (47). As can be seen in Fig. 6, 52% of the ^{32}P-labeled 60–70S RNA of MMTV-S (from C3H) hybridized to the DNA from "early" mammary tumors, while under identical conditions the hybridization value to the DNA from livers of these same animals reached saturation at approximately 42%. This implies a nucleic acid sequence homology of approximately 80% between the horizontally (milk) transmitted MMTV-S and the vertically transmitted MMTV-L. A similar nucleic acid sequence relationship between the horizontally and vertically transmitted MMTV variants of the C3H mouse was obtained by competitive hybridization experiments. Increasing amounts of the RNA of MMTV(C3H) and of MMTV(C3Hf) were added to the hybridization reaction between ^{3}H-MMTV(C3H) 60–70S RNA and C3H mammary tumor DNA. The hybrid formation is almost completely (94%) inhibited by adding MMTV(C3H) RNA, while addition of the same amount of MMTV (C3Hf) RNA inhibits the hybrid formation by only 67% (Fig. 5C).

The fidelity of the ribonuclease-resistant ^{3}H-RNA·DNA hybrids described were analyzed for thermal stability on hydroxylapatite (48). As shown in Fig. 7, no difference in Te$_{1/2}$ (temperature at which half of the hybrid was eluted from hydroxylapatite) was observed between the ribonuclease-resistant hybrids formed between the DNA from RIII, C3H, or GR mammary tumors and the ^{3}H-labeled 60–70S RNA from MMTV (RIII).

The mammary tumors of the three strains of mice examined (GR, RIII, and C3H) contain approximately the same number of MMTV proviral sequences. This was determined with the assumption that the outcome of the competition hybridizations was not affected by a varying ratio of rate constants for the DNA·RNA and DNA·DNA renaturations, owing to varying cellular DNA: viral RNA ratios. Employing this assumption, the cellular DNA:viral RNA ratio at half-maximal hybridization is directly proportional to the number of proviral sequences per haploid cellular genome (49). From the formula given by Tonegawa et al. (50), and assuming the molecular complexity of MMTV 60–70S RNA is 8×10^6, the number of MMTV proviral copies is approximated at seven to nine per haploid cellular genome in the RIII, GR, and C3H mouse mammary tumor cell. If the molecular complexity of the MMTV 60–70S RNA is approximately 2.4×10^6, as was demonstrated for the 60–70S RNA of RSV (51,52),

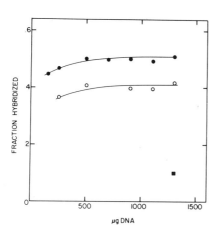

FIG. 6. Saturation hybridization between ^{32}P-60–70S RNA of MMTV(C3H) and DNA from "early" mammary tumors (•) and livers (o) of the same tumor-bearing C3H-A^{vy} mice. A total of 2,000 cpm of ^{32}P-60–70S RNA of MMTV(C3H) was hybridized to increasing amounts of cellular DNA fragments, with increasing volume (therefore increasing DNA·RNA ratios while keeping the DNA concentration constant) to maintain cellular DNA Cot values of 40,000. The hybrids were then dissolved in 2 × SSC (0.3 M NaCl and 0.03 M Na citrate) to 200 μg DNA per milliliter. Half of this solution was treated with 50 μg/ml RNase A and 100 U/ml RNase T$_1$ for 45 min at 37°C, after which both aliquots were assayed for TCA-precipitable radioactivity. The fraction of input radioactive viral RNA that entered into an RNase-resistant ^{32}P-RNA·DNA hybrid is plotted versus micrograms of DNA added to the hybridization mixture. Calf thymus DNA (■)was used as control DNA.

then the frequency of MMTV proviral sequences would be about three times higher, i.e., approximately 23–30 copies per haploid cellular genome.

General Comments

The viral genomes of the horizontally transmitted variants of the mouse mammary tumor virus of the mouse strains GR, RIII, C3H, and A appear to be at least 95% homologous as analyzed by molecular competitive hybridization. This technique considers the total genome of the RNA tumor virus and avoids inconclusive

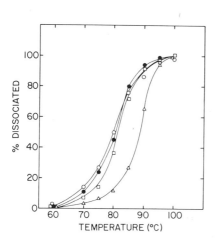

FIG. 7. Thermal stability of hybrids formed between ^{3}H-60–70S RNA of MMTV(RIII) and DNA from mammary tumors of the mouse strains RIII (•), GR (□), and C3H (o). The hybridizations between the ^{3}H-60–70S MMTV(RIII) RNA and 600 μg DNA fragments were performed to cellular DNA Cot values of 40,000 followed by treatment with RNase as described (45). The reaction mixtures were diluted to a DNA concentration of 50 μg/ml in 0.12 M sodium phosphate (pH 6.8) and analyzed by hydroxylapatite (45). The percentage of dissociation of the hybridized radioactive RNA bound to the column in a RNA:DNA hybrid is given versus elution temperature. The thermal dissociation of the DNA:DNA hybrid of RIII mammary tumor DNA (△) after reassociation to a cellular DNA Cot value of 40,000 and analyzed by chromatography on hydroxyapatite is given for comparison.

results that may arise because of the use of incomplete or preferential cDNA transcripts.

The similarity in nucleic acid sequences of the horizontally transmitted MMTVs is reflected in the similarity of their virulence and antigenic composition (5,12,53). The similarity in nucleic acid sequence of the MMTV(GR), which is transmitted by both milk and vertically via gametes (54), to the horizontally transmitted MMTVs of the other mouse strains studied is particularly interesting. The outcome of the molecular hybridization assay, as used, is confident within approximately 5%; differences in nucleic acid sequences smaller than 5% could therefore exist but would not be detected in our assay.

The difference in nucleic acid sequences between the horizontally and vertically transmitted MMTV variants of the C3H mouse is approximately 25%, as measured both by saturation hybridization (Fig. 6) and competition hybridization (Fig. 5). The nucleic acid sequence differences of the RNAs of the C3H MMTV transmitted as a germinal provirus and the C3H MMTV transmitted via an alternate mechanism such as nursing is in accord with the difference in virulence (5,12) of these variants.

MASON-PFIZER VIRUS

MPV was isolated from a carcinoma of the breast of a rhesus monkey and has been successfully propagated by cocultivation of the original mammary tumor tissue with rhesus mixed embryo cells (7,55). Host range studies have shown the virus to be also capable of replicating in rhesus embryonic lung, chimpanzee lung, human mixed embryo cell cultures, and an established human lymphocyte cell line, NC37 (56). MPV possesses morphological features of both the types B and C oncornaviruses, yet in certain features is morphologically distinct from both classes (Table 1) (7,57). Recently, there have been reports that viruses morphologically and immunologically similar to MPV have been isolated from certain rhesus (58,59) and human (60–71) cell lines.

The biochemical and biophysical properties of MPV are characteristic of RNA tumor viruses. The virus has a buoyant density in sucrose of 1.16 g/ml (72). It has a 60–70S RNA (72) which contains polyadenylate sequences of 200 nucleotides (73). The RNA-instructed DNA polymerase of MPV resembles that of the MMTVs with respect to a Mg^{++} divalent cation requirement, but appears to be immunologically distinct from the polymerases of other known RNA tumor viruses (38,74,75).

Analysis of MPV Proteins

We present here a characterization of the proteins and glycoproteins of MPV and their locations within the virion. Those viron-associated proteins which may be coded for by the virus genome were identified by growing the virus in different cell types (76).

MPV was first grown in CMMT cells (a mixed culture of the original rhesus carcinoma cells plus rhesus embryo cells). Cells were incubated with medium containing ^{3}H-amino acids, and the proteins of the virus produced were analyzed by SDS polyacrylamide gel electrophoresis (PAGE). Radioactively labeled virus was employed to eliminate the possibility that any of the proteins detected originated from extracellular components of the growth medium (e.g., glycoproteins of fetal calf serum). The virus sample was extensively purified by polyethylene glycol precipitation, two equilibrium centrifugations followed by a single velocity sedimentation. The result of the SDS-PAGE analysis of MPV proteins is shown in Fig. 8A (open circles). The apparent molecular weights of virion polypeptides were calculated from their relative mobilities using the known molecular weights of the marker proteins. The major viral polypeptide exhibited a molecular weight of 27,000 (p27) confirming previous observations (63,77,78). In addition to the p27 protein, five other major proteins were clearly recognizable (76) with molecular weights of 10,000 (p10), 12,000 (p12), 14,000 (p14), 20,000 (p20), and 68,000 (p68). The polypeptide pattern observed for MPV was different from that observed for C-type oncornaviruses (79) and the MMTVs from several strains of mice (Fig. 2).

Glycoproteins of MPV

In order to identify the glycoproteins of MPV, virus grown in CMMT was doubly labeled with ^{3}H-glucosamine and ^{14}C-amino acids, and purified by two density gradient centrifugations and one velocity sedimentation; virus-associated proteins were then analyzed by SDS-PAGE (Fig. 8A). It is evident that the protein gp68 contains the highest level of ^{3}H-glucosamine label coincident with ^{14}C-amino acid label and represents the major virion glycoprotein. Occasionally in some viral preparations an additional minor glycoprotein with a molecular weight of 75,000 (gp75) was observed. At present it is unclear whether gp68 and gp75 represent two distinct proteins or the same protein with varying degrees of glycosylation. In addition to gp68, another viral protein, gp20, appears to contain a low but significant level of ^{3}H-glucosamine label and therefore may constitute a minor glycoprotein of MPV. Correcting for differences in molecular weight and number of molecules per virion, it appears that gp68 is approximately 15 times more heavily labeled with glucosamine than gp20. A small peak of ^{3}H-glucosamine label found in a low-molecular-weight component ($<$10,000) (Fig. 8) does not coelectrophorese with any discrete ^{14}C-amino acid-labeled polypeptides and may represent glycolipid or glycopeptide.

Effect of Ultracentrifugation on MPV Proteins

It has been demonstrated that the major 70,000 glycoprotein (gp70) of Friend leukemia virus (FLV) can be released from the virus by shearing forces produced during high-speed centrifugation, ultrasonication, or osmotic shock (80). To determine whether any proteins were selectively lost during purification, MPV proteins were analyzed by SDS-PAGE at each stage of the purification. The

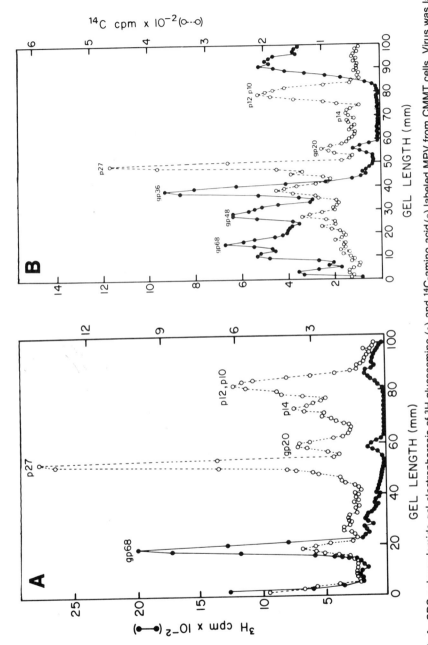

FIG. 8. A: SDS-polyacrylamide gel electrophoresis of ^{3}H-glucosamine (●) and ^{14}C-amino acid (○) labeled MPV from CMMT cells. Virus was labeled and purified by polyethylene glycol (PEG) precipitation, two equilibrium density gradient centrifugations, and one velocity sedimentation as described (76). **B:** SDS-polyacrylamide gel electrophoresis of proteins of MPV grown in NC-37 cells and doubly labeled with ^{3}H-glucosamine (●) and ^{14}C-amino acids (○). The differentially labeled viruses were copurified (76).

results are shown in Fig. 9. It is evident that the proteins p10, p12, p14, gp20, p27, and gp68 are in the same relative proportion at all steps in the purification, suggesting that these proteins are part of the virion structure. Futhermore, the major MPV glycoprotein, gp68, does not appear to be lost during the purification procedure.

Polypeptide Composition of MPV Grown in Other Primate Cells

In order to determine which virion-associated proteins may be coded for by the virus genome, MPV was grown in two additional primate cell types: one rhesus and one human. Those proteins present in virions, regardless of cell type of origin, is a strong indication that they are coded for by the virion. MPV originally derived from the CMMT cell line was grown in NC-37 human lymphoblast cells and rhesus foreskin cells (Rhfs). Coelectrophoresis of proteins of virions grown in CMMT and NC-37 cells revealed that proteins p10, p12, p14, gp20, p27, and gp68 were present in both preparations with no detectable difference in the migration of any of these proteins (76). Identical results are seen for MPV grown in Rhfs cells. However, two glycoproteins, gp36 and gp48, represent major proteins of MPV grown in NC-37 cells (Fig. 8B). These two proteins do not appear to be present in Rhfs-grown MPV, which exhibits a polypeptide pattern more similar to that for CMMT-grown MPV (Fig. 8A). To determine whether proteins gp36 and gp48 from NC-37-grown MPV represent virion proteins or proteins contributed by the host cell, MPV derived from NC-37 cells was propagated in human amnion cells (AV-3). Polypeptides of MPV from AV-3 cells were subsequently analyzed by SDS-PAGE. Except for protein gp36 (which was replaced by a peak at 40,000d) no qualitative difference was observed in the protein patterns of MPV grown in AV-3 or NC-37 cells. A summary of the above results is given in Table 6.

Localization of Viral Proteins in the Virion

The location of MPV proteins within the virion was investigated by using iodination catalyzed by the enzyme lactoperoxidase. Viral proteins exposed to the external environment are labeled by this technique. Purified MPV grown in CMMT cells was iodinated by lactoperoxidase either before or after disruption with the non-ionic detergent NP-40. Intact virus iodinated to high specific activities apparently did not undergo a significant alteration in structure, since such preparations rebanded at the density of untreated virus, i.e., 1.17 g/ml. If purified virions were first disrupted with NP-40 and subsequently iodinated, the polypeptide pattern of SDS gels were very similar to polypeptides of MPV labeled *in vivo* with ^{3}H-amino acids. When intact virus was first iodinated and then disrupted and analyzed by SDS-PAGE, the polypeptide pattern was significantly altered. The data are summarized in Table 7. It is apparent that the extent of labeling has significantly decreased for all viral proteins with the exception of gp68. These results indicate that gp68 represents the major external protein of the virion (76).

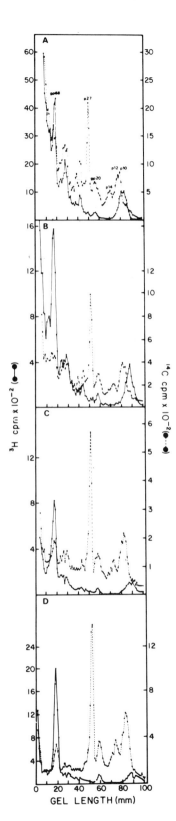

FIG. 9. SDS-polyacrylamide gel electrophoresis of ^{3}H-glucosamine (•) and ^{14}C-amino acid (○) labeled MPV at different stages of purification. Viruses were copurified from CMMT cells and analyzed by SDS-PAGE at various stages of purification as described (76). **A**: PEG precipitation alone. **B**: PEG plus one equilibrium density centrifugation. **C**: PEG plus two equilibrium density centrifugations. **D**: PEG plus two equilibrium density centrifugations followed by one velocity sedimentation.

TABLE 6. *Polypeptides of MPV [a]from different cell types*

	Presence of polypeptide in four cell types			
Protein	CMMT	NC-37	Rhfs	AV-3
p10	+[b]	+	+	+
p12	+	+	+	+
p14	+	+	+	+
gp20	+	+	+	+
p27	+	+	+	+
gp36	−	+	−	±
gp48	−	+	±	+
gp68	+	+	+	+
gp75	±	±	±	±

[a]Virus purified by polyethylene glycol precipitation, double equilibrium banding followed by velocity sedimentation (76).
[b]+, present in virion. −, absent from virion.
±, present occasionally in viral preparations.

General Comments

These experiments enabled us to identify six distinct and reproducible polypeptides associated with Mason-Pfizer virions. The molecular weights of these proteins based on SDS-PAGE analysis are: 10,000 (p10), 12,000 (p12), 14,000 (p14), 20,000 (gp20), 27,000 (p27), and 68,000 (gp68). The SDS-PAGE polypeptide gel pattern for MPV is different from that of both mammalian types B and C viruses. Furthermore, none of the above proteins was selectively lost during extensive purification of the virus and are present in the same relative proportions regardless of the cell type from which the virus originated. These results suggest that these six proteins are virus coded and not derived from host cell components.

TABLE 7. *Iodination of MPMV proteins before and after disruption*

	Total ^{125}I (cpm)		
Protein	Intact	Disrupted	Intact/disrupted[a]
gp68	16,050 (61)[b]	9,800 (10)	1.00
p27	3,600 (14)	44,150 (45)	0.05
gp20	3,800 (14)	14,300 (15)	0.22
p14	1,200 (5)	9,100 (9)	0.10
p10–12	1,600 (6)	20,000 (21)	0.05

[a]Normalized to 1.00 for protein p68.
[b]Numbers in parentheses signify relative percentages of each protein of the total protein peaks (76).

MPV RNA Structure

The RNA of most oncornaviruses is a highly structured 60–70S molecule that can be dissociated to 30–40S subunits and smaller RNAs utilizing various denaturing conditions (81,82). We report here an analysis of the structure of MPV RNA and demonstrate its similarity to the RNA structure of that of other oncornaviruses such as avian myeloblastosis virus (82) and Rauscher murine leukemia virus (MuLV).

Characterization of the RNAs of MPV and MuLV was derived from electrophoresis in mixed agarose-polyacrylamide gels. Culture media containing ^{3}H-labeled MPV and ^{32}P-MuLV were mixed, the viruses copurified, and the viral RNAs coextracted. The 60–70S RNAs were isolated on glycerol gradients and subjected to electrophoresis in 1.8% polyacrylamide gels containing 0.5% agarose (Fig. 10). By comparing the relative electrophoretic mobilities of vesicular stomatitis virus RNA and NC37 ribosomal 28S and 18S RNAs, the molecular weights of MPV and MuLV RNAs were estimated to be 8×10^6 (83). This must be taken, however, as an "apparent" molecular weight, as we are dealing with a highly structured molecule.

Studies were undertaken to determine the subunit structure of MPV and MuLV 60–70S RNAs by stepwise dissociation with formamide. RNA (60–70S) from ^{3}H-uridine-labeled MPV and ^{32}P-labeled MuLV were extracted and copurified. Partial dissociation of both MPV and MuLV RNA occurred after treatment with 10% formamide (Fig. 11A), whereas complete dissociation was achieved with 40% formamide (Fig. 11B). Disaggregation of the viral RNAs by heating at 80°C for 2.5 min yielded essentially the same result as 40% formamide (Fig. 11C). The molecular weights of the subunits of MPV and MuLV were similar and were estimated to be 2.8×10^6 (83).

To determine if the time interval between virus release from cells and tissue culture fluid collection affects the size of RNA subunits, ^{3}H-uridine-labeled MPV was harvested at either 2- or 24-hr intervals. The viral RNAs isolated from culture fluids from both 2- and 24-hr harvests had similar sedimentation values (60–70S). After treatment with 40% formamide the 60–70S RNA from virus of 2-hr collections yielded a major RNA subunit with a sedimentation coefficient of 30S. Identical treatment (with 40% formamide) of 60–70S RNA from virus of 24-hr collections, however, yielded a heterogeneous array of small RNA molecules; this suggests a rapid degradation of RNA within virions after release from cells, a phenomenon that has been found for other oncornaviruses. Treatment of 60–70S RNA from virus of 2-hr collections with 10% and 20% formamide revealed intermediate RNA structures between 65S and 30S (83). Similar treatment of 60–70S RNA from virus of 24-hr collections, however, yielded more heterogeneous peaks with much lower sedimentation values. Heating the 60–70S RNA from virus of 2-hr collections at 80°C for 2.5 min yielded RNA subunit structures similar to those obtained with 40% formamide.

To characterize any low-molecular-weight RNAs associated with MPV RNA, purified ^{3}H-MPV 60–70S RNA from 2-hr viral harvests was heated at 80°C for

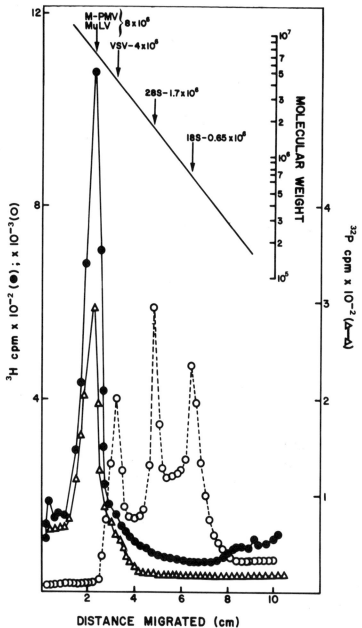

FIG. 10. Polyacrylamide gel electrophoresis of MPV and MuLV high-molecular-weight RNA. ^{3}H-MPV was grown in CMMT cells, and ^{32}P-MuLV in NIH-Swiss 3T3 cells. RNAs were prepared by the addition of ^{3}H-uridine or ^{32}P to the tissue culture medium in roller bottle cultures. Pooled tissue culture fluid was clarified by centrifugation at 6,500 g for 10 min and stored at –80°C until use. Virus was precipitated from the tissue culture fluids by polyethylene glycol. The virus precipitate was collected by centrifugation, resuspended, and centrifuged through 20% glycerol in TNE. Viral RNA was extracted and layered onto a linear 10–30% glycerol gradient in TNE and centrifuged for 3.5 hr at 40,000 rpm in an SW41 rotor at 4°C. The 60–70S RNA regions were pooled and precipitated. The RNAs were resuspended in electrophoresis buffer and analyzed by polyacrylamide gel electrophoresis, as described (83).

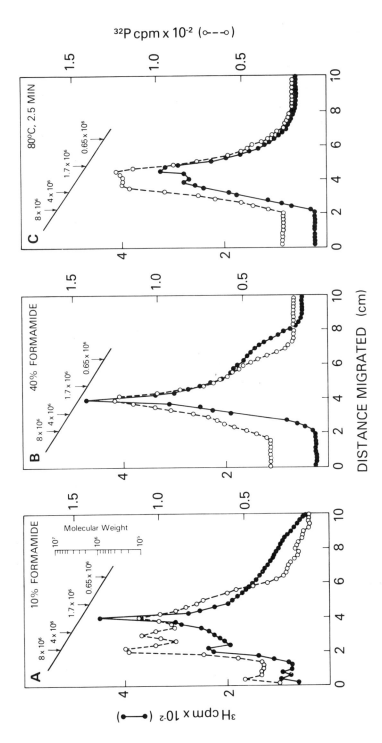

FIG. 11. Stepwise dissociation of MPV and MuLV high-molecular-weight RNA by formamide and heat. ³H-MPV RNA (●) and ³²P-MuLV RNA (○), isolated as described in Fig. 10, were denatured with (**A**) 10% formamide for 10 min at 37°C or (**B**) 40% formamide for 10 min at 37°C, or by (**C**) heating at 80°C for 2.5 min. The resultant dissociation products were analyzed by mixed agarose polyacrylamide gel electrophoresis (83).

2.5 min and electrophoresed on a 10% polyacrylamide gel. When compared to ^{32}P cellular 4S and 5S RNA markers, three small RNAs with molecular weights of 2.5×10^4, 3.5×10^4, and 10^5 were evident (83). These molecular weights were calculated to correspond to approximate sedimentation coefficients of 4S, 4.5S, and 7S, respectively, and are similar in size to those found in Rous sarcoma virus (84). The 4S, 4.5S, and 7S were present in ratios of 8:3:4 and represented approximately 4%, 1.5%, and 2%, respectively, of the total counts per minute of the original 60–70S RNA molecule.

The stepwise dissociation of MPV 60–70S RNA by limited formamide treatment suggests that the RNA subunits of MPV may be linked by differentially stable hydrogen-bonded regions. Similar results were obtained by Travnicek and Riman (82) and the 60–70S RNA of avian myeloblastosis virus. The studies reported here demonstrate the similarities of MPV RNA to the RNAs of known avian and mammalian RNA tumor viruses in terms of size, subunit structure, and associated RNAs.

Nucleotide Sequence Relationships Between MPV RNA and RNA of Other Oncornaviruses

Viruses recently isolated from cultures of various rhesus tissues are morphologically and immunologically related to MPV. Cell lines producing these particles have been established from a normal rhesus lactating mammary gland (X381) and from normal rhesus placental tissue (58,59). Isolates from a number of human cells have also been reported that exhibit a morphology similar to MPV, immunologically cross react with MPV, and have at least partial nucleic acid sequences in common with MPV. These cell lines include HeLa clones as described by Gelderblom, Bauer, and colleagues (60–62), AO cells (63), and a variety of other cell lines (64–71). Some of these cell lines, however, have been shown to contain HeLa cell markers (85).

We have undertaken studies (86) that showed little or no detectable differences in nucleic acid sequences among the RNAs of MPV, X381, and RNA isolated from the cytoplasm of HeLa (60) and AO (63) cell lines producing particles morphologically similar to MPV. No MPV-related sequences, however, were found in the RNA or DNA of two clones of HeLa cells obtained from the American Type Culture Collection. No detectable nucleic acid sequence homology was observed between MPV 60–70S RNA and the RNAs of a variety of types B and C viruses.

Hybridization of MPV RNA to DNA from MPV-Infected Cells

MPV 60–70S RNA from virus grown in NC-37 cells was purified and iodinated *in vitro* to a specific activity of approximately $2–5 \times 10^7$ cpm/μg (86). This RNA was 100% acid-precipitable, 99% sensitive to ribonuclease, and banded as a sharp peak in cesium sulfate at a density of 1.63 g/ml. Iodinated MPV RNA was hybridized to DNA (at a concentration of 3 mg/ml) purified from MPV-infected NC-37 cells for various amounts of time (Table 8). The hybrids were assayed for ribonuclease resistance. The cellular DNA exhibited a $Cot_{1/2}$ of approximately 3,000, indicating that the MPV-related proviral information is in the nonrepeated class of DNA and is present at approximately one to two copies per haploid cellular genome. The same $Cot_{1/2}$ was obtained using tritiated MPV 60–70S RNA prepared as previously described (83). The hybridization with [125]I 60–70S RNA achieved a maximum hybridization of greater than 60% at a Cot of 75,000, while less than 6% hybridization was observed with the DNA of either uninfected NC37 cells or *E. coli* (Table 8). This assured us that the vast majority of ^{125}I-RNA used in these studies was MPV-specific and did not contain significant amounts of RNA or DNA of NC37 cells—the cells in which the virus was grown.

To develop conditions for a sensitive competitive hybridization assay, however, it is important to determine the minimum amount of DNA from MPV-infected NC37 cells needed to obtain maximum hybridization. Therefore increasing amounts of DNA from MPV-infected NC37 cells (at a constant DNA concentration of 5 mg/ml) were annealed to a constant amount of ^{125}I MPV 60–70S RNA. The annealing reactions were incubated at 68°C to a Cot of 35,000 and analyzed for ribonuclease sensitivity; 0.3 mg was the lowest input of DNA that gave maximal hybridization with the amount of [125]I 60–70S MPV RNA used. This DNA:RNA ratio (i.e., 0.3 mg DNA from MPV-infected NC37 cells and 2,000 cpm ^{125}I MPV 60–70S RNA) was therefore employed in the competitive molecular hybridization experiments described below.

TABLE 8. *Hybridization of MPV* [125]*I 60–70S RNA to DNA of MPV-infected NC37 cells*

Cellular DNA	Cot	% Hybrid-ization
NC37, MPV-infected	100	4.1
	600	14.4
	1,000	19.9
	5,000	32.8
	10,000	40.3
	50,000	55.4
	75,000	64.0
NC-37, uninfected	10,000	4.6
	75,000	5.1
E. coli	10,000	4.1
	75,000	3.2

One thousand counts of [125]I 60–70S MPV RNA was annealed to 1 mg of cellular DNA as described (86). The hybridization mixture was incubated for appropriate periods to achieve the desired Cots.

Competitive Molecular Hybridizations

Various amounts (0.1–1,000 ng) of unlabeled MPV 60–70S RNA were added
to the standard hybridization reactions between ^{125}I MPV 60–70S RNA and
DNA from MPV-infected NC37 cells. Approximately 95% of the [125]I 60–70S
RNA from MPV was competed out with 400 ng unlabeled MPV RNA (Fig. 12,
closed circles). The midpoint of this curve was obtained with an input of 6.3 ng
MPV RNA. When the same competition reaction was performed using cytoplasmic RNA from NC37 cells infected with MPV (Fig. 12, open circles), competition was again observed to a level of approximately 95%, but this time with an
input of 10^5 ng of cellular RNA. The midpoint of this competition reaction was
achieved at approximately 9,500 ng of competitor RNA. A comparison of the
midpoints using viral versus cytoplasmic competitor RNA indicates that approximately 0.07% of the total cytoplasmic RNA of MPV-infected cells is MPV-
related. This is in good agreement with the percentage obtained using Crt analysis
of the hybridization between cytoplasmic RNA and ^{3}H-cDNA made from MPV
RNA (87). A small amount of competition was observed with competitor RNA
from uninfected NC37 cells up to an input of 5×10^5 ng RNA (Fig. 12,
triangles). This competition may be due in part to the 4, 4.5, and 7S RNAs
associated with the 60–70S MPV genome (83).

The competition of the hybridization between the ^{125}I MPV RNA and the
DNA of MPV-infected cells was then used to determine the extent of relatedness,
if any, between MPV RNA and the 60–70S RNAs of types B and C RNA tumor

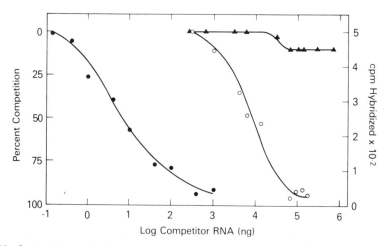

FIG. 12. Competitive molecular hybridization of the MPV genome. [125]I-60–70S MPV RNA
(2,000 cpm) was hybridized to 300 μg DNA from MPV-infected NC37 cells. Increasing
amounts of unlabeled viral of cytoplasmic RNAs were added to this reaction. The samples
were incubated at 68°C in 0.12 M sodium phosphate (pH 6.8), 0.4 M NaCl, 0.1% SDS, and
0.05 M EDTA to a Cot of 35,000, and then were assayed for acquisition of RNase resistance
as described (86). ●, MPV 60–70S RNA. ○, cytoplasmic RNA from MPV-infected NC37 cells. ▲,
cytoplasmic RNA from uninfected NC37 cells.

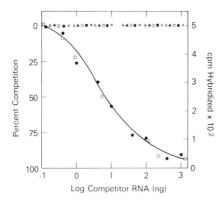

FIG. 13. Competition of the MPV genome with viral RNAs. Hybridizations between ^{125}I-MPV 60–70S RNA and DNA of MPV-infected NC37 cells were as described in the legend to Fig. 12. Competition reactions were performed using viral RNA as competitor from: ●, MPV; ○, X-381; Δ, MMTV-RIII; ▲, GPV-B; □, SSV-1; ■, AMV; X, MuLV(Rauscher).

viruses. No competition was detected using viral RNA (0.1–1,000 ng) from the following C-type viruses examined: avian myeloblastosis virus, MuLV (Rauscher), and simian sarcoma virus (Fig. 13). Furthermore, no competition of hybridization was observed using 0.1–1,000 ng viral RNA from the RIII MMTV, or B-GPV (Fig. 13).

A virus (X381) morphologically similar to MPV was isolated from a cultured rhesus lactating mammary gland (58). To determine the extent of nucleic acid sequence homology between MPV and X381, 0.1–1,000 ng of X381 RNA was added to the standard MPV competition hybridization reaction. As can be seen in Fig. 13, unlabeled X381 RNA (open circles) showed the same degree of competition as the homologous unlabeled MPV RNA (closed circles). It can therefore be concluded that X381 and MPV share at least 95% sequence homology.

Experiments were then undertaken (86) to determine the relatedness between MPV and morphologically similar isolates produced from HeLa (60) and AO (63) cells. Sufficient quantities of unlabeled 60–70S RNA from particles produced by these cell lines could not be obtained because of their low level of virus production. We therefore sought to determine if any MPV-related sequences could be found in the cytoplasmic RNA of these cells. Increasing amounts of cytoplasmic RNA (10^2 to 5×10^5 ng) were introduced into the hybridization reaction between ^{125}I-MPV RNA and the DNA from MPV-infected NC37 cells. As shown in Fig. 14, greater than 90% competition was obtained using the RNA from the HeLa clone described by Gelderblom et al. (60), and at least 85% competition was obtained with the RNA from the AO cell line (63). Two to five times more cytoplasmic RNA from these two lines was required to reach the 50% point of the competition curve, compared with RNA from the NC37 cells producing MPV. These two cell lines therefore contain RNA that is at least 90% related to the RNA of MPV. No MPV-related information was found, however, in the RNA purified from two clones of HeLa cells (CCL2 and CCL2.1) obtained from the American Type Culture Collection (Fig. 14).

The presence of MPV information in the RNA of one clone of HeLa cells (60) and its absence from two others may be explained by one of two

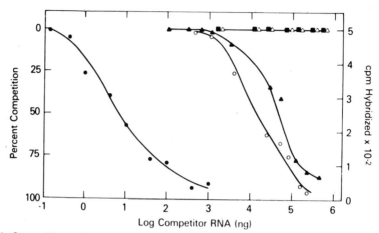

FIG. 14. Competitive molecular hybridization of the MPV genome with cellular RNA as competitor. Competition hybridizations were performed as described in the legend to Fig. 12. The following cellular RNAs were used as competitor RNA: ●, MPV 60–70S RNA; ○, cytoplasmic RNA from HeLa cells (60); ■, cytoplasmic RNA from HeLa cells (American Type Culture Collection CCL2); Δ, cytoplasmic RNA from HeLa cells (American Type Culture Collection CCL2.1); ▲, cytoplasmic RNA from AO cells (63).

alternatives. First, the MPV-related information is present in the DNA of all HeLa cells and has been activated in certain clones; and second, the viral information is not in the DNA of all HeLa clones, and some clones contain MPV information which may have been introduced by laboratory manipulation. To ascertain which is correct, ^{125}I-MPV 60–70S RNA was annealed to $300\mu g$ nuclear DNA from the three clones of HeLa cells in question; the hybridization reaction was incubated to a Cot of 35,000. Significant hybridization (greater than 80% of the control hybridization to MPV-infected NC37 cells) was detected with the clone of HeLa cells (60) producing MPV-related particles, although no MPV-related sequences were detected in the DNA of the two HeLa clones from the American Type Culture Collection. This finding (86) supports the second explanation stated above.

Hybridization of ^{125}I-MPV RNA to the DNA of Various Species

The lack of appreciable hybridization of MPV ^{125}I-RNA to the DNA of normal NC37 cells and two clones of HeLa cells demonstrates that MPV is not an "endogenous" virus of humans; i.e., the entire genome is not present as a provirus in the DNA of all cells of the species. ^{125}I-MPV 60–70S RNA shows a low degree of hybridization to normal rhesus tissue (Table 9). The explanation for this finding is currently under investigation. It appears therefore that MPV, while indigenous to rhesus monkeys (88–90), is not an "endogenous" virus of that species (90). Table 9 also demonstrates that MPV is not an "endogenous" virus of any of the 11 other species tested, nor is it appreciably related in nucleic acid sequences to an "endogenous" virus of any of these species.

TABLE 9. *Hybridization of MPV ^{125}I 60–70S RNA to cellular DNA of various species*

Source	%Hybridization[a]
Human (NC37 cells infected with MPV)	59.4
Human (NC37 cells, uninfected)	6.7
Human (liver)	6.9
Monkey (rhesus)	13.1
Cat	1.0
Chicken	6.3
Cow	6.9
Dog	5.1
Guinea pig	4.3
Hamster	5.0
Mouse	3.2
Pig	2.2
Rabbit	4.9
Rat	3.6
Sheep	6.4

[a]Hybridizations were performed as described (86).

General Comments

The technique of competitive molecular hybridization used in these studies considers the entire viral RNA genome and avoids inconclusive results that may result if incomplete or preferential cDNA transcripts are employed. Numerous reports have appeared recently concerning the detection of viruses morphologically related to MPV in a variety of human cell lines including clones of HeLa (60) and AO (63) cells. The AO cells in question have been reported to contain HeLa-like markers (85). The greater than 90% sequence homology between MPV RNA and the RNA from these cells, and the lack of any detectable MPV-related information in the RNA or DNA of two clones of HeLa cells from the American Type Culture Collection, provide evidence that at least some isolates may be the result of either viral or cellular contamination.

The fact that MPV is not an "endogenous" virus of humans does not mean that any of the MPV-related isolates reported (60, 63–71) are not human isolates. The possibility has not been ruled out that MPV is being transmitted in either rhesus or human populations by some mechanism other than as a germinal provirus. There are lines of evidence that in fact support this possibility in rhesus monkeys. MPV-related proviral sequences have been found (90) in the DNA of certain organs of rhesus monkeys, while the DNA of other organs of the same monkeys do not contain these particular sequences.

BIOCHEMICAL STUDIES OF THE BUdR-INDUCED GUINEA PIG VIRUS

Halogenated pyrimidine deoxynucleotides have been useful (91) for the *in vitro* induction of RNA tumor viruses in a variety of mammalian cells. In the case of either normal or leukemic guinea pig cells, induction with BUdR or IUdR leads to the production of oncornavirus particles that are morphologically and biochemically similar to known RNA tumor viruses (8–11,92). Based on preliminary morphological findings and the presence of high-molecular-weight RNA and reverse transcriptase, the BUdR-induced guinea pig virus (GPV) was initially described as a typical C-type virus (8,9,93). Subsequent studies asserted that the BUdR-induced GPV shares morphological properties of both B- and C-type viruses (10,94). Recently, however, it was demonstrated (11) that the BUdR-induced GPV is extremely similar morphologically to the B-type mouse mammary tumor virus. For example, the BUdR-induced GPV particles bud from the plasma membrane with a complete nucleoid; the mature particles may have an eccentric, electron-dense nucleoid; and negatively stained particles exhibit protruding spikes on the outer membrane, similar to those seen on MMTV (Table 1). Intracytoplasmic A-particles, another feature of cells producing MMTV, are present in BUdR-induced guinea pig cells. We present here biochemical and biophysical properties of the virus particles (B-GPV) released by guinea pig cells after BUdR induction, and compare them to those of MuLV, MMTV, and MPV.

Density of B-GPV

Isopycnic centrifugation in sucrose of ^{32}P-GPV and ^{3}H-amino acid-labeled MMTV resulted in an average buoyant density value of 1.18 g/ml for both. Equilibrium density centrifugation of ^{32}P-GPV and ^{3}H-uridine-labeled MuLV resulted in a buoyant density value of 1.18 g/ml for ^{32}P-GPV and 1.16 g/ml for ^{3}H-MuLV (95). Equilibrium density centrifugation in CsCl of ^{32}P-GPV, ^{3}H-MMTV, and ^{3}H-MuLV resulted in buoyant density values of 1.21 g/ml for GPV and MMTV, and 1.17 g/ml for MuLV (Table 4).

High-Molecular-Weight RNA of B-GPV

The RNA complex of the BUdR-induced GPV has been reported to be "larger" than that of MuLV, as determined by sedimentation analysis (92). Sedimentation analysis of ^{3}H-labeled B-GPV RNA on a 10–30% glycerol gradient revealed (95) a high-molecular-weight RNA with a sedimentation value of 60–70S and variable amounts of 28S and lower-molecular-weight RNA. After alcohol precipitation of the 60–70S ^{3}H-labeled RNA, this RNA was redissolved and analyzed by mixed agarose-polyacrylamide gel electrophoresis and shown to have an "apparent" (83) molecular weight of 8×10^6 (95). The same value has been found in this laboratory for the molecular weight of the 60–70S RNA complexes of MPV, MMTV, and MuLV using identical conditions of electrophoresis. Denaturation (82,83) of this HMW-RNA complex releases a ^{3}H-RNA with a molecular weight of approximately 2.6×10^6, as well as lower-molecular-weight RNAs. These studies indicate the HMW-RNA of B-GPV is comparable to the RNA of several oncornaviruses with respect to its apparent weight and subunit structure (95).

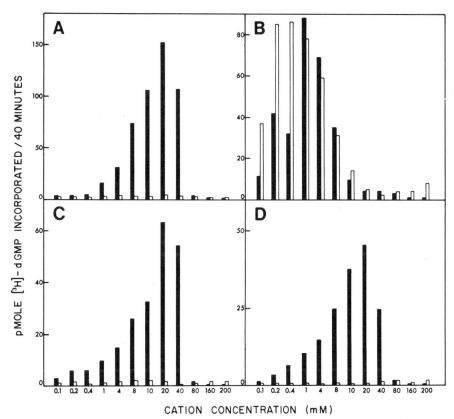

FIG. 15. DNA polymerase activity of various oncornaviruses as a function of Mg++ (closed bars) or Mn++ (open bars) concentration in the reaction mixture. Virus concentrates were disrupted with 2% NP-40 and used in a DNA polymerase assay using the synthetic template poly rC:oligo dG as described (95). The results are expressed as picomoles of ^{3}H-dGTP incorporated into a rC:dG polymer in a 40-min reaction versus the indicated cation concentration. All reactions were linear through the 40-min time point. **A**: MMTV(RIII). **B**: MuLV (Rauscher). **C**: B-GPV. **D**: MPV.

Cation Preference of the B-GPV DNA Polymerase

Characterization of the mammalian B- and C-type virus reverse transcriptases by their cation preference was previously reported (35,37,38,74,96). The reverse transcriptases of the MMTVs and of MPV were reported to prefer the Mg^{++} cation, while the reverse transcriptases of the mammalian C-type viruses have been reported to prefer Mn^{++}. To determine the similarity or difference in the cation preferences for these viruses, titrations over a 2,000-fold range of Mg^{++} and Mn^{++} were performed with B-GPV, MMTV, MPV, and MuLV. The results are illustrated in Fig. 15. It is clear that B-GPV (Fig. 15C), MMTV (Fig. 15A), and MPV (Fig. 15D) DNA polymerases have a strict Mg^{++} preference, using the template poly rC:oligo $dG_{(10-12)}$, with a Mg^{++} optimum at approximately 20 mM. The greatest difference between these viruses and the type-C MuLV (Fig. 15B) is obtained using 0.2–0.4 mM Mn^{++} for MuLV.

Competitive Molecular Hybridization

Radioactively labeled 60–70S RNA of B-GPV was used in competitive molecular hybridization assays to determine if any nucleic acid sequence homology is shared with the RNA of other oncornaviruses (95). Increasing amounts of unlabeled viral RNAs were added to the hybridization reaction between radioactive B-GPV 60–70S RNA and DNA from normal guinea pigs. No inhibition of this hybrid formation was induced by adding the unlabeled viral RNAs of MPV, MMTV, MuLV, or hamster sarcoma virus (Fig. 16) up to a cellular DNA: competitor viral RNA ratio of 100:1. Addition of increasing amounts of unlabeled B-GPV RNA, however, resulted in an increasing inhibition of the hybrid formation (to a maximum of 90%).

Assuming that the rate constants for the DNA:RNA hybridization and DNA:DNA renaturation are independent of the cellular DNA:viral RNA ratio, then the cellular DNA:viral RNA ratio at half maximal hybridization is directly proportional to the number of proviral sequences per haploid cellular genome (49). From the formula given by Tonegawa et al. (50), and assuming a B-GPV genome molecular weight of 8×10^6, the number of B-GPV proviral sequences can be calculated to be 83 per haploid genome. If the molecular weight

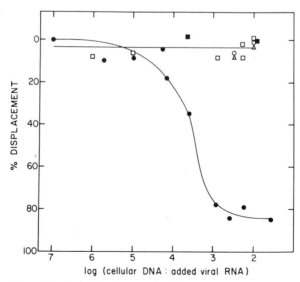

FIG. 16. Competition of the hybridization reaction between radioactive 60–70S B-GPV RNA and DNA from spleens of guinea pigs. Unlabeled competitor RNAs were: GPV (●), MMTV(C3H) (□), MuLV (○), hamster sarcoma virus (Δ), or MPV (■). The hybridizations were performed to a cellular DNA Cot value of 40,000 and assayed as described (95).

of the genome is assumed to be 2.4 × 10⁶ (52), then approximately 250–275 copies of B-GPV proviral sequences are present per haploid cellular genome.

No hybridization above intrinsic RNase resistancy of the ³H 60–70S GPV RNA was obtained if the radioactively labeled 60–70S GPV RNA was hybridized to various mammalian DNAs (other than guinea pig DNA) up to a cellular Cot value of 10⁵ (Table 10). This is evidence that B-GPV is not considerably related to an "endogenous" virus of any of the seven species examined (95).

General Comments

The classification of RNA tumor viruses was originally based on their morphology (1). The virus particles detected in BUdR-induced guinea pig cells are similar to the B-type MMTV in many stages of morphogenesis. The buoyant density of B-GPV is 1.18 g/ml in sucrose and 1.21 g/ml in CsCl; these values are identical to the buoyant density values of the B-type MMTV and distinct from those of the C-type viruses. Moreover, the DNA polymerases of B-GPV and MMTV prefer Mg⁺⁺ to Mn⁺⁺ in a poly rC:oligo dG templated assay. Biochemical and biophysical properties such as buoyant density and cation preference in a DNA polymerase assay, however, are only two of the numerous properties of RNA tumor viruses. Therefore until more evidence becomes available, B-GPV should be characterized as an endogenous guinea pig virus with several morphological and biochemical features similar to the murine type B MMTVs.

TABLE 10. *Hybridization of ³H B-GPV 60–70S RNA to cellular DNA*

Source	Fraction hybridized
Mouse (RIII)	0.09
Rat	0.13
Cat	0.11
Dog	0.10
Calf	0.08
Baboon	0.12
Human	0.10
Guinea pig	0.73
E. coli	0.13
No DNA added	0.12

Cellular DNA fragments (600 μg) and 2,000 cpm ³H 60–70S RNA were incubated in 4 × SSC (0.6 M NaCl and 0.06 M Na citrate), 0.1% SDS, and 3 μg yeast RNA in a volume of 100 μl until a cellular Cot of 100,000 was reached. The hybridization mixture was then transferred to 4 ml 2 × SSC (0.3 M NaCl and 0.03 M Na citrate). The sample was divided in half, and ribonuclease A was added to one aliquot to 50 μg/ml. Both aliquots were incubated at 37°C for 45 min and then assayed for TCA-precipitable radioactivity. The fraction hybridized was calculated by dividing the value of the RNase-treated sample by the value of the untreated sample (95).

CONCLUDING COMMENTS

The distribution of proviral sequences in the species of isolation for each of the agents reported on here is of interest (**Table 4**). The B-GPV appears to be a true "endogenous virus;" i.e., it is transmitted as a germinal provirus and is present in at least one copy per haploid genome in every cell of the animal. As shown here, B-GPV is present at a frequency of approximately 85–275 copies per haploid genome. The MMTVs of the C3H, GR, and RIII mouse strains are present at much lower proviral copy numbers (**Table 4**). The horizontally transmitted MMTV of the C3H mouse is not a true endogenous virus, however, for while its entire genome is present as a provirus in mouse mammary tumor cells approximately 25% of the viral genome appears to be absent in cells of certain normal organs of the same tumor-bearing animal (Fig. 6) (45). On the opposite end of the spectrum is the Mason-Pfizer virus. Many normal rhesus tissues examined show that the entire MPV genome is not present as a provirus. MPV does appear to be, however, a virus indigenous to the rhesus population (88) and therefore may be maintained via some infectious process. This is evidenced by the fact that certain organs of some rhesus monkeys contain MPV-proviral information (90). Even in cells experimentally infected with MPV, MPV-proviral sequences are present at only one or two copies per haploid genome (86).

The lack of detectable sequence homology among B-GPV, MPV, and MMTV is of interest in light of a similar lack of appreciable sequence homology among type C viruses of various species (97–101). The lack of any detectable difference in the nucleic acid sequences of the RNAs of the horizontally transmitted MMTVs of RIII, C3H, GR, and A strains of mice is in contrast, however, with the great deal of nucleic acid sequence divergence observed within the murine type C viruses (99,102,103).

The mouse mammary tumor viruses, Mason-Pfizer virus (and morphologically similar isolates), and the BUdR-induced guinea pig virus share several structural and biochemical properties (Tables 1 and 4; Fig. 15). These include: (a) the presence of intracytoplasmic A-particles in infected cells; (b) a complete nucleoid at budding; (c) an eccentric nucleoid in the mature particle; (d) a virion density of 1.21 g/ml in CsCl; and (e) a viral DNA polymerase activity with a Mg^{++} cation preference. Whereas any one of these criteria may not be sufficient to distinguish these viruses from the mammalian C-type or the intracisternal A-type particles, the combination of the above five distinguishing characteristics surely merits consideration of a common grouping of these agents.

REFERENCES

1. Bernhard, W. (1960): The detection and study of tumor viruses with the electron microscope. *Cancer Res.*, 20:712–727.
2. Gross, L. (1970): *Oncogenic Viruses.* Pergamon Press, Oxford.
3. Perk, K., and Dahlberg, J. E. (1974): Murine intracisternal A type particles fail to separate from the membrane of the endoplasmic reticulum. *J. Virol.*, 14:1304–1306.
4. Bittner, J. J. (1936): Some possible effects of nursing on the mammary gland tumor incidence in mice. *Science*, 84:162.
5. Bentvelzen, P. (1972): The biology of the mouse mammary tumor virus. *Int. Rev. Exp. Pathol.*, 11:259–297.

6. Dalton, A. (1972): Further analysis of the detailed structure of type B and C particles. *J. Natl. Cancer Inst.,* 48:1095–1099.
7. Chopra, H. C., and Mason, M. M. (1970): A new virus in a spontaneous mammary tumor of a rhesus monkey. *Cancer Res.,* 30:2081–2086.
8. Hsiung, D. G. (1972): Activation of guinea pig C-type virus in cultured spleen cells by 5-bromo-2'-deoxyuridine. *J. Natl. Cancer Inst.,* 49:567–570.
9. Nayak, D. P., and Murray, P. R. (1973): Induction of type C virus in cultured guinea pig cells. *J. Virol.,* 12:177–187.
10. Rhim, J. D., Duh, F. G., Cho, H. Y., Wuu, K. D., and Vernon, M. L. (1973): Activation by 5-bromo-2'-deoxyuridine of particles resembling guinea pig leukemia virus from guinea pig nonproducer cells. *J. Natl. Cancer Inst.,* 51:1327–1331.
11. Dahlberg, J. E., Perk, K., and Dalton, A. J. (1974): Virus-like particles induced in guinea pig cells by 5-bromo-2'—deoxyuridine are morphologically similar to murine B-type virus. *Nature (Lond.),* 249:828–830.
12. Nandi, S., and McGrath, C. M. (1973): Mammary neoplasia in mice. *Adv. Cancer Res.,* 17:353–414.
13. Lasfargues, E. Y., Moore, D. H., Murray, M. R., Haagensen, C. D., and Pollard, E. C. (1959): Production of the milk agent in cultures of mouse mammary carcinoma. *J. Biophys. Biochem. Cytol.,* 5:93–96.
14. Lasfargues, E. Y., Murray, M. R., and Moore, D. H. (1960): Cultivation of the mouse mammary carcinoma virus. *Natl. Cancer Inst. Monogr.,* 4:151–166.
15. Sanford, K. K., Andervont, H. B., Hobbs, G. L., and Earle, W. R. (1961): Maintenance of the mammary tumor agent in long-term cultures of mouse mammary carcinoma. *J. Natl. Cancer Inst.,* 26:1185–1191.
16. Sykes, J. A., Whitescarver, J., and Briggs, L. (1968): Observations on a cell line producing mammary tumor virus. *J. Natl. Cancer Inst.,* 41:1315–1327.
17. Parks, W. P., and Scolnick, E. M. Murine mammary tumor cell clones with varying degrees of virus expression. *Virology,* 55:163–173.
18. Parks, W. P., Scolnick, E. M., and Kozikowski, E. H. (1974): Dexamethasone stimulation of murine mammary tumor virus expression: A tissue culture source of virus. *Science,* 184:158–160.
19. Yagi, M. J. (1973): Cultivation and characterization of Balb/cfC3H mammary tumor cell lines. *J. Natl. Cancer Inst.,* 51:1849–1855.
20. Keydar, J., Gilead, Z., Hartman, J., and Ben Shaul, Y. (1973): In vitro production of mouse mammary tumor virus in a mouse mammary tumor ascites line. *Proc. Natl. Acad. Sci. U.S.A.,* 70:2983–2987.
21. Fine, D. L., Plowman, J. K., Kelley, S. P., Arthur, L. O., and Hillman, E. A. (1974): Enhanced production of mouse mammary tumor virus in dexamethasone-treated 5-iododeoxyuridine-stimulated mammary tumor cell cultures. *J. Natl. Cancer Inst.,* 52:1886.
22. Cardiff, R. D., Blair, P. B., and Nakayama, P. (1968): In vitro cultivation of mouse mammary tumor virus: Detection of MTV production by radioisotope labeling and identification by immune precipitation. *Proc. Natl. Acad. Sci. U.S.A.,* 59:895–902.
23. McGrath, C. M. (1971): Replication of mammary tumor virus in tumor cell cultures: Dependence on hormone-induced cellular organization. *J. Natl. Cancer Inst.,* 47:455–467.
24. Dickson, C., Haslam, S., and Nandi, S. (1974): Conditions for optimal MTV synthesis in vitro and the effect of steroid hormones on virus production. *Virology,* 62:242–252.
25. Cardiff, R. D. (1973): Quantitation of mouse mammary tumor virus (MTV) virions by radioimmunoassay. *J. Immunol.,* 111:1722–1729.
26. Kimball, P. C., Boehm-Truitt, M., Schochetman, G., and Schlom, J. (1976): Characterization of mouse mammary tumor viruses from primary tumor cell cultures. I. Immunological and structural studies. *J. Natl. Cancer Inst.,* 56:111–117.
27. Kimball, P., Michalides, R., Colcher, D., and Scholm, J. (1976): Characterization of mouse mammary tumor viruses from primary tumor cell cultures. II. Biochemical and biophysical studies. *J. Natl. Cancer Inst.,* 56:119–124.
28. Verstraetem, A. A., Hageman, Ph. C., and Kwa, H. G. (1973): A radioimmunoassay for MTV-antigens. *Eur. J. Cancer,* 9:155–157.
29. Parks, W. P., Howk, R. S., Scolnick, E. M., Oroszlan, S., and Gilden, R. V. (1974): Immunochemical characterization of two major polypeptides from murine mammary tumor virus. *J. Virol.,* 13:1200–1210.

30. Feldman, H., and Rodbard, D. (1971): Chapter 7. In: *Principles of Competitive Protein-Binding Assays*, edited by W. Odell and W. Daughday, pp. 158–199. Lippincott, Philadelphia.

31. Green, R. W., Bolognesi, D. P., Schafer, W., Pister, L., Hunsmann, G., and Noronha, F. (1973): Polypeptides of mammalian oncornaviruses. I. Isolation and serological analysis of polypeptides from murine and feline C-type viruses. *Virology*, 56:565–579.

32. Strand, M., and August, J. T. (1973): Structural proteins of oncogenic ribonucleic acid viruses. Interspec II, a new interspecies antigen. *J. Biol. Chem.*, 248:5627–5633.

33. Sherr, C. J., Fedele, L. A., Benveniste, R. E., and Todaro, G. J. (1975): Interspecies antigenic determinants of the reverse transcriptases and P30 proteins of mammalian type-C viruses. *J. Virol.*, 15:1440–1448.

34. Mora, P. T., McFarland, V. W., and Luborsky, S. W. (1966): Nucleic acid of the Rauscher mouse leukemia virus. *Proc. Natl. Acad. Sci. U.S.A.*, 55:438–445.

35. Spiegelman, S., Burny, A., Das, M. R., Keydar, J., Schlom, J., Travnicek, M., and Watson, K. (1970): Synthetic DNA-RNA hybrids and RNA-RNA duplexes as templates for the polymerases of the oncogenic RNA viruses. *Nature (Lond.)*, 228:430–432.

36. Goodman, N. C., and Spiegelman, S. (1971): Distinguishing reverse transcriptase of an RNA tumor virus from other known DNA polymerases. *Proc. Natl. Acad. Sci. U.S.A.*, 68:2203–2206.

37. Howk, R., Rye, L., Killeen, L., Scolnick, E., and Parks, W. (1973): Characterization and separation of viral DNA polymerase in mouse milk. *Proc. Natl. Acad. Sci. U.S.A.*, 70:2117–2121.

38. Dion, A. S., Vaidya, A. B., and Fout, G. S. (1974): Cation preferences for poly rC:oligo dG directed DNA synthesis by RNA tumor viruses and human milk particulates. *Cancer Res.*, 34:3509–3515.

39. Schlom, J., and Spiegelman, S. (1971): Simultaneous detection of reverse transcriptase and high molecular weight RNA unique to oncogenic RNA viruses. *Science*, 174:840–843.

40. Schlom, J., Michalides, R., Kufe, D., Hehlamn, K., Spiegelman, S., Bentvelzen, P., and Hageman, P. (1973): A comparative study of the biologic and molecular basis of murine mammary carcinoma: A model for human breast cancer. *J. Natl. Cancer Inst.*, 51:541–551.

41. Watson, D. H. (1962): Electron micrographic counts on PTA-sprayed virus preparations. *Biochim. Biophys. Acta*, 61:321–331.

42. Hageman, P., Calafat, J., and Daams, J. H. (1972): The mouse mammary tumor viruses. In: *RNA Viruses and Host Genome in Oncogenesis*, edited by P. Emmelot and P. Bentvelzen, pp. 283–308. North American Elsevier, New York.

43. Varmus, H. E., Bishop, J. M., Nowinski, R. C., and Sarkar, N. (1972): Mammary tumor virus specific nucleotide sequences in mouse DNA. *Nature [New Biol.]*, 238:189–191.

44. Varmus, H., Quintrell, N., Medeiros, E., Bishop, J. M., Nowinski, R. C., and Sarkar, N. H. (1973): Transcription of mouse mammary tumor virus genes in tissues from high and low tumor incidence mouse strains. *J. Mol. Biol.*, 79:663–679.

45. Michalides, R., and Schlom, J. (1976): Relationship in nucleic acid sequences between mouse mammary tumor virus variants. *Proc. Natl. Acad. Sci. U.S.A.*, 72:4635–4639.

46. Heston, W., and Vlahakis, G. (1968): C3H-A^{vy}-A high hepatoma and high mammary tumor strain of mice. *J. Natl. Cancer Inst.*, 40:1161–1166.

47. Hilgers, J. H. M., Theuns, G. J., and Van Nie, R. (1973): Mammary tumor virus (MTV) antigens in normal and mammary tumor-bearing mice. *Int. J. Cancer*, 12:568-576.

48. Neiman, P. E., Wright, S. E., McMillin, C., and MacDonnell, D. (1974): Nucleotide sequence relationships of avian RNA tumor viruses: Measurement of the deletion in a transformation-defective mutant of Rous sarcoma virus. *J. Virol.*, 13:837–846.

49. Wright, S. E., and Neiman, P. E. (1974): Base-sequence relationships between avian ribonucleic acid endogenous and sarcoma viruses assayed by competitive ribonucleic acid-deoxyribonucleic acid hybridization. *Biochemistry*, 13:1549–1554.

50. Tonegawa, S., Steinberg, C., Dube, S., and Bernardi, A. (1974): Evidence for somatic generation of antibody diversity. *Proc. Natl. Acad. Sci. U.S.A.*, 10:4027–4031.

51. Duesberg, P. H., and Vogt, P. K. (1973): Gel electrophoresis of avian leukosis and sarcoma viral RNA in formamide: Comparison with other viral and cellular RNA species. *J. Virol.*, 12:594–599.

52. Billeter, M. A., Parsons, J. T., and Coffin, J. M. (1974): The nucleotide sequence complexity of avian tumor virus RNA. *Proc. Natl. Acad. Sci. U.S.A.*, 71:3560–3564.

53. Blair, P. B. (1971): Strain specificity in mouse mammary tumor virus virion antigens. *Cancer Res.*, 31:1473–1477.

54. Bentvelzen, P. (1974): Host-virus interactions in murine mammary carcinogenesis. *Biochim. Biophys. Acta,* 355:236–259.

55. Mason, M. M., Bogden, A. E., Illievski, V., Esber, H. J., Baker, J. R., and Chopra, H. C. (1972): History of a rhesus monkey adenocarcinoma containing virus particles resembling oncogenic RNA viruses. *J. Natl. Cancer Inst.,* 48:1323–1331.

56. Jensen, E. M., Zelljadt, I., Chopra, H. C., and Mason, M. M. (1970): Isolation and propagation of a virus from a spontaneous mammary carcinoma of a rhesus monkey. *Cancer Res.,* 30:2388–2393.

57. Kramarsky, B., Sarkar, N. H., and Moore, D. H. (1971): Ultrastructural comparison of a virus from a rhesus monkey mammary carcinoma with four oncogenic RNA viruses. *Proc. Natl. Acad. Sci. U.S.A.,* 68:1603–1607.

58. Ahmed, M., Korol, W., Schidlovsky, G., Vidrine, J., and Mayyasi, S. (1973): Detection of Mason-Pfizer monkey virus in normal monkey mammary tissue and embryonic cultures. *Proc. Am. Assoc. Cancer Res.,* 14:34.

59. Yeh, J., Ahmed, M., Lyles, J., Larson, D., and Mayyasi, S. A. (1975): Competition radioimmunoassay for Mason-Pfizer monkey virus: Comparison with recent isolates. *Int. J. Cancer,* 15:632–639.

60. Gelderblom, H., Bauer, H., Ogura, H., Wigand, R., and Fischer, A. B. (1974): Detection of oncornavirus-like particles in HeLa cells. I. Fine structure and comparative morphological classification. *Int. J. Cancer,* 13:246–253.

61. Bauer, H., Daams, J. H., Watson, K. F., Molling, K., Gelderblom, H., and Schafer, W. (1974): Oncornavirus-like particles in HeLa cells. II. Immunological characterization of the virus. *Int. J. Cancer,* 13:254–261.

62. Watson, K. F., Molling, K., Gelderblom, H., and Bauer, H. (1974): Oncornavirus-like particles in HeLa cells. III. Biochemical characterization of the virus. *Int. J. Cancer,* 13:262–267.

63. Parks, W. P., Gilden, R. V., Bykovsky, A. F., Miller, G. G., Zhadanov, V. M., Soloviev, V. D., and Scolnick, E. M. (1973): Mason-Pfizer virus characterization: A similar virus in a human amniotic cell line. *J. Virol.,* 12:1540–1547.

64. Bykovsky, A. F., Miller, G. G., Yershov, F. I., Ilyin, K. V., and Zhadanov, V. M. (1973): B-type oncornaviruses isolated from continuous human cancer cell lines. *Arch. Gesamte Virusforsch.,* 42:21–35.

65. Graffi, V. A., Bierwolf, D., Widnaier, R., Bender, E., Wunderlich, V., Rudolph, M., Mothes, E., Niezabitowski, A., and Papsdorf, G. (1974): In der gewebekultur zuchtbares oncornavirus in malignen permanenten menschlichen zellinien vom embryo einer krebskranken frau. *Dtsch. Gesamte Wesen,* 29, H. 32, 1489–1498.

66. Hooks, J., Gibbs, C. J., Jr., Chopra, H., Lewis, M., and Gajdusek, D. C. (1972): Spontaneous transformation of human brain cells grown in vitro and description of associated virus particles. *Science,* 176:1420–1422.

67. Ilyin, K. V., Bykovsky, A. F., and Zhandov, V. M. (1972): An oncornavirus type-B from human larynx carcinoma cells. *Vopr. Virusol.,* 17:494–499.

68. Ilyin, K. V., Bykovsky, A., and Zhandov, V. M. (1973): An oncornavirus isolated from human cancer line. *Cancer,* 32:89–96.

69. Miller, G. G., Zhdanov, V. M., Lozinsky, T. F., Volkova, M. Y., Ilyin, K. V., Golubev, D. B., Irlin, I. S., and Bykovsky, A. F. (1974): Production of an oncornavirus by the continuous human cell line, Detroit-6. *J. Natl. Cancer Inst.,* 52:357–364.

70. Zhdanov, V. M., Soloviev, V. D., Bektemirov, T. A., Filatov, F. P., and Bykovsky, A. F. (1972): Isolation of a leukovirus from a continuous tumor cell line. *Arch. Gesamte Virusforsch.,* 39:309–316.

71. Zhdanov, V. M., Soloviev, V. D., Bektemirov, T. A., Ilyin, K. V., Bykovsky, A. F., Mazurenko, N. P., Irlin, I. S., and Yershov, F. I. (1973): Isolation of oncornaviruses from continuous human cell cultures. *Intervirology,* 1:19–26.

72. Schlom, J., and Spiegelman, S. (1971): DNA polymerase activities and nucleic acid components of virions isolated from a spontaneous mammary carcinoma of a rhesus monkey. *Proc. Natl. Acad. Sci. U.S.A.,* 68:1613–1617.

73. Gillespie, D., Marshall, S., and Gallo, R. C. (1972): RNA of RNA tumor viruses contains

poly A. *Nature [New Biol.]*, 236:227–231.

74. Abrell, J. W., and Gallo, R. C. (1973): Purification, characterization and comparison of the DNA polymerases from two primate RNA tumor viruses. *J. Virol.*, 12:431–439.

75. Yaniv, A., Ohno, T., Kacian, D., Colcher, D., Witkin, S., Schlom, J., and Spiegelman, S. (1974): Serological analysis of reverse transcriptase of the Mason-Pfizer monkey virus. *Virology*, 59:335–338.

76. Schochetman, G., Kortright, K., and Schlom, J. (1976): Mason-Pfizer monkey virus: Analysis and localization of virion proteins and glycoproteins. *J. Virol.*, 16:1208–1219.

77. Nowinski, R. C., Fleissner, E., and Sarkar, N. H. (1972): Structural and serological aspects of the oncornaviruses. *Perspect. Virol.*, 8:31–60.

78. Tronick, S. R., Stephenson, J. R., and Aaronson, S. A. (1974): Immunological properties of two polypeptides of Mason-Pfizer monkey virus. *J. Virol.*, 14:125–132.

79. Bolognesi, D. (1974): Structural components of RNA tumor viruses. *Adv. Virus Res.*

80. Moennig, V., Frank, H., Hunsmann, G., Schneider, J., and Schafer, W. (1974): Properties of mouse leukemia viruses. VII. The major glycoprotein of Friend leukemia virus; isolation and physiochemical properties. *Virology*, 61:100–111.

81. Duesberg, P. H. (1968): Physical properties of Rous sarcoma virus RNA. *Proc. Natl. Acad. Sci. U.S.A.*, 60:1511–1518.

82. Travnicek, M. E., and Riman, J. (1973): Subunits of oncornavirus high molecular weight RNA. I. Stepwise conversion of 60S AMV (avian myeloblastosis virus) RNA to subunits. *Biochem. Biophys. Res. Commun.*, 53:217–223.

83. Schochetman, G., and Schlom, J. (1975): RNA subunit structure of Mason-Pfizer monkey virus. *J. Virol.*, 15:423–427.

84. Faras, A. J., Garapin, A. C., Levinson, W. E., Bishop, J. M., and Goodman, H. M. (1973): Characterization of the low-molecular weight RNAs associated with the 70S Rous sarcoma virus. *J. Virol.*, 12:334–342.

85. Nelson-Rees, W. A., Zhdanov, V. M., Hawthorne, P. K., and Flandermeyer, R. R. (1974): HeLa-like marker chromosomes and type-A variant glucose-6-phosphate dehydrogenase isoenzyme in human cell cultures producing Mason-ofizer monkey virus-like particles. *J. Natl. Cancer Inst.*, 53:–757.

86. Colcher, D., Drogan, W., and Schlom, J. (1976): Mason-Pfizer RNA genome: Relationship to the RNA of morphologically similar isolates and other oncornaviruses. *J. Virol.*, 17:705–712. *publication.*)

87. Colcher, D., Spiegelman, S., and Schlom, J. (1974): Sequence homology between the RNA of Mason-Pfizer monkey virus and the RNA of human malignant breast tumors. *Proc. Natl. Acad. Sci. U.S.A.*, 71:4975–4979.

88. Ahmed, M., Schidlovsky, G., Korol, W., Vidrine, G., and Cicmanec, J. L. (1974): Occurrence of Mason-Pfizer monkey virus in healthy rhesus monkeys. *Cancer Res.*, 34:3504–3508.

89. Ahmed, M., Martin, D., Yeh, J., Schidlovsky, G., Korol, W., and Mayyasi, S. (1974): Biological characterization of oncornaviruses present in rhesus placental cultures. *Proc. Am. Assoc. Cancer Res.*, 15:44.

90. Colcher, D. M., Schochetman, G., and Schlom, J. (1975): Mason-Pfizer monkey virus (MPMV): A horizontally transmitted oncornavirus of rhesus monkeys. In: *Proceedings of the American Association of Cancer Research*, p. 22.

91. Lowy, D. R., Rowe, W. P., Teich, N., and Hartley, J. W. (1971): Murine leukemia virus: High frequency activation in vitro by 5-iododeoxyuridine and 5-bromodeoxyuridine. *Science*, 174:155–156.

92. Murray, P. R., and Nayak, D. P. (1974): Characterization of bromodeoxyuridine-induced endogenous guinea pig virus. *J. Virol.*, 14:679–688.

93. Gross, P. A., Fong, C. K. Y., and Hsiung, G. D. (1973): Characterization of guinea pig C-type virus. *Proc. Soc. Exp. Biol. Med.*, 143:367–370.

94. Rhim, J. P., Wuu, K. D., Vernon, M. L., and Huebner, R. J. (1974): Induction of guinea pig leukemia-like virus from cultured guinea pig cells. *Proc. Soc. Exp. Biol. Med.*, 147:323–330.

95. Michalides, R., Schlom, J., Dahlberg, J., and Perk, K. (1976): Biochemical properties of the bromodeoxyuridine-induced guinea pig virus. *J. Virol.*, 16:1039–1050.

96. Scolnick, E., Rands, E., Aaronson, S. A., and Todaro, G. J. (1970): RNA-dependent DNA polymerase activity in five RNA viruses: Divalent cation requirements. *Proc. Natl. Acad. Sci. U.S.A.*, 67:1789–1796.

97. Kang, C. Y., and Temin, H. M. (1973): Lack of sequence homology among RNAs of avian leukosis-sarcoma viruses, reticuloendotheliosis viruses, and chicken endogenous RNA-directed DNA polymerase activity. *J. Virol.*, 12:1314–1324.

98. Quintrell, N., Varmus, H. E., and Bishop, J. M. (1974): Homologies among the nucleotide sequences of the genomes of C-type viruses. *Virology*, 58:568–575.

99. East, J. L., Knesek, J. E., Chan, J. C., and Dmochowski, L. (1975): Quantitative nucleotide sequence relationships of mammalian RNA tumor viruses. *J. Virol.*, 15:1396–1408.

100. Gillespie, D., and Gallo, R. C. (1975): RNA processing and RNA tumor virus origin and evolution. *Science*, 188:802–811.

101. Benveniste, R. E., and Todaro, G. J. (1974): Evolution of type C viral genes. I. Nucleic acid from baboon type C virus as a measure of divergence among primate species. *Proc. Natl. Acad. Sci. U.S.A.*, 71:4513–4518.

102. Haapala, D. K., and Fischinger, P. J. (1973): Molecular relatedness of mammalian RNA tumor viruses as determined by DNA RNA hybridization. *Science,* 180:972–974.

103. Chattopadhyay, S. K., Lowy, D. R., Teich, N. M., Levine, A. S., and Rowe, W. P. (1974): Evidence that the AKR murine-leukemia-virus genome is complete in DNA of the high-virus AKR mouse and incomplete in the DNA of the ''virus-negative'' NIH mouse. *Proc. Natl. Acad. Sci. U.S.A.*, 71:167–171.

Breast Cancer: Trends in Research and Treatment, edited by J. C. Heuson, W. H. Mattheiem, and M. Rozencweig. Raven Press, New York © 1976.

Roundtable Discussion: Virology

Chairman: A. Billiau

Billiau: We have heard very convincing evidence pertaining to mice and monkeys, and Dr. Schlom also presented some stringent data, I think, suggesting the presence of virus genetic material in human breast cancers. Dr. Bentvelzen, perhaps you could briefly summarize what you think about the possible presence of viral proteins in human breast cancer. Do you think the time is far off when we might be able to detect such proteins, and what techniques do you think should be used?

Bentvelzen: There have been some reports in the literature that breast cancer patients either had some proteins which are related to those of the mouse mammary virus or have immunological reactions to those proteins. Three different laboratories have found a certain category of breast cancer patients displaying an immunological reaction: in particular, a cellular reaction to a glycoprotein with a molecular weight of 50,000 which was derived from breast cancer tissue.

Those cellular reactions were determined by two different techniques. The first is the rather cumbersome and very tricky leukocyte-migration inhibition test. When leukocytes are taken from an unstimulated individual, they usually start to wander in the tissue culture system, whether the antigen is present or not. On the other hand, when leukocytes are taken from a sensitized individual and the antigen is added, migration is then completely inhibited. According to Maurice Black, inhibition of leukocytes by the glycoprotein could be demonstrated in 30% of breast cancer patients. The second and far more reliable technique, at least in our hands, is leukocyte stimulation. If the particular antigen is added to leukocytes from an unsensitized individual, nothing happens in terms of DNA synthesis—it will be at background levels. However, under similar conditions, leukocytes from a sensitized individual show a remarkable increase in DNA synthesis, and this proves to be a very specific marker.

It was found in several laboratories that not only do leukocytes display their reactions to that particular glycoprotein, but there is a similar reaction, in both tests, with the mouse mammary tumor virus. It is assumed now that the glycoprotein is related to a glycoprotein of the mouse virus which has a molecular weight of 52,000. However, I know of no laboratory that has yet tested leukocytes from patients against the mouse glycoprotein 52,000—they have taken the whole virus. Some more tests are needed, although it looks promising.

Lastly, it was reported by Müller in Dresden that approximately 25% of his patients have antibodies which react with a line of mouse mammary tumors in the immunofluorescence test, which is even more tricky than the leukocyte migration inhibition test. He was convinced that he had something specific, because the reaction could be blocked by absorption with the mouse virus.

In order to evaluate these findings fully, we must first look at the model system for human breast cancers, the mouse mammary tumor system. In the mouse mammary virus virion, various proteins have been identified according to their molecular weights. Besides these glycoprotein of molecular weight 52,000 (which we call GP52), there is another glycoprotein (M.W. 60,000); the location of the other two glycoproteins (M.W. 36,000 and 10,000) that have been found is not yet known. In the core there is a very predominant protein with M.W. 28,000 and of course RNA and reverse transcriptase.

We then looked at mammary tumor cells and the glycoprotein 52,000 was found in them; it was detected with monospecific antisera by means of membrane immunofluoresence or by cytotoxicity tests. We also now know for sure that in the cytoplasm there is an accumulation of an antigen in granular form with a molecular weight of 28,000, the protein that is in the core. Unique transplantation antigens have been clearly demonstrated on the cell surface, especially by transplantation experiments, which are completely new and which differ from one tumor to the other.

That is a very important discovery because there has always been such a big fuss made about unique transplantation antigens in chemically induced tumors, and this has been regarded as evidence against the viral origin of those tumors; but clearly in these virally induced tumors you find those unique antigens. There is also some evidence that there is a common antigen for all of those tumors which is probably coded for by the virus but is not present in the virus particle itself. We have been looking at the immunological reactions of mice with and without tumors and virus expression. Especially in tumor-bearing mice of various categories where there is a virus involved, antibodies are present against both P28 (a protein of M.W. 28,000), which can be found by using immunofluorescence on acetone-fixed cultures, and glycoprotein 52, which is present on the cell surface. There were also antibodies against the nonvirion antigen that is common to all those tumors. Those antibodies are not cytotoxic; and even by concentrating them and adding a large amount of complement, cells were not killed. As far as cell-mediated immunity goes, we have also seen that there is a cytotoxic reaction of mice to mammary tumor cells. One very interesting phenomenon was that when we incubated tumor cells with serum from tumor-bearing mice using normal leukocytes as controls, we got a very strong cytotoxic reaction with the tumor cells. This might mean that the serum (presumably the antibodies) could trigger a cytotoxic reaction against tumor cells. We found also indications for cellular reactivity against the virus in tumor-bearing mice with the leukocyte adherence inhibition assay and the lymphocyte blastogenesis test.

What are we doing with all this information—with the knowledge that there might be a virus involved in mice or in man? We have already started vaccination programs, and I have worked for several years with formolized virus as well as with live virus. As you might anticipate one would never use attenuated or formolized viruses in man; it is not ethical. We have made preparations of the mouse glycoprotein 52,000, injected mice with a single shot, and tested those mice for reactivity to mammary tumor cells against virus. They showed very strong reactivity in the antibody and the cellular immunity response; they can also kill tumor cells in *in vivo* experiments.

We used the GR mouse, which develops mammary tumors very early (in human terms, a 25-year-old girl with mammary cancer) and which releases virus continuously. We immunized these mice with GP52 from mammary tumor virus, and after 30 days took lymphocytes, mixed them with tumor cells, and then transplanted them into syngeneic mice. There was a 100% take within 2 months in the controls.

If the tumor cells are mixed with normal lymphocytes, there is also a 100% take; with a very high number of normal lymphocytes, there is even acceleration of tumor growth-immune stimulation of tumor growth, which is significant. This has also been reported by Prehn. If the lymphocytes of the immunized animals are used, you get no take whatsoever, indicating that there is a poor cytotoxic activity in those vaccinated mice. We have now been working on this for almost a year, and these mice have not yet developed tumors. I am afraid that they develop some autoimmune phenomenon, because there is expression of endogenous virus in various organs, which might be fatal. We are also now trying to isolate the nonvirion antigen. Perhaps in the future we can immunize mice with nonvirion tumor antigen and achieve just as good prophylaxis as we had in this experiment.

Vakil: There was no evidence from our retrospective cohort study in Toronto to relate risk of breast cancer to the experience of being breast-fed, since breast-fed women had a breast cancer experience remarkably similar to those who had never been breast-fed. Therefore this observation did not support the hypothesis of viral transmission via maternal milk. How do the viral oncologists explain the excess of breast cancer in certain human families?

Burny: You heard, in Dr. Hilgers' talk, that endogenous viruses are involved in the mouse mammary tumor system, and although as Dr. Bentvelzen explained there is an immune reaction of the host, it looks like the endogenous virus can propagate and move from one generation to the other. In this very specific case, there is some kind of an autoimmune disease going on, for which the basic, classic distinction of the immune system—respecting the self and not the nonself—does not seem like holding true. So part of the answer is that maybe in some families there is integration of some viral information that would express itself with high frequency. However, we do not necessarily have to limit ourselves to endogenous viruses because indeed it is well established in several systems that exogenous viruses are involved. The first system in which it was suggested was 3 years ago in leukemia, lymphoma, and Hodgkin's disease in man (the work of Spiegelman's group). They showed that if they prepared a cDNA of what they call "a viral fraction"—an extract of a tumor where viral particles should be if they are present—and then look for viral sequences in normal tissues of leukemic patients or in normal tissues of normal patients, they do not find them. If they first hybridize their probe on normal DNA they take out much of the cDNA so there are normal sequences in the viral ones. In a second step if they hybridize what is left, in what did not hybridize they get hybridization to the DNA of a tumor, but not if they hybridize to the DNA of a normal cell. So that shows that in this system there are DNA sequences information present in a transformed tumor cell and not present in a normal cell, so then it presents itself as being due to an infectious agent. That was the first type of experiment done on a putative exogenous virus using man as the experimental system. After that, last year a report came out saying that the same thing applied in the avian leukemia system. Also if you look at tumors or leukemic cells induced by recent field isolates of viruses, you come to the conclusion that there are DNA sequences in the transformed cells that are viral-related and not present in normal cells. Again therefore, in the field leukemia of the avian animal, there is a process that looks like an infection. Recently in bovine leukemia, it was shown that the same situation pertains. If you get cDNA in the bovine leukemia virus and hybridize to normal DNA, you get something like 10–15% hybridization; if you go to the DNA of the tumor of leukemic cells you get something like 60–65% hybridization, which is about the best one can get owing to experimental difficulties. So, in addition to the endogenous viruses, which could very well explain a family incidence, exogenous viruses are well known in some systems and may play a role. As Dr. Schlom pointed out, in the MPMV studies they are carrying out in his laboratory and in some others, there is also information tending to show that the MPMV sequences are present in some organs of some monkeys.

In conclusion, it looks like the whole picture of viral induction of tumors and of viral transformation might turn out to be very complicated, with endogenous viruses, exogenous viruses, and maybe both at the same time playing a role. Now, if exogenous viruses have anything to do with family occurrence of cancer, then one has to think of genetic transmission of specific defects in that family, of physiological conditions, environmental conditions which could explain that a given genotype leads to lack of resistance to a virus that might very well be an exogenous one. I think that all these are possibilities.

Thiry: Have you any opinion on the identity of the virus which contaminates some HeLa lines? Is this virus identical or only similar to Mason-Pfizer virus?

Schlom: If we look at the DNA of HeLa cells from which this virus was supposedly reported, it is certainly there as is the whole genome of Mason-Pfizer virus. However, if you look in HeLa cells in the American Type Culture Collection there is no Mason-Pfizer-related information in the DNA of those cells.

Thiry: Do you know whether immunological tests using Mason-Pfizer antigen have been performed in women with breast cancer?

Schlom: This virus is relatively new, and its protein structure has just recently been elucidated. These proteins are now being prepared in such a form that we can make monospecific antisera, etc., and this is obviously a line of investigation that we and others are pursuing.

In reference to a previous question that you raised with Dr. Bentvelzen about MTV antigens or viral antigens and human breast cancer, there is a very important area of work that has just been started. This is a human breast tumor cell line called the 734B, which was just isolated and characterized as a true human breast tumor cell line and is producing particles that have all the biochemical properties I mentioned for RNA tumor viruses. In those studies Drs. Rich and McGrath are finding nucleic acid sequences and proteins that are related to the mouse mammary tumor virus: and although this work needs confirmation and extension, it is definitely a very exciting area.

Heuson: Is there yet a clearly defined line of research that could lead in the short or medium term to the detection of virus-derived markers that might indicate a high risk of developing breast cancer in a given woman?

Schlom: Work is being done in leukocyte migration inhibition in Dr. Maurice Black's laboratory and by Drs. Hollings and Heuberman at the National Cancer Institute in Bethesda using cell-mediated immunity in viral antigens. Until now it has been very difficult to obtain good clean viral antigen preparations for the mouse mammary tumor viruses because they have been obtained from milk and tumor homogenates. Now we have cell culture sources of these viruses and can make nice clean viral preparations, purify the proteins, make monospecific antisera, and start these studies. The same is true of the Mason-Pfizer virus, so I think we will know within a few years whether we are looking at something real.

Rich: In view of the fact that 734B also appears to have some similarities with human breast tumors, I wonder if the homology that you discussed between mouse mammary tumor virus in human tumors and Mason-Pfizer virus in human tumors, represents the same genomic information. Also is there a relationship between MPMV and murine mammary tumor virus?

Schlom: There is a 95% chance that we are looking at two different kinds of virus information in those human breast tumors.

Rich: How do the H_2 factors determining susceptibility of C-type virus oncogenicity compare to those which appear to govern mammary tumor?

Hilgers: I could not have answered that question in the way that I can now had you asked it a few months ago. During the spring and summer of this year there have been some very important breakthroughs in the field of how viruses induce new antigens, mostly work with LCM and ectromelia virus. Let me explain it to you in the anti-V system. I told you that anti-V interferes with H_2D and TL molecules on the cell surface, thereby exposing new antigenic specificities on these normal major transplantation antigens. So apart from viral tumor antigens, there are also new antigens on normal transplantation components induced by that virus, depending on the haplotype for which other specificities appear. The Australians have shown that the cellular immunity induced by these viruses against certain diseases is to these new antigens on normal transplantation molecules, whereas it is thought that human immunity is mainly due to the viral antigens. So the situation that only the immune response to the viral antigens might play a role in determining susceptibility is not valid any more; cellular immunity to the new antigens may play an important role. If you find common tumor antigen on a particular tumor, it does not necessarily mean that virus has induced it; it can be induced by another agent, by a chemical, etc. So finding common tumor antigens is not necessarily a prerequisite for a viral etiology, and we should be very well aware of this fact. This might be an introduction to the next session on the immunological defense mechanisms—that we are still at the very beginning of understanding what is happening in the model systems.

Breast Cancer: Trends in Research and Treatment, edited by J. C. Heuson,
W. H. Mattheiem, and M. Rozencweig. Raven Press, New York © 1976.

Introduction: Immunology

J. Wybran

One piece of indirect evidence that immune factors may indeed play a role in human breast cancer is the very important observation made by the pathologist Berg, who showed that there is a correlation between good prognosis and the presence of sinus histocytosis of the lymph nodes. Is there any other evidence or factors that may also suggest to us that the immune system is important in human breast cancer? Is the very long course of the disease in these patients such a factor which may be discussed later on? Is it a factor that there may be a high incidence of cancer patients in the same family, suggesting some immune deficiency?

Later on in this section we examine the evidence for specific immunity against breast cancer. We may also have some discussion about the hypothesis that human breast cancer patients have, in fact, a defect in their immunosurveillance system that is reflected by a decreased general nonspecific immunity. Another way of looking at breast cancer—and this is really a new departure—is that we may also think of hormone dependence of the immune system, and indeed there are recent reports showing that female hormones can influence the immune response. Lastly, we are going to discuss immunotherapy. We know how complex the immune system is when defense mechanisms are involved. Both cells and antibodies are responsible for killing tumor cells, and I am relatively sure there are other factors. We know that antibodies can be cytotoxic in the presence of complement to tumor cells, killing those tumor cells. We also know that antibodies in the presence of normal mononuclear cells (they have been termed K-cells because we do not yet know if they are lymphocytes or monocytes) can kill tumor cells. Another system of killing is more direct, involving both T- and B-lymphocytes; there is also the macrophage system. Then there are other cells which do not produce a positive immune response toward the tumor but induce a negative response; these are the suppressor cells. Other factors which are a product of the immune response, and which also play a negative role in tumor immunity are the blocking factors, which in some cases may be antigen-antibody complexes, or in other cases just shedding of antigens of the tumor cells. Finally there are the lymphocytotoxins, products of activated lymphocytes.

Therefore when we deal with immunotherapy we must find the right balance in order to push the immune system in the direction of killing the tumor cells, but also avoid pushing it into the negative factors which are the suppressor cells and blocking factors.

Breast Cancer: Trends in Research and Treatment, edited by J. C. Heuson,
W. H. Mattheiem, and M. Rozencweig. Raven Press, New York © 1976.

Immune Response to a Syngeneic
Rat Mammary Adenocarcinoma

Zoltan J. Lucas

Department of Surgery, Stanford University, Stanford, California 94305

A central dogma of tumor biology is that tumor-bearing hosts respond immuno-logically to tumor-associated neoantigens of syngeneic and autochthonous tumors (1–3). Various tests demonstrating death of tumor target cells *in vitro* serve to detect these reactions (4–7). In general, however, the responses detected by *in vitro* cytotoxicity tests cannot be correlated with an increased survival advantage to the host (8,9). Their general ineffectiveness in eliminating the tumor poses a perplexing question. Our philosophical approach to this problem is to investigate thoroughly each facet of the host response to a syngeneic tumor and compare it to the responses in allogeneic animals to the same tumor as well as to kidney or skin grafts.

Nonimmunologists generally do not appreciate the extraordinary complexity of the immune response to a cellular antigen. It involves the interaction of several different cell types in four discrete phases: antigen recognition (afferent phase), lymphocyte activation and clonal replication (central phase), differentiation into effector cells (effector phase), and the generation of inhibitory or feedback events (autoregulatory phase). Figure 1 portrays our operational view of the immune response to a cellular antigen. This description is synthesized from reported immune reactions to different antigens and does not imply that all these steps have been demonstrated for any one antigen. A similar analysis with detailed references has been presented (10). The immune response begins when antigen-sensitive cells (ACS) contact antigenic determinants. The initial contact is mediated through surface receptors on lymphocytes: immunoglobulin IgG or IgM for B-lymphocytes and an undefined structure for T-lymphocytes. Current investiga-tions suggest that IgM-producing B-lymphocytes, which are capable of responding to complex antigens without the participation of other antigen-sensitive cells, undergo extensive proliferation on the initial contact with antigen. Large numbers of antibody plaque-forming cells appear in the spleen within 4 days, and shortly thereafter specific IgM antibody is in the serum. Similar events occur with antigen-sensitive T-lymphocytes, which after clonal replication differentiate into a variety of T-effector cells (cytotoxic lymphocytes, augmentor cells, lymphokine-

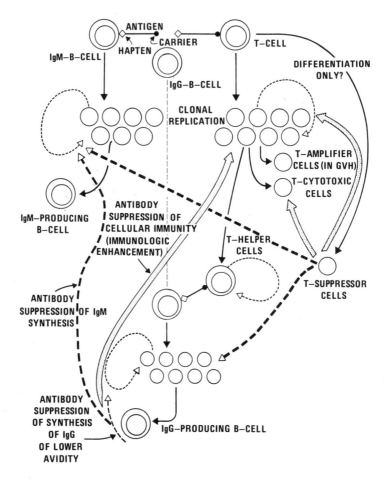

FIG. 1. Current operational view of the immune response to a complex cellular antigen.

secreting cells, helper T-cells). Both types of differentiated effector cells share a short half-life. After approximately 5–7 days sufficient T-helper cells have been generated in the continuous presence of antigen so that IgG-producing B-cells, requiring simultaneous presentation of antigen and specific T-helper cells, are activated into clonal replication, resulting in IgG antibody 4 days later.

A single antigenic determinant actually induces many different antibodies; they react with the determinant with varying avidities, presumably owing to differences in the primary amino acid sequences. As the immune response progresses, however, the antibodies produced become more homogenous. Ultimately only antibodies with the highest avidity for the antigen are produced. IgM antibody and IgG antibody of low avidity disappear because the cells that produce them are relatively short-lived. Also there is a failure to generate new effector cells capable of making these antibodies from the available "memory" cells. This inhibition is an example of the autoregulatory phase of the immune response, occurring as IgG antibodies of the highest avidity sequester antigen and suppress antibody synthesis of the IgM class and the less-avid types of IgG antibody (antibody-mediated suppression of antibody synthesis). Autoregulation of antibody of cellular or T-cell-mediated immunity also occurs. Serum from an animal dying of a tumor, if injected simultaneously with live tumor cells into another syngeneic animal, caused rapid death. This phenomenon, called *immunologic enhancement* (because tumor growth was enhanced), is now attributed to inhibition of the cellular immune response, which if not totally abrogating the tumor is at least effective in decreasing tumor growth. Autoregulatory events mediated by T-lymphocytes have recently been detected also. Suppressor T-cells are observed some 10 days after immunization with soluble antigen, and inhibit the generation of IgM- and IgG-producing cells and of T-effector cells capable of causing graft-versus-host (GVH) disease. Our immediate objective is to define quantitatively these phases of the immune response to a specific syngeneic transplantable mammary adenocarcinoma in rats.

EXPERIMENTAL SYSTEM

Biologic Characteristics of the 13762 Tumor

The rat mammary adenocarcinoma 13762A (obtained from Dr. Arthur Bogden, Mason Research Institute Tumor Bank, Worcester, Mass.) originated in 7,12-dimethylbenz(a)anthracene (DMBA)-treated Fischer 344 rats as a solid tumor and was converted to ascites form by intraperitoneal passage. The ascitic tumor, referred to as MTA, was maintained in 2-month old Fischer female rats by serial intraperitoneal transfer of 2×10^7 cells every 10–12 days.

MTA cells grow rapidly in the peritoneal cavity of syngeneic rats, as shown by a temporal study quantitating tumor cells after injection of 2×10^7 cells into syngeneic and allogeneic animals (11) (Fig. 2). In syngeneic animals growth proceeded exponentially, with a doubling time of approximately 18 hr. When approximately 10^9 cells were produced within 10–12 days, the animal died. In BN and LBN rats the same number of injected tumor cells grew rapidly for 4 days before decreasing. Allogeneic and semiallogeneic animals (LBN) survived tumor injection. The maximum number of tumor cells obtained in nonsyngeneic animals was 2×10^8 cells, representing four doublings in 4 days before tumor growth was stopped. Rejection began abruptly at 4 days but thereafter proceeded rapidly; more than half of the tumor cells were killed in the next 4 days. The 13762A tumor is weakly immunogenic in syngeneic animals. Animal death occurs after injections of as few as 10 MTA cells. In addition, immunization with three injections of irradiated tumor cells does not protect animals against even 10 viable tumor cells (11).

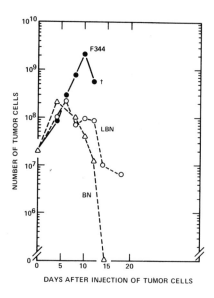

DAYS AFTER INJECTION OF TUMOR CELLS

FIG. 2. Comparisons of MTA growth kinetics in syngeneic Fischer and allogeneic LBN and BN rats following intraperitoneal injections of 2×10^7 cells. Tumor cells in the peritoneal exudate obtained by washing with 50 ml Earle's balanced salt solution were microscopically quantitated. Fischer rats died between 13 and 15 days; allogeneic animals survived the tumor injection. (From Fortner et al., Ref. 11.)

Detection of Cytotoxic Cells in Spleens of Tumor-Inoculated Animals

The cytotoxicity of spleen cells at various times after injection with 2×10^7 MTA cells is detected by enumerating the tumor cells remaining in microassay wells after incubation with immune lymphocytes. Target cells are MTA cells adapted for growth in monolayer culture (MTM cells) (11). Residual target cell enumeration is from the ^{86}Rb incorporated intracellularly after equilibration with a precisely defined amount of extracellular ^{86}Rb. This technique is based on the principle that normal cells maintain their intracellular potassium concentration within narrow limits and that ^{86}Rb is metabolized like potassium under tracer conditions. Only adherent viable cells incorporate ^{86}Rb from the external medium. The accuracy and simplicity for quantitating plastic-adherent target cells by this method have been established (12). Its application to cell-mediated cytotoxicity (CMC) is comparable to techniques utilizing ^{51}Cr release from prelabeled cells or to direct microscopic counting of residual target cells (13). Figure 3 illustrates the CMC activity of spleens from animals injected at various times. In spite of good precision with the ^{86}Rb assay (usual standard error of quadruplicate samples for any one animal is 3%), marked day-to-day variation in cytotoxicity occurred. Each point in Fig. 3A represents the spleen cells for a single animal. The spread illustrates differences that appear to be characteristic of this tumor. To check for animal variation, lymphocytes from pools of spleens of five animals immunized at various times were tested for their cytotoxicity. Figure 3B shows that the kinetic patterns of CMC from pooled animals are similar to those of individual animals (Fig. 3A), but that the standard errors (S_x) for values on days 8, 10, and 12 are less (S_x of 8.4, 6.9, and 6.3, respectively, for individual animals, and 4.9, 4.9, and 3.3, respectively, for the pooled animals).

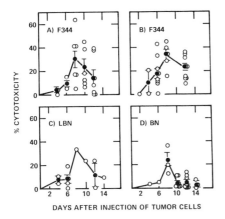

FIG. 3. Cytotoxicity of spleen cells following injection of 2 × 10⁷ MTA cells. **A:** Fischer rats. **B:** MTA-HP injected into Fischer rats (11). **C:** MTA injected into LBN rats. **D:** MTA injected into BN rats. Each *open circle* in **A, C,** and **D** represents spleen cells from a single animal. *Open circles* in **B** represent a single experiment of pools of five animal spleens. Each *closed circle* represents the mean value ±1 S.E.M. (From Fortner et al., ref. 11.)

Cytotoxic lymphocytes are also produced after injecting MTA into allogeneic animals. The same kinetic pattern in splenic CMC activity occurs in LBN (Fig. 3C) and BN (Fig. 3D) animals, as in syngeneic rats, even though the allogeneic animals begin to reject the tumor by days 4 – 6 (Fig. 2).

Specificity of the Cytotoxic Response

Unrelated syngeneic mammary tumor (3230 AC tumor) and syngeneic Fischer fibroblast targets tested the specificity of CMC activity of spleen cells from immunized animals. Sensitization was performed with MTM, MTA, 3230 AC, and Fischer spleen cells. CMC was determined 10 days later on MTM, 3230 AC, and Fischer fibroblast targets. As indicated in Table 1, cells from animals immunized with MTM or MTA cells killed the MTM target better than the 3230

TABLE 1. *Cytotoxicity of spleen lymphocytes in reciprocal sensitization*

Tested on	Cytotoxicity of lymphocytes sensitized against four cell types[a]			
	MTM	MTA	3230 AC	Fischer spleen
MTM				
a	63 ± 7	58 ± 3	21 ± 5	0
b	—	42 ± 3	6 ± 3	—
3230 AC				
a	11 ± 2	48 ± 6	80 ± 12	0
b	—	29 ± 3	16 ± 3	—
Fischer fibroblast				
b	—	16 ± 3	7 ± 3	—

From Fortner et al., ref. 11.

[a]Spleen cells were from one F-344 animal each immunized with 10⁷ cells of the indicated types 10 days earlier. The cells were adsorbed on plastic petri dishes. The T/E ratio was 40:1, and the incubation time 40 hr. Values are mean percent cytotoxicity ± one S.E.M.

AC or Fischer fibroblast targets. Similarly, animals immunized with the 3230 AC mammary tumor killed that target better than either MTM or Fischer fibroblasts. Animals injected with Fischer lymphocytes did not kill either tumor target.

IN VITRO SENSITIZATION

A recurrent vexing problem with this experimental system was the difficulty in reproducibly obtaining sensitized effector cells by immunization *in vivo*. Coexisting blocking or suppressor factors that accompany the response *in vivo* also affect the cytotoxicity of *in vivo* generated effector cells (14–16). This complexity has prompted researchers to explore simpler ways of sensitizing lymphocytes against foreign cellular antigens. In 1965 Ginsberg and Sachs pioneered the development of techniques permitting sensitization of unprimed lymphocytes on monolayers of xenogeneic fibroblasts (17). We therefore investigated the *in vitro* sensitization technique to provide a standardized population of cytotoxic lymphocytes to the transplantable syngeneic adenocarcinoma.

In vitro sensitization was achieved by incubating 30×10^6 syngeneic spleen cells on monolayers of 3,000-r irradiated MTM cells on 60 mm diameter petri dishes in 4 ml RPMI-1640 with 10% agammaglobulinemic horse serum, 5×10^{-5} M mercaptoethanol, 2 mM glutamine, and antibiotics (18). On the fifth day nonadherent cells were removed by vigorous washing; the bulk of the tumor cells were separated from the spleen cells by sedimentation on a Ficoll-isopaque gradient and were reincubated on plastic petri dishes. Average recovery of viable lymphocytes was 15% of the number initially added. The technique is presented in Fig. 4.

Kinetics of Primary In Vitro Sensitization

Unprimed lymphocytes placed on irradiated MTM cells and removed at daily intervals were tested in microassay wells at a lymphocyte/target ratio of 40:1 after 20 hr of incubation. Cytotoxicity is detected in low amounts on day 2, becomes significantly larger on day 3 (33%), and is still increasing on day 5 (Fig. 5), the last day that cells are tested for cytotoxicity (18).

Reproducibility of Primary In Vitro Sensitization Technique

Varying numbers of lymphocytes were generated on irradiated MTM cell monolayers for 5 days and tested in the microassay. Figure 6A, presenting the results of one experiment, shows that target death is detectable with a lymphocyte/tumor ratio of 8:1, and increases linearly to a limiting lymphocyte number of approximately 2.4×10^5 cells per well (40:1 ratio), where a maximum of 40–60% of the targets are killed during the 20- and 41-hr assay incubation times, respectively.

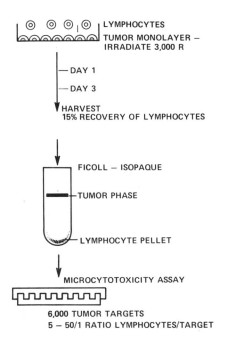

FIG. 4. Technique of *in vitro* generation of specifically cytotoxic lymphocytes.

Figure 6B demonstrates the reproducibility from several experiments. The values define essentially the same linear relationship seen within the single experiment shown in Fig. 6A and indicate saturation at the same number of effector cells, approximately 2.4×10^5. This approximates the lymphocyte population necessary to attain confluent coverage of the assay well surface. Additional lymphocytes pile atop each other and may not make contact with the target monolayer since the plates are not rocked (13,18).

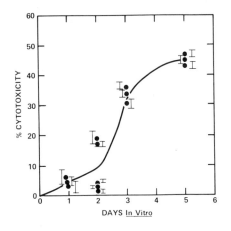

FIG. 5. Kinetics of *in vitro* sensitization of syngeneic spleen cells on MTM tumor cells. Points represent the mean and 1 S.E.M. of quadruplicate samples. (From Kuperman et al., ref. 18.)

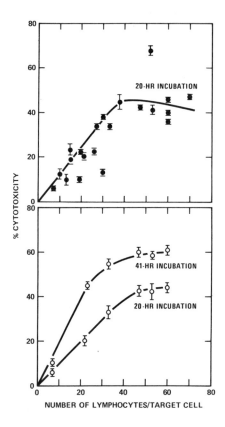

FIG. 6. Stoichiometry of CMC with *in vitro* syngeneic sensitized cells. **Bottom:** Results of one experiment with quadruplicate samples with lymphocytes obtained 5 days after *in vitro* cultivation on MTM cells. Standard errors are indicated by the cross bars. **Top:** Results of five experiments done at different times with 5-day sensitized syngeneic spleen cells. (From Kuperman et al., ref. 18.)

DEVELOPMENT OF MEMORY AND SUPPRESSOR FUNCTIONS MODULATING CELLULAR CYTOTOXICITY

After sensitization with organ or tumor allografts, CMC characteristically exists for only a limited time. It appears after 4 days, peaks 2–4 days later, and then abruptly decreases. The disappearance in allogeneic systems is thought to be related to successful rejection of the graft, when antigen is no longer present. However, as demonstrated above, a similar sequential response, which occurs in animals bearing nonrejected syngeneic tumors, ultimately kills the host. The fall in CMC reactivity in the face of persistent antigen has been interpreted as a regulatory control process normal to the immune response. Feedback control on cellular immunity to organ and tumor grafts by specific immunoglobulins has been described (immunologic enhancement) and more recently has also been found with "suppressor" T-cells. Suppressor cell activity has been found to affect GVH reactions, the generation of cytotoxic effector cells from mixed lymphocyte cultures, and mitogenesis by phytohemagglutinin (19–22).

Operational definitions of the possible cells involved are essential in studying such complex cell interactions. We now present our initial attempts at operationally defining cytotoxic, memory, and suppressor cell activities, and demonstrate the sequential changes they undergo on inoculation of Fischer rats with the 13672A tumor.

Operational Definition of Memory Cells Based on a Higher and Faster Cytotoxic Response in In Vitro Culture Compared with Unprimed Cells

Spleen cells from Fischer rats bearing MTA tumors for various times (primed cells) were placed on irradiated MTM targets for different lengths of time and the resultant cytotoxicity of the surviving lymphocytes on MTM determined and compared with that of similarly handled spleen cells from nonimmunized animals (unprimed cells). As shown in Fig. 7, cytotoxicity is generated faster from spleen cells of animals injected with tumor 3–10 days earlier than from unprimed cells (23). In addition, the cytotoxic activity of the primed cells is higher than that of unprimed cells at all times during the *in vitro* culture period. The higher cytotoxic response of *in vivo* primed cells is taken as a "memory" index. Cells from animals primed 12 days earlier did not show this response; instead, they demonstrated a lower cytotoxicity than unprimed cells (Fig. 7, panel labeled 12 days). Although 12-day primed cells have a slight initial cytotoxic effect, the *in*

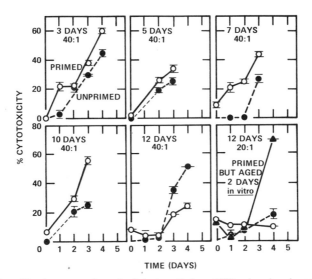

FIG. 7. Kinetics of *in vitro* generation of cytotoxic cells from MTA-primed and unprimed Fischer spleen cells on direct incubation on sensitizing monolayers. *Open circles,* cells from animals previously injected with 2 × 10⁷ viable tumor cells at the times specified at the top of each insert. *Solid circles,* cells from unprimed animals. *Triangles,* 12-day primed spleen cells incubated for 48 hr without targets before transfer to a sensitizing monolayer. Standard error for four replicate samples is indicated by the brackets. The scale on the ordinate represents the duration of *in vitro* culture before the surviving lymphocytes were tested for cytotoxicity. All assays were for 20 hr. Effector/target cell ratio is indicated in each panel. Each panel represents spleen cells pooled from five animals injected with tumor at the specified times cultured *in vitro* for 1–4 days. (From Kuperman et al., ref. 23.)

vitro culture results in loss of this activity within 2 days and markedly less generation of new cytotoxicity compared to the unprimed cells. This suggests that 12-day spleen cells either have lost memory activity or contain suppressor factor(s) capable of inhibiting the anamnestic response.

Assuming that memory cells should be long-lived even in the absence of antigen, we incubated 12-day primed cells on petri dishes without targets for 2 days and determined the effect this had on their subsequent ability to generate a cytotoxic response *in vitro*. Results (Fig. 7, lower right panel) show that, whereas unaged 12-day primed cells generate less cytotoxicity than unprimed cells, those aged for 2 days develop a high degree of cytotoxicity (closed triangles: 63% cytotoxicity on the fourth day of *in vitro* culture).

Adoptive Transfer of Immune Spleen Cells into Irradiated, Syngeneic, Nontumor-Bearing Hosts

The complex cytotoxicity patterns generated *in vivo*—in part due to blocking and/or suppressor factors and in part to the simultaneous presence of cytotoxic, memory, and possibly the putative suppressor cells—make the definition of memory cells based on direct transfer tests highly tenuous. Since *in vitro* culture appeared to reduce the suppressive effect in 12-day spleen cells, we reasoned that longer incubation in a better nutritional environment but in the absence of tumor antigen might eliminate all but memory cells for MTM. Spleen cells pooled from five Fischer rats bearing MTA tumors for various times were administered intravenously into the syngeneic irradiated rats. Five days later the spleen cells from the adoptively transferred animals were incubated for 1–3 days on MTM monolayers and the generation of cytotoxic cells compared with similarly handled lymphocytes from unprimed animals. Figure 8 shows that the generation of cytotoxic cells from primed animals is still higher and faster than from unprimed animals. In addition, Fig. 8 shows that the cytotoxicity present in the cells primed for 8, 10, and 12 days disappears during the 5 days in the tumor-free host. These cells show increased cytotoxicity only after 2 days of incubation *in vitro,* contrasting with the directly tested primed cells, which showed increased cytotoxicity at 24 hr. Also, the data illustrated in the last panel in the bottom row of Fig. 8 confirm results of *in vitro* experiments demonstrating loss of the suppressive effect of 12-day cells on incubation of the primed cells in an antigen-free environment. These results are interpreted as indicating the existence of three populations of cells in the immune spleen: (a) fully differentiated cytotoxic cells that are eliminated by 5 days in an antigen-free environment; (b) suppressor cells that are similarly eliminated; and (c) memory cells that survive in the absence of antigens both *in vivo* and *in vitro* (23).

Operational Definition of Suppressor Cells Based on Inhibition of In Vitro Generation of Cytotoxicity

The above experiments compared primed and unprimed cells separately incubated on sensitizing tumor monolayers. Direct evidence of the interaction between

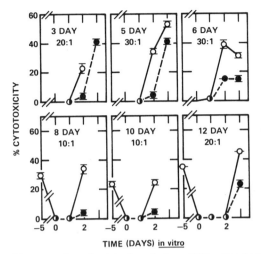

TIME (DAYS) in vitro

FIG. 8. Kinetics of *in vitro* generation of cytotoxic cells from MTA-primed and unprimed spleen cells after 5-day adoptive transfer in irradiated syngeneic animals. *Open circles,* cells from animals injected with 2×10^7 viable tumor cells at the time specified. *Solid circles,* cells from nonimmunized animals. On the ordinate –5 is the day the spleens were removed from the tumor-bearing animal and injected into the irradiated recipients. Each panel represents spleen cells pooled from five animals injected with tumor at the specified times, transferred to an irradiated host for 5 days, and then cultured 0–3 days. (From Kuperman et al., ref. 23.)

cytotoxic cell precursors and suppressor cells was sought by mixing approximately equal numbers (1.5×10^7) of primed and unprimed cells at the initiation of *in vitro* sensitization. Results of cytotoxicity were compared with those of primed and unprimed cells incubated at twice (3×10^7) the concentration of each type in the mixed cell experiments. If the cytotoxicities of the primed and unprimed cells were additive, the mixture should demonstrate lysis of the sum of one-half the primed and unprimed values (Table 2, tabulated under "expected"). The data show a biphasic response. Sensitizing cultures containing cells from animals primed 5–11 days earlier are 7–17% higher than the expected value. These are significant at p values of 0.03–0.01. Twelve days after tumor inoculation, however, the mixed cultures show a marked decrease in lytic activity. Four of five mixtures containing 11- or 12-day primed cells had 8–22% less lytic activity than expected. These were significant at p values of 0.03–0.001 (23).

Operational View of the Events Occurring on Days 1–12 After High-Dose MTA Tumor Inoculation in Syngeneic Animals

Figure 9 summarizes the operational definitions of cytotoxic and memory cells and the suppressor and recruitment phenomena. These definitions are based on comparisons of CMC assay results, which are scored by the percent of target cells

TABLE 2. *Influence of primed cells on cytotoxicity of in vitro generated cytotoxic cells*

Duration of *in vivo* priming	% Cytotoxicity on MTM target cells[a]					
			Mixture			
	Primed	Unprimed	Observed	Expected	Δ[b]%	p[c]
2 days	25 ± 2	16 ± 3	26 ± 4	21 ± 3	+6	ns
5 days	63 ± 2	55 ± 4	71 ± 1	59 ± 3	+12	<0.03
7 days	26 ± 3	9 ± 5	32 ± 4	18 ± 4	+14	<0.03
8a days	24 ± 2	19 ± 2	39 ± 3	22 ± 2	+17	<0.01
8b days	26 ± 1	25 ± 1	33 ± 1	26 ± 1	+7	<0.01
9 days	15 ± 2	20 ± 3	10 ± 4	17 ± 3	−7	ns
10 days	76 ± 1	55 ± 3	80 ± 1	63 ± 2	+17	<0.03
11 days	11 ± 4	12 ± 1	4 ± 1	12 ± 3	−8	<0.025
12a days	16 ± 4	16 ± 2	27 ± 1	16 ± 3	+11	<0.01
12b days	16 ± 2	8 ± 2	4 ± 2	12 ± 2	−8	<0.001
12c (40 hr)[d]	65 ± 2	72 ± 1	46 ± 3	68 ± 2	−22,	<0.03
12d	42 ± 2	44 ± 2	34 ± 3	43 ± 2	−9	<0.03

From Kuperman et al., ref. 23.
[a]Concurrent sensitization of mixed lymphoid cells. Immunizing dose, 2 × 10⁷ MTA cells. Mean percent cytotoxicity (relative to targets plus nonimmune lymphocytes) ± 1 S.E.M.
[b]Difference between observed and expected cytotoxicities (calculated as described in the text).
[c]p (determined by the Mann Whitney U test), comparing the observed and expected values of cytotoxicity.
[d]Values in parentheses indicate duration of cytotoxicity assay.
All other assays are at 20 hr.

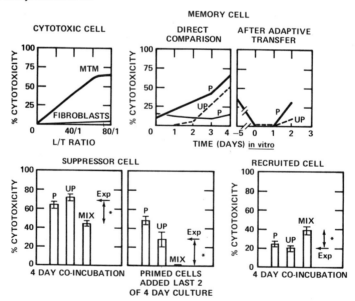

FIG. 9. Operational definitions of various cell functions related to cell-mediated cytotoxicity to a syngeneic tumor. See text for explanation.

killed rather than by quantitating lytic activity in the actual number of cytotoxic cells. Thus it is difficult to define parameters that quantitatively reflect changes in the numbers of any of the above-defined cells. Despite this limitation, one may obtain a qualitative impression of the sequence of development of these functional lymphoid cell populations by a kinetic plot of the indirect measurements. Figure 10 compares the indirect measures of the actual cytotoxicities from *in vivo* primed cells tested directly in the CMC assay (from Fig. 3A), the differences at Day 1 between primed and unprimed cells for memory cells defined by direct testing in *in vitro* sensitization (from Fig. 7), the differences at day 2 between primed and unprimed cells after 5 days' adoptive transfer for memory cells without contaminating cytotoxic and suppressor cells (from Fig. 8), and the differences between observed and expected cytotoxicity in the mixed cell experiments on sensitizing monolayers for suppression or recruitment (Table 2). Memory cells precede the development of differentiated cytotoxic cells and persist at high levels even at 12 days, when the cytotoxic cell response is waning. Cytotoxic cells appear on day 4, peak at day 8, and decrease on days 10–12, when suppressor cell function abruptly appears. The decrease in cytotoxic cells seems to result from two events: (a) the 2- to 3-day half-life of differentiated cytotoxic cells (23), and (b) failure of their continued generation from memory cells. The latter coincides with the appearance of suppressor cells (23).

IMPLICATIONS FOR CLINICAL APPLICATION

This review of our investigations offers evidence for the existence of several subpopulations of lymphocytes in spleens of syngeneic tumor-bearing animals. Cytotoxic and memory cells coexist from approximately the 4th and 10th days after inoculation with 10^7 tumor cells; memory and suppressor cells coexist from the 10th to 12th days. Later times were not examined with this inoculation dose. The suppressor cells appear to inhibit the conversion of memory to effector cells.

These observations have a bearing on projected clinical immunotherapy programs planning to use "immune" lymphocytes from patients recovered from a particular histologic type of cancer (24), relatives or household contacts of the patient—assuming that the contacts were exposed to the oncogeneic agent and are immune (25), or lymphocytes sensitized or "activated" *in vitro* (24). First, one would have to utilize defined populations of cytotoxic cells contaminated by little or no suppressor activity. This is impossible at present because there are no tests for defining suppressor cells in human systems. That potential harm could accrue to patients injected with suppressor cells is evident from current preliminary experiments in my laboratory measuring growth of subcutaneously injected 13762 cells after mixing with various lymphocyte populations. Lymphocytes from spleen or lymph nodes of animals inoculated 7 days earlier caused a marked reduction in the rate of tumor growth (but did not prevent ultimate death) relative to lymphocytes from nontumor-bearing animals. In contrast, tumors injected with spleen cells with animals 14 days after tumor inoculation grew much faster than the

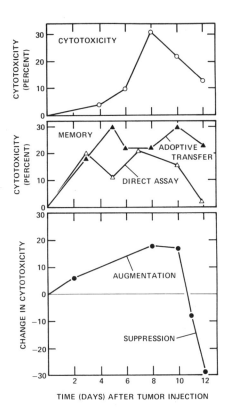

FIG. 10. Appearance of spleen lymphoid cell populations related to cellular cytotoxicity after high-dose intraperitoneal inoculation of rat mammary adenocarcinoma 13762 A. (From Kuperman et al., ref. 23.)

control tumor. Although preliminary, these results provide practical confirmatory observations on the anticipated risks and are not merely theoretical.

Second, one would anticipate a temporally limited effectiveness in injecting cytotoxic lymphocytes. This results from not only the innately short half-life of cytotoxic cells, but also because suppressor cell activity, if present in the patient, would prevent differentiation of any memory cells in the injected cells, just as they prevent conversion of the patient's own memory cells.

Thus far there are few if any aspects of the immune response to tumors that are qualitatively different from the response to allogeneic organ transplants. At a first approximation, we may consider the appearance of suppressor cell function an autoregulatory mechanism to shut down the primary cytotoxic response to a foreign antigen, which in most cases would have been successfully eliminated. We must first learn why the tumor is not eliminated by the primary cytotoxic response that eliminates allogeneic organ grafts, as well as devise methods to separate the various functionally different subpopulations of lymphocytes before successful application of specific immunotherapy is likely to yield clinical benefit. The immunologist's task ahead, then, is challenging but solvable.

ACKNOWLEDGMENTS

The author is grateful to the Williams & Wilkins Company, Baltimore, Maryland, for permission to utilize the following figures and tables previously published in the *Journal of Immunology:* Figures 2, 3, 5 through 8, and 10, and Tables 1 and 2.

The secretarial assistance of Ms. Judith Whitsell in the preparation of this manuscript is gratefully acknowledged.

This work was supported by Contract No. NI4-CB-33905 from the National Institutes of Health.

REFERENCES

1. Klein, G., Sjogren, H. O., Klein, E., and Hellstrom, K. E. (1960): Demonstration of resistance against methylcholanthrene-induced sarcomas in the primary autochthonous host. *Cancer Res.,* 20:1561–1576.
2. Attia, M. A., De Ome, K. B., and Weiss, D. W. (1965): Immunology of spontaneous mammary carcinomas in mice. II. Resistance to a rapidly and slowly developing tumor. *Cancer Res.,* 25:451–457.
3. Jagarlamoody, S. M., Aust, J. C., Tew, R. H., and McKhann, C. F. (1971): In vitro detection of cytotoxic cellular immunity against tumor-specific antigens by radioisotopic technique. *Proc. Natl. Acad. Sci. U.S.A.,* 68:1346–1350.
4. Brunner, K. T., Mauel, J., Rudolf, H., and Chapuis, B. (1970): Studies of autograft immunity in mice. I. Induction, development and in vitro assay of cellular immunity. *Immunology,* 18:501–515.
5. Green, H., Barrow, P., and Goldberg, B. (1969): Effect of antibody and complement on permeability control in ascites tumor cells and erythrocytes. *J. Exp. Med.,* 110:699–713.
6. Moller, E. (1965): Contact-induced cytotoxicity by lymphoid cells containing foreign isoantigens. *Science,* 147:873–879.
7. Hellstrom, K. E., and Hellstrom, I. (1970): Immunologic enhancement as studied by cell culture techniques. *Annu. Rev. Microbiol.,* 24:373–398.
8. Howell, S. B., Dean, J. H., Esber, E. C., and Law, L. W. (1974): Cell interactions in adoptive immune rejection of a syngeneic tumor. *Int. J. Cancer,* 14:662–674.
9. Howell, S. B., Esber, E. C., and Law, L. W. (1974): Cellular immunity in mice with simian virus 40-induced mKSA tumors: Comparison of three assays of tumor immunity. *J. Natl. Cancer Inst.,* 52:1361–1363.
10. Lucas, Z. J. (1976): Immunobiology of tissue transplantation. In: *Scientific Basis for Reconstructive Surgery,* edited by L. Vistnes and D. Kernahan. Little, Brown and Co., New York *(in press).*
11. Fortner, G. W., Kuperman, O., and Lucas, Z. J. (1975): Immune response to a syngeneic mammary adenocarcinoma. I. Comparison of kinetics of tumor cell growth and cytotoxic responses in syngeneic and allogeneic rats. *J. Immunol.,* 115:1269.
12. Walker, S. M., and Lucas, Z. J. (1972): Cytotoxic activity of lymphocytes. I. Assay for cytotoxicity by rubidium exchange at isotopic equilibrium. *J. Immunol.,* 109:1223–1232.
13. Lucas, Z. J., and Walker, S. M. (1974): Cytotoxic activity of lymphocytes. III. Standardization of measurement of cell-mediated lysis. *J. Immunol.,* 113:209–224.
14. Hellstrom, I., Sjogren, H. O., Warner, G., and Hellstrom, K. E. (1971): Blocking of cell-mediated tumor immunity by sera from patients with growing neoplasms.*Int. J. Cancer,* 7:226–237.
15. Baldwin, R. W., Price, M. R., and Robins, R. A. (1972): Blocking of lymphocyte-mediated cytotoxicity for rat hepatoma cells by tumor-specific antigen-antibody complexes. *Nature[New Biol],* 238:185–186.
16. Bonavida, B. (1974): Studies on the induction and expression of T cell-mediated immunity. II. Antiserum blocking of cell-mediated cytolysis. *J. Immunol.,* 112:1308–1321.
17. Ginsberg, H., and Sachs, L. (1965): Destruction of mouse and rat embryo cells in tissue culture

by lymph node cells from unsensitized rats. *J. Cell. Comp. Physiol.,* 66:199–220.

18. Kuperman, O., Fortner, G. W., and Lucas, Z. J. (1975): Immune response to a syngeneic mammary adenocarcinoma. II. In vitro generation of cytotoxic lymphocytes. *J. Immunol.,* 115:1277.

19. Peavy, D. L., and Pierce, C. W. (1974): Cell-mediated immune responses in vitro. I. Suppression of the generation of cytotoxic lymphocytes by concanavalin A and concanavalin A-activated spleen cells. *J. Exp. Med.,* 140:356–369.

20. Kirchner, H., Herberman, R. B., Glaser, M., and Lavrin, D. H. (1974): Suppression of in vitro lymphocyte stimulation in mice bearing primary Moloney sarcoma virus-induced tumors. *Cell. Immunol.,* 13:32–40.

21. Folch, H., and Waksman, B. H. (1974): The splenic suppressor cell. I. Activity of thymus-dependent adherent cells: changes with age and stress. *J. Immunol.,* 113:127–139.

22. Folch, H., and Waksman, B. H. (1974): The splenic suppressor cell. II. Suppression of the mixed lymphocyte reaction by thymus-dependent adherent cells. *J. Immunol.,* 113:140–144.

23. Kuperman, O., Fortner, G. W., and Lucas, Z. J. (1975): Immune response to a syngeneic mammary adenocarcinoma. III. Development of memory and suppressor functions modulating cellular cytotoxicity. *J. Immunol.,* 115:1282.

24. Morton, D. L. (1972): Immunotherapy of cancer. *Cancer,* 30:1647–1655.

25. Yonemoto, R. H., and Terasaki, P. I. (1972): Cancer immunotherapy with HLA-compatible thoracic duct lymphocyte transplantation. *Cancer,* 30:1438–1443.

Breast Cancer: Trends in Research and Treatment, edited by J. C. Heuson, W. H. Mattheiem, and M. Rozencweig. Raven Press, New York © 1976.

Roundtable Discussion: Immunology

Chairman: J. Wybran

Tubiana: There is a significant difference between the survival rate of patients receiving postoperative radiotherapy and those having surgery alone. Secondly, in some of the groups mentioned by Dr. Stjernswärd, the type of surgery used was not the same—it is not a direct comparison between surgery and another type of surgery plus radiotherapy. I would not like to leave the reader with the feeling that there is always a worse survival rate when patients have been submitted to surgery plus radiotherapy.

Lastly, I would like to make another point. It is true that there has been some discussion from a therapeutic point of view. Data have been shown indicating that immunotherapy might be useful, and it is well known that when the tumor is of good prognosis there is an immunological reaction, which has been described by many workers. A few years ago Dr. Basky showed that after surgery there is reactivation of immunological defenses and in particular of the cytotoxic effect of lymphocytes. More recently Drs. Basky and Manners published data showing that after a radiotherapy course the cytotoxicity of the lymphocytes is reactivated, and that furthermore this reactivation occurs earlier and stronger than after surgery alone. In some cases radiotherapy might play a useful role, but I would certainly not say that is so in all cases. Indeed I would caution that in some cases radiotherapy might be detrimental when there is no residual disease. Do not misunderstand me to say that where there is some residual disease that anything I have said has clinical relevance. I want to remove that idea for one reason. We recently began studying another breast cancer, the R3230, and we find that it has an entirely different set of immunological parameters. I wish to convey to you the feeling that one has to consider the experimental system as very unique. There are certain host-tumor virus external-factor interrelationships that modify the system, and I do not know if either my system or any other is translatable to the human. Furthermore, I am not sure, in working with an outbred population of species such as the human (who do not have similar genetic inbreeding as do rats and mice) that you are not compounding the difficulty. In the human situation you have many different immune or host-tumor responses, whereas we are looking for a unique host-tumor response. I think that this must be constantly kept in mind, that perhaps many patterns will show up in the human system, whereas in the rat and mouse model systems you can get one, two, three, four "pure responses."

Daehnfeldt: Could you please give further information concerning the sexual hormone influence on immunity—whether there is stimulation or inhibition?

Wybran: There are not many studies in this field. To my knowledge there are three types of studies in humans: One type shows by individual tests that stilbestrol can inhibit or decrease the PHA responsiveness. The second type shows that gonadotropins can also decrease the PHA responsiveness, and we usually assume (rightly or wrongly) that PHA responsiveness is a correlate of cell-mediated immunity *in vivo.* Lastly, women who receive oral contraceptives have a decreased immunity—their lymphocytes do not react very well to PHA, suggesting once again that there may be a decrease in cell-mediated immunity. On the other hand, women who have received progesterone on a chronic basis for a year or so have an increased DNCB sensitization, showing that there might be a booster of cell-mediated immunity. These are only very preliminary results, but they might be very important in understanding the relationship between human breast cancer and immunity.

Kenis: I would like to add that the paper by Margary and Baum in 1971 showed that there was increased phagocytic activity by diethylstilbestrol. There are also studies showing that in patients responding to hormone therapy, the blood leukocytes, which were decreased at the time of progressive disease, increased after additional hormone or castration.

Stjernswärd: There is also the work in mice showing that orchidectomy significantly protected them against the spontaneous tumor and the transplanted one. There are also the data of Mailer from the United States approximately 4 years ago; he claimed that he found a correlation between lymphocyte count and responsiveness to a given hormone therapy.

Wybran: Dr. Lejeune, what is the role of macrophage and monocyte in animal models or in human breast cancer?

Lejeune: The only thing I can say is that there is now evidence of macrophages inside mammary carcinomas; and in several models, including melanoma and lymphoma, there is evidence that macrophages are the main effector cells for rejection of the tumor. It seems that for the most part it is nonspecific; but as far as this discussion is concerned, I would like to comment on the so-called stimulation of macrophages. I think it is very dangerous to assume, for example, that an increased phagocytic ability of the macrophages means that they function better in the sense that they can better reject tumor cells. It is sometimes completely the opposite. There are several studies which show that if you increase the phagocytose of antigen by macrophage, you reduce the immune reaction. I think it is very interesting that if you irradiate macrophages you decrease the phagocytic ability, and those irradiated macrophages are better for inducing an immune response in animal models.

Stjernswärd: Eccles and Alexander measured immunogenicity, metastasizing ability, and macrophage involvement in transplantable tumor in an experimental rat system. They found that the tumors that are immunogenic do not metastasize and have a high macrophage content; the ones that are not immunogenic do metastasize and there is no macrophages. The macrophage count can be 0–6% and B-macrophages approximately 4%. Alexander's group will publish data on humans with evidence correlating metastases and macrophage content in the primary tumor.

Wybran: Is there a place for immunotherapy in adjuvant therapy since in this instance a minimal number of tumor cells are being dealt with? Clinical results in acute leukemia are highly suggestive of a positive effect of immunotherapy.

Blonk-Van der Wijst: Until now there have been some studies on immunotherapy with only a few patients in an advanced stage of disease after failure of other therapy. The question now is—can we use immunotherapy in a primary stage? Anderson, Gally, and Wood in Glasgow studied the effects of irradiated cancer cells as a part of first treatment of cancer of the breast when the residual cancer was small. The treatment was given immediately after mastectomy and radiotherapy to 16 patients with prognostically unfavorable cancer. Twelve are still alive at periods of 43–74 months. One survivor had many metastases; the other had no biochemical, clinical, radiological, or scintigraphic signs of disseminated disease. This study is perhaps promising for a trial and for using immunotherapy as adjuvant therapy or in cases of small tumors.

Kenis: There are many data in animals showing that BCG may have some good effect after surgery—for instance, in the case of mammary tumor in rats—and there are recent papers showing that in cases where it is impossible to get cures by surgery alone or BCG alone, the mixture of both therapies gives a high proportion of cures. (This was published by Sparks and his group in December 1974.) It was also interesting that recently Pimm and Baldwin demonstrated that BCG can even increase the survival of mice or delay the growth of a rat's tumor transplanted to nude mice. Thus in a case where there are no T-cells BCG may delay growth of the tumor. There was work done many years ago at the Bordet Institute by Piessens showing that BCG given after oophorectomy in rats with DMBA-induced tumor may delay recurrence of the tumor; when BCG is given at another time, it may enhance the growth of the tumor.

Wybran: There is a trial going on at the moment in the M. D. Anderson Hospital where they have compared two groups of approximately 50 patients with advanced breast cancer disease. Both groups received chemotherapy, but in one group BCG was added. After 2 years 50% of the patients in the group on chemotherapy alone died, whereas only 2 or 4 of 50 patients died in the group receiving immunotherapy also.

Breast Cancer: Trends in Research and Treatment, edited by J. C. Heuson, W. H. Mattheiem, and M. Rozencweig. Raven Press, New York © 1976.

Introduction: Experimental Models

L. M. van Putten

I would like to discuss very briefly the function of models in cancer research. One of the functions is to detect mechanisms in animal tumors, with the obvious consequence that it will be necessary later to verify that the mechanism detected is also operative in one of the human tumors. In addition, models have been used to define modes of therapy and to detect cytostatic drugs. The whole screening system is based on models, and there the function of the model is not to simulate a clinical tumor but to have an optimal efficiency for detecting drugs. As we progress in chemotherapy, we find more and more complex situations; we use combined therapies, combined modalities. The question is: do we have suitable models for that?

Is there any suitable model for mammary tumors? If we look at a traditional therapy form such as surgery, which has been discussed for decades, we find that there is no experimental model that has the properties which simulate the problems of human mammary tumor: the early lymph node metastases and late appearance of hematogenic metastases. Even if we had one such model, it would not be enough. We have many patients with cancer, and one model of a transplantable tumor in an inbred strain may simulate the situation of a single patient but not all, and therefore we can never predict. These types of considerations make us sometimes despair of the usefulness of extending models further. Nevertheless, we can see that some models are obviously suffering from the fact that we do not have enough of them. One example of this is melanoma. The most widely used mouse melanoma is now number B16, which is insensitive to DTIC, the drug which seems in clinical studies to be the most promising one. Therefore we can see that this tumor alone cannot predict the usefulness of cytostatic drugs. Does that imply that such a model is useless? It may be that since we find no response to DTIC in approximately 60–70% of melanomas in man that this one melanoma also does not respond; we cannot exclude that there is a possibility of response to other drugs. Therefore it is more encouraging to see that in the last few years a number of models for colon tumors have been developed in which the first indications are that the patterns of response to cytostatic drugs may not be too dissimilar from what is found in patients. At least a number of these tumors seem to respond to 5FU to the nitrosoureas, and to cyclophosphamide as the best agents. That in itself shows some promise that for some tumors, models can be found which may have some predictive value.

In the course of this discussion you will read about models for mammary tumors from this point of view, but let me end by looking further ahead. What we would like to do is to give a combined treatment with all modalities to a patient whose tumor we know may have one of a number of properties, and to predict the usefulness of that therapy in a model. We can do that by analyzing each separate component, but the combination can never be tested unless we have the complete model. When I enumerate the properties of that model you will realize that our hopes of ever getting it are very remote. It should be (1) a slow growing tumor, which shows spontaneous metastases to lymph nodes, hematogenic metastases, (2) moderately antigenic, (3) responsive to at least four steroid hormones, in a fraction of the cases, and to insulin. In that sense we can more or less define the properties we know now, which a fraction of these models must fulfill. We must have a large enough number of variations of this model to cover a limited number of the variations in man, and at the moment we have only a few models that fulfill three or four of these demands; therefore, much work remains to be done if we are to look forward to the possibility of testing combined therapy in models. However, this should not detract from the usefulness of models in analyzing mechanisms of response. This is an aspect for which the models are obviously useful if it is later confirmed that similar mechanisms are operative at least in the clinical disease with which we are dealing.

Breast Cancer: Trends in Research and Treatment, edited by J. C. Heuson,
W. H. Mattheiem, and M. Rozencweig. Raven Press, New York © 1976.

Hormone Dependency of Rat Mammary Tumors

J. C. Heuson,* N. Legros,* J. A. Heuson-Stiennon,† G.
Leclercq,* and J. L. Pasteels†

*Service de Médecine et Laboratoire d' Investigation Clinique,
Institut Jules Bordet, Brussels; and †Laboratoire d' Histologie,
Faculté de Médecine, Université Libre de Bruxelles, Brussels, Belgium*

There are two kinds of mammary tumors of the rat that are used as experimental models. The first are transplantable tumors (1,2) and the others are chemically induced (3,4). Both are of interest for studying hormone dependency. For lack of space, however, we consider only the rat mammary tumor induced by the carcinogen 7,12-dimethylbenz(a)anthracene (DMBA). This model is readily available and has been and still is the subject of numerous studies. It lends itself to investigations of hormone sensitivity in regard to tumor growth (3,5–7) as well as the various phases of tumor induction (3,8,9).

METHOD OF TUMOR INDUCTION

Tumor induction is usually carried out in female Sprague-Dawley rats. A single gastric instillation or intravenous injection (10) of the carcinogen (4) is given at the critical age of 50 days. Tumors begin to appear within 6 weeks of treatment and are found in 70–100% of rats by 3 months (4). They have the histopathological features of adenocarcinomas (3).

MAIN APPLICATIONS

Two major fields in which this model proved useful are (a) in the study of mechanisms underlying hormone dependency of the tumors, and (b) in the screening of new compounds with potential antitumor activity. These two applications are discussed in succession. It is not the purpose of this chapter to be exhaustive but rather, after providing a general background, to present current studies of our laboratories and discuss applications of potential interest.

HORMONE DEPENDENCY

The DMBA-induced adenocarcinomas undergo total or partial regression after ovariectomy or hypophysectomy (3), induction of alloxan diabetes (11), or administration of various hormones (3,5,12) or hormone antagonists (9,13,14). On the other hand, their growth rate is enhanced by the administration of insulin (7), prolactin (15,16), or progesterone (6,17). In ovariectomized rats estrogens are known to reactivate tumor growth, but only when insulin (11) and prolactin (18) are present. The mechanisms underlying these effects are not yet clearly understood. Thus one of the questions so far unanswered is what ovarian hormone or hormones are responsible for maintenance of tumor growth in the intact animal, the withdrawal of which by ovariectomy induces tumor regression. The following experiment was devised to investigate this problem.

EFFECT OF ESTROGENS AND PROGESTERONE AFTER OVARIECTOMY

Groups of tumor-bearing rats were ovariectomized. Some received subcutaneous injections of 17 β-estradiol at various dosages. Total tumor surface per rat was measured in each experimental group before and 6 weeks after treatment. The results expressed as ratios of these measurements are given in Fig. 1. Normal tumor growth in nonovariectomized animals as well as the expected tumor regression after ovariectomy are represented on the left part of the graph. The right part

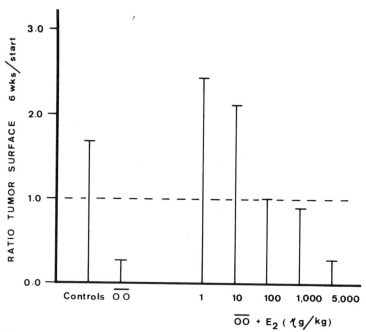

FIG. 1. Effect of increasing doses of estradiol-17β on rat mammary tumor growth in ovariectomized animals (oo). The period of observation was 6 weeks; seven matched groups of 12 rats were constituted by block randomization of the animals according to size and number of tumors. Statistical analysis with the Wilcoxon test on the paired differences, two-tailed, yields the following levels of significance: $\overline{oo}$ vs. controls, $p < 0.01$; $\overline{oo}$, E_2 (1 or 10 μg/kg) vs. $\overline{oo}$ $p <$ 0.01; $\overline{oo}$, E_2 (5,000 or 1,000 μg/kg) vs. $\overline{oo}$, E_2 (1 μg/kg), $p < 0.01$.

depicts the effect of increasing doses of estradiol given to ovariectomized animals from the time of operation. The smaller doses were very effective in restoring tumor growth, while the larger supraphysiological doses were distinctly inhibitory. The biphasic effect of estrogens is reminiscent of that observed in breast cancer patients in whom small physiological doses are said to stimulate tumor progression (19), whereas administration of large doses represents one of the most effective treatments of the disease. Mechanisms have been proposed to explain this biphasic effect on rat tumors, among which are stimulation of prolactin secretion by low doses of estrogens and inhibition of the growth-enhancing effect of prolactin by large doses (16).

Progesterone is a second ovarian hormone that proved equally effective in restoring tumor growth in ovariectomized rats (Fig. 2). Remarkably, tumors growing under the stimulating effect of either estrogens or progesterone display totally different histological features (Fig. 3). Estradiol-stimulated tumors closely

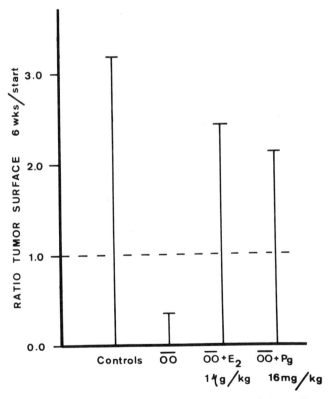

FIG. 2. Effect of estradiol-17β, (1 μg/kg) and progesterone (16 mg/kg) on rat mammary tumor growth in ovariectomized animals ($\overline{oo}$). The period of observation was 6 weeks; there were four matched groups (Fig. 1) of 12 rats. Statistical analysis with the Wilcoxon test on the paired differences, two-tailed, yields the following levels of significance: $\overline{oo}$ vs. controls, $p < 0.01$; $\overline{oo}$, E$_2$ (1 μg/kg) vs. $\overline{oo}$, $p = 0.02$; $\overline{oo}$, Pg (16 mg/kg) vs. $\overline{oo}$, $p < 0.05$.

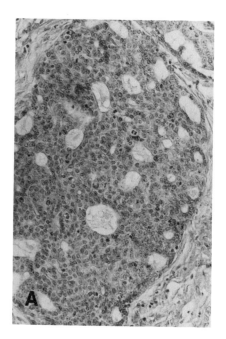
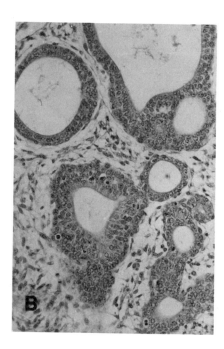

FIG. 3. A: Typical aspect of a tumor growing in an ovariectomized rat receiving estradiol-17β (1 μg/kg). The picture is similar to that seen in tumors from control nonovariectomized rats. The cells are actively proliferating, round, and closely packed over wide areas containing a fair number of alveolar structures. **B.** Characteristic aspects of a tumor growing in an ovariectomized rat receiving progesterone (16 mg/kg). The tumor tissue is made up of cavities surrounded by a regular wall most often composed of a double layer of large cuboidal cells. Hematoxylin and eosin stain.

resemble tumors growing in nonovariectomized, untreated rats. The cells are actively proliferating, round, and closely packed over wide areas containing a fair number of alveolar structures. In sharp contrast, progesterone-stimulated tumors have totally different cytological and histological characteristics. The tumor tissue is made up of variably sized cavities surrounded by a regular wall most often composed of a double layer of large cuboidal cells.

It therefore appears that the usual structure of the DMBA tumors in nonovariectomized rats is predominantly determined by estrogens, which are the main hormones produced by the ovaries of virgin rats. Large doses of progesterone in the absence of ovarian estrogens profoundly distort the architecture of the tumor tissue. This may result either from proliferation of distinct, progesterone-dependent cell clones or from a special configuration of the tumor tissue induced by the differentiating effect of progesterone. These alternative hypotheses are worth further investigation.

HORMONAL EFFECTS IN ORGAN CULTURE

Organ cultures of DMBA tumors were carried out to analyze the effect of various hormones on DNA synthesis and histological appearance. Cultures were maintained for 4 days in the chemically defined medium 199 at 37°C in an atmosphere of 95% O_2 and 5% CO_2. Hormones were added either singly or in combination at the following final concentrations: insulin 10 μg/ml, prolactin (ovine) 5 μg/ml, progesterone 1 μg/ml, and estradiol 1 μg or 1 ng/ml. Deoxyribonucleic acid (DNA) synthesis was measured by ^{3}H-thymidine incorporation into DNA and was expressed as disintegrations per minute (dpm) per microgram of DNA-P.

Effects on DNA Synthesis

In accordance with our previous findings (20), insulin enhanced DNA synthesis to a considerable though variable extent in a majority of tumors, while it was ineffective in some "insulin-independent tumors" (Fig. 4). The insulin-independent tumors also proved to be totally insensitive to all other hormones tested.

A second characteristic feature was the stimulating effect of the combination of

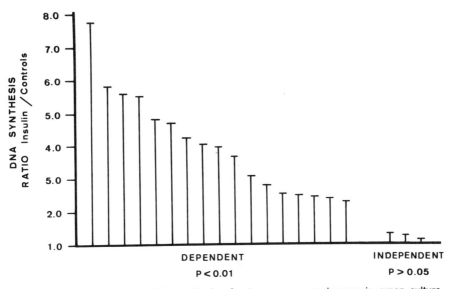

FIG. 4. Effect of insulin on DNA synthesis of rat mammary carcinomas in organ culture. Explants were cultured for 4 days in the chemically defined medium 199; insulin was added at the concentration of 10 μg/ml. DNA synthesis was measured by the incorporation of ^{3}H-thymidine into DNA during a 1-hr pulse at the end of the 4-day cultures, and the results were expressed as disintegrations per minute (dpm) per microgram of DNA-P. Twenty tumors were studied. Analysis of variance revealed that in 17 cases insulin significantly increased thymidine ^{3}H-incorporation over the control values ("insulin-dependent," $p < 0.01$) and was ineffective in three cases ("insulin-independent," $p > 0.05$).

prolactin and progesterone in the presence of insulin. This was observed in approximately two-thirds of the tumors tested (Fig. 5). Either hormone alone was distinctly less effective. The stimulating effect of prolactin alone has already been reported (21,22). Finally, it was found that estradiol in combination with prolactin and in the presence of insulin was inhibitory in 4 out of 10 tumors (Fig. 6), an observation that is in agreement with other reports (21,22).

These *in vitro* results can be reconciled with known facts about hormonal control of growth of the DMBA tumors. Thus it is well known that most tumors are insulin- and prolactin-dependent *in vivo* (7,15,16). Progesterone also stimulates their growth, as described above. The case of estrogens is more complex. While small physiological doses of estrogens restore tumor growth in ovariectomized rats, large pharmacological doses as used in cultures are inhibitory (see above); these doses possibly interfere with the stimulating effect of prolactin at the tumor tissue level as demonstrated in organ culture and already suggested by *in vivo* experiments (16).

Effects on Tumor Tissue Differentiation

The histological appearance of the tumors studied was that of papillary or cribriform carcinomas. Secretory activity was occasionally observed. There was

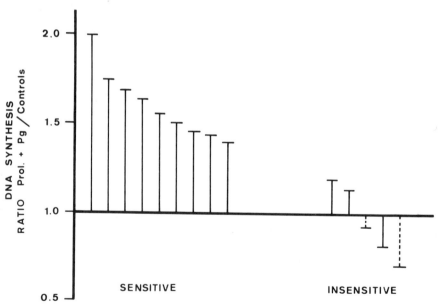

FIG. 5. Effect of prolactin plus progesterone, in the presence of insulin, on DNA synthesis of rat mammary carcinomas in organ culture. Hormones were added at the following concentrations: insulin 10 μg/ml, ovine prolactin 5 μg/ml, and progesterone 1 μg/ml. DNA synthesis was measured as in Fig. 4. Insulin-independent tumors (- - - - -) were insensitive to the combination of prolactin and progesterone, whereas 9 of the 12 insulin-dependent tumors (————) were sensitive to the combination of prolactin and progesterone (analysis of variance; $p < 0.05$).

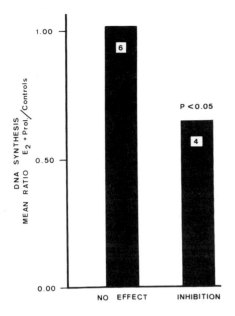

FIG. 6. Effect of prolactin plus estradiol-17β, in the presence of insulin, on DNA synthesis of rat mammary carcinomas in organ culture. Hormones were added at the following concentrations: insulin 10 μg/ml, ovine prolactin 5 μg/ml, and estradiol-17β 1 μg or 1 ng/ml. DNA synthesis was measured as in Fig. 4. All 10 tumors studied were insulin-dependent; in four, DNA synthesis was inhibited by the combination of prolactin and estradiol-17β (analysis of variance, $p < 0.05$).

no histological characteristic that enabled us to predict hormone responsiveness *in vitro*.

After 4 days of culture, tumors that were insulin-dependent for DNA synthesis required insulin for full maintenance of the preculture histological features; insulin-free cultures displayed regressive changes, with shrunken cytoplasm and nuclei, and no typical glandular pattern (Fig. 7A). Addition of prolactin and insulin induced considerable and characteristic changes (Fig. 7B). Cells were large and well organized around glandular cavities. Signs of secretory activity were obvious and were mainly visible as lipid droplets at the apical part of the cells. Addition of progesterone to the combination of insulin-prolactin completely suppressed the differentiating effect of the latter. Insulin-independent tumors (based on DNA synthesis) were fully maintained in insulin-free cultures.

In conclusion, the rat mammary tumor retains the capacity of the normal mammary tissue to differentiate and to undergo secretory changes under the proper hormonal stimuli (23). Noteworthy is the demonstration of the inhibitory effect of progesterone on the prolactin-insulin induction of secretory activity, an effect that has not yet been reported to occur in normal mammary tissue *in vitro*.

USE OF DMBA TUMORS FOR SCREENING NEW DRUGS

In view of apparent similarities between human breast cancer and the DMBA rat mammary tumor, this experimental model appears suitable for screening new drugs potentially active in breast cancer treatment. Examples of screening applications as performed in our laboratory follow.

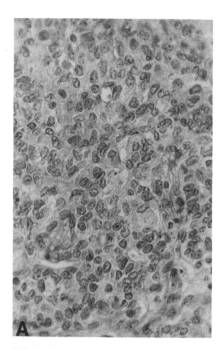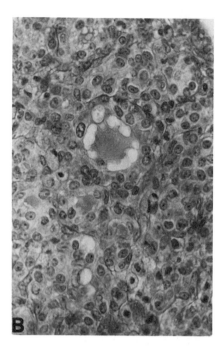

FIG. 7. Four-day organ culture of a rat mammary carcinoma. **A:** Culture without hormone. The cytoplasm and nuclei are shrunken, and no glandular pattern is observed. **B.** Culture in the presence of insulin plus prolactin. Cells are large and well organized around glandular cavities; signs of secretory activity are obvious and are mainly visible as lipid droplets at the apical part of the cells.

Antiprolactin Drugs

In view of its known prolactin dependence, it seemed appropriate to test prolactin inhibitors in the DMBA tumor model. CB 154 (2-Br-α-ergocryptine) was selected because it is a potent inhibitor of prolactin release in different animal species including rats and man. It was indeed found to be inhibitory on rat mammary tumor induction (9) and growth (Fig. 8) (24). This observation led us to undertake a clinical trial of CB154 in postmenopausal patients with advanced breast cancer (25). This trial was entirely negative, suggesting that prolactin might not play a role in human breast cancer that is as important as that in the experimental model.

Estrogen Antagonists

Two estrogen antagonists—nafoxidine (Upjohn) and tamoxifen (ICI, Great Britain)—that compete with the binding of estrogens to their target-tissue-specific receptors were tested in the rat model. Both proved effective in reducing tumor growth (Fig. 9). They were therefore subjected to clinical trials in advanced breast cancer. Nafoxidine was extensively studied by the EORTC Breast Cancer Coop-

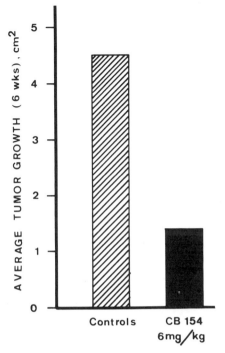

FIG. 8. Effect of CB154 on rat mammary tumor growth. The period of observation was 6 weeks, and there were 15 matched pairs (Fig. 1). Wilcoxon test on the paired differences, two-tailed: $p < 0.05$.

erative Group in randomized trials (26–28) and was found to be at least as effective as the best of the known hormonal treatments, i.e., ethinyl estradiol. Tamoxifen was tried by Cole et al. (29) and later by Ward (30), and was found effective and apparently devoid of any significant side effects. It has become one

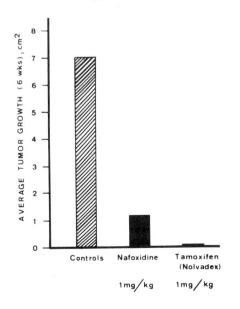

FIG. 9. Effect of nafoxidine and tamoxifen on rat mammary tumor growth. The period of observation was 6 weeks, and there were three matched groups (Fig. 1) of 12 rats. Wilcoxon test on the paired differences, two-tailed: nafoxidine vs. controls, $p < 0.05$; tamoxifen vs. controls, $p < 0.01$.

of the agents used in the combination chemotherapy trials of the EORTC Breast Group as reported by Engelsman and Mattheiem elsewhere in this volume.

Analogue of Gonadotropin-Releasing Hormone

Compound A-43818 (Abbott) is another drug recently subjected to screening. It is an analogue of the synthetic gonadotropin-releasing hormone (GnRH) that unexpectedly was found by Rippel et al. (31) to inhibit ovarian activity in the ewe. The results of the experiment are presented in Fig. 10. It is clear from the graph that A-43818 induced tumor regression, although to a lesser extent than ovariectomy, and that it might be worth testing it in human breast cancer. The endocrine mechanism of action of this compound is currently being studied.

Screening in Relation to Presence of Estrogen Receptors in Tumors

The rat mammary tumor as well as human breast cancer contains cytoplasmic estrogen receptors that bind estrogenic molecules. The estrogen-receptor complex is then translocated into the nucleus and interacts with the chromatin (32). Therefore a cytotoxic agent linked to an estrogenic molecule might, under certain conditions, follow the same route and act selectively on cancers containing estrogen receptors. Examples of such molecules are presented in Fig. 11. The screening of these molecules involves assessment of their *in vitro* affinity for the

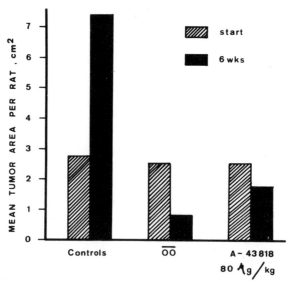

FIG. 10. Effect of A-43818 on rat mammary tumor growth. The period of observation was 6 weeks, and there were matched groups (Fig. 1) of 12 rats. Wilcoxon tests on the paired differences, two-tailed: ovariectomy vs. controls, $p < 0.01$; A-43,818 vs. controls, $p < 0.01$; A-43,818 vs. ovariectomy, $p < 0.02$.

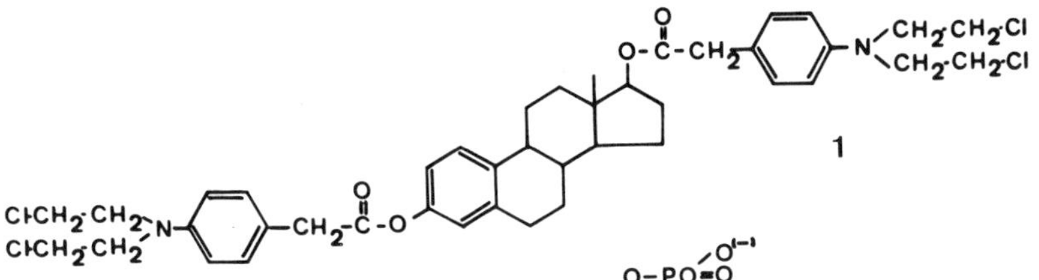

FIG. 11. Chemical structure of various estrogens linked with cytotoxic agents. **1:** Estradiol mustard (NSC-112259). **2:** Estracyt® (Leo 299; NSC-89199). **3, 4,** and **5** compounds produced by Dr. H. Hamacher (University of Tübingen, Germany).

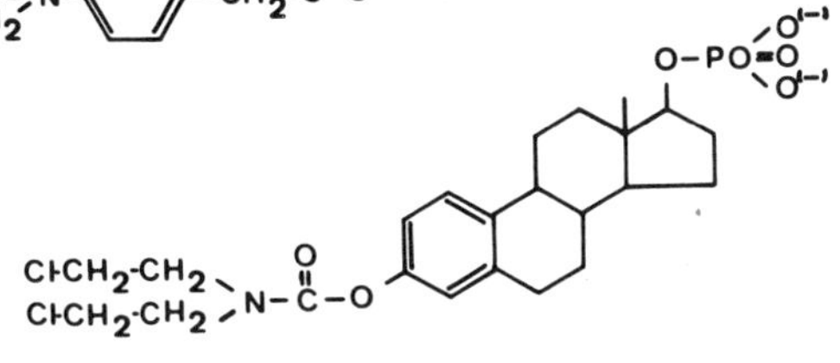

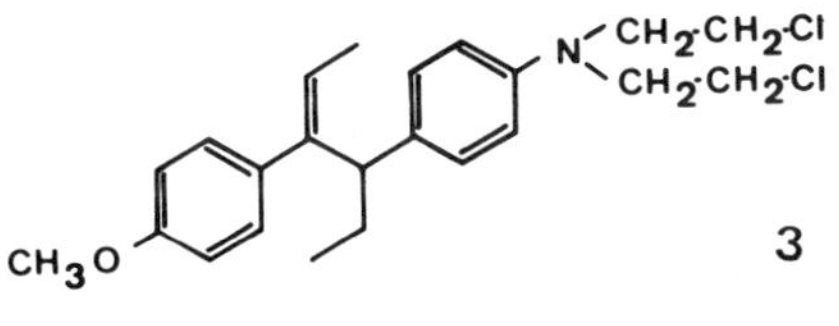

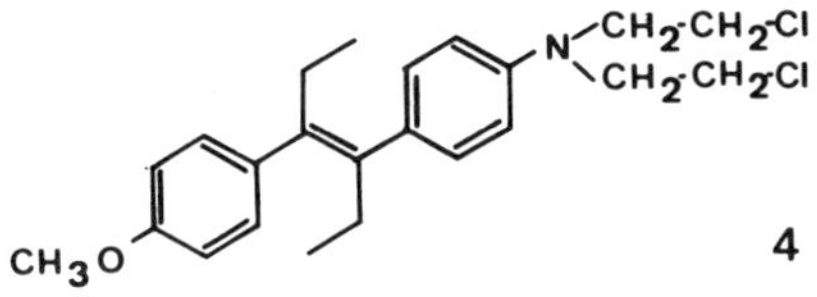

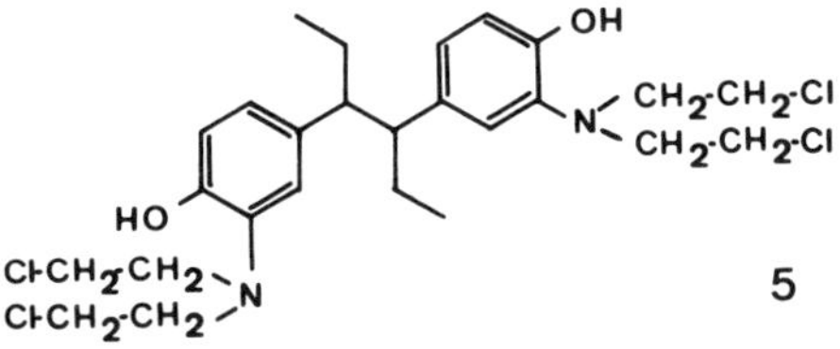

specific estrogen receptors and stability in biological media, followed by therapeutic trials in the rat tumor model. Experiments based on this scheme are in progress.

CONCLUSION

This overview of some recent works on the DMBA-induced mammary tumor of the rat indicates that this animal model is of value for improving our knowledge of the hormone dependence mechanisms of breast tumors, and based on this improved knowledge is useful in selecting and screening new compounds of potential value in the treatment of breast cancer.

ACKNOWLEDGMENTS

This work was supported by grants from the "Fonds Cancérologique de la Caisse Générale d'Epargne et de Retraite de Belgique" and was performed in part under contract of the Ministère de la Politique Scientifique within the framework of the Association Euratom, University of Brussels, University of Pisa.

REFERENCES

1. Hilf, R., Michel, I., Bell, C., Freeman, J. J., and Borman A. (1965): Biochemical and morphological properties of a new lactating mammary tumor line in the rat. *Cancer Res.,* 25:286–299.
2. Segaloff, A. (1966): Hormones and breast cancer. *Recent Prog. Horm. Res.,* 22:351–379.
3. Huggins, C., Briziarelli, G., and Sutton, H., Jr. (1959): Rapid induction of mammary carcinoma in the rat and the influence of hormones on the tumors. *J. Exp. Med.,* 109: 25–41.
4. Huggins, C., Grand, L. C., and Brillantes, F. P. (1961): Mammary cancer induced by a single feeding of polynuclear hydrocarbons and its suppression. *Nature (Lond.),* 189:204–207.
5. Huggins, C., Moon, R. C., and Morii, S. (1962): Extinction of experimental mammary cancer. I. Estradiol-17β and progesterone. *Proc. Natl. Acad. Sci. U.S.A.,* 48:379–386.
6. Jabara, A. G. (1967): Effects of progesterone on 9,10-dimethyl-1,2- benz(a)anthracene-induced mammary tumours in Sprague-Dawley rats. *Br. J. Cancer,* 21:418–429.
7. Heuson, J. C., Legros, N., and Heimann, R. (1972): Influence of insulin administration on growth of the 7,12- dimethylbenz(a)anthracene-induced mammary carcinoma in intact, oophorectomized, and hypophysectomized rats. *Cancer Res.,* 32:233–238.
8. Jabara, A. G., and Harcourt, A. G. (1971): Effects of progesterone, ovariectomy and adrenalectomy on mammary tumours induced by 7,12-dimethylbenz(a)anthracene in Sprague-Dawley rats. *Pathology,* 3:209–214.
9. Heuson, J. C., Waelbroeck, C., Legros, N., Gallez, G., Robyn, C., and L'Hermite, M. (1971/72): Inhibition of DMBA-induced mammary carcinogenesis in the rat by 2-Br-α-ergocryptine (CB 154), an inhibitor of prolactin and by nafoxidine (U-11, 100 A), an estrogen antagonist. *Gynecol. Invest.,* 2:130–137.
10. Huggins, C., Morii, S., and Grand, L. C. (1961): Mammary cancer induced by a single dose of polynuclear hydrocarbons. *Ann. Surg.,* 154:315–318.
11. Heuson, J. C., and Legros, N. (1972): Influence of insulin deprivation on growth of the 7,12-dimethylbenz(a)anthracene-induced mammary carcinoma in rats subjected to alloxan diabetes and food restriction. *Cancer Res.,* 32:226–232.
12. Teller, M. N., Stock, C. C., and Bowie, M. (1966): Effects of 17α-thioestradiol, 2 estradiol analogs, and 2 androgens on 7,12-dimethylbenz(a)anthracene-induced rat mammary tumors. *Cancer Res.,* 26:2329–2333.
13. Terenius, L. (1971): Anti-oestrogens and breast cancer. *Eur. J. Cancer,* 7:57–64.
14. DeSombre, E.R., and Arbogast, L. Y. (1974): Effect of the antiestrogen CI 628 on the growth of rat mammary tumors. *Cancer Res.,* 34:1971–1976.
15. Pearson, O. H., Llerena, O., Llerena, L., Molina, A., and Butler, T. (1969): Prolactin-dependent rat mammary cancer: A model for man? *Trans. Assoc. Am. Physicians,* 82:225–238.
16. Meites, J. (1972): Relation of prolactin and estrogen to mammary tumorigenesis in the rat. *J. Natl. Cancer Inst.,* 48:1217–1224.
17. Huggins, C., and Yang, N. C. (1962): Induction and extinction of mammary cancer. *Science,* 137:257–262.
18. Sterental, A., Dominguez, J. M., Weissman, C., and Pearson, O. H. (1963): Pituitary role in the estrogen dependency of experimental mammary cancer. *Cancer Res.,* 23:481–484.
19. Pearson, O. H., West, C. D., and Hollander, V. P. (1954): Evaluation of endocrine therapy for advanced breast cancer. *J.A.M.A.,* 154:234–239.

20. Heuson, J. C., Coune, A., and Heimann, R. (1966): Cell proliferation induced by insulin in organ culture of the rat mammary carcinoma. *Exp. Cell Res.,* 45:351–360.
21. Welsch, C. W., and Rivera, E. M. (1972): Differential effects of estrogen and prolactin on DNA synthesis in organ cultures of DMBA-induced rat mammary carcinoma. *Proc. Soc. Exp. Biol. Med.,* 139:623–626.
22. Lewis, D., and Hallowes, R. C. (1974): Correlation between the effects of hormones on the synthesis of DNA in explants from induced rat mammary tumours and the growth of the tumours. *J. Endocrinol.,* 62:225–240.
23. Hallowes, R. C., Wang, D. Y., and Lewis, D. J. (1973): The lactogenic effects of prolactin and growth hormone on mammary gland explants from virgin and pregnant Sprague-Dawley rats. *J. Endocrinol.,* 57:253–264.
24. Heuson, J. C., Waelbroeck-Van Gaver, C., and Legros, N. (1970): Growth inhibition of rat mammary carcinoma and endocrine changes produced by 2-Br-α-ergocryptine, a suppressor of lactation and nidation. *Eur. J. Cancer,* 6:353–356.
25. European Breast Cancer Group (1972): Clinical trial of 2-Br-α-ergocryptine (CB 154) in advanced breast cancer. *Eur. J. Cancer,* 8:155–156.
26. E.O.R.T.C. Breast Cancer Group (1972): Clinical trial of nafoxidine, an oestrogen antagonist in advanced breast cancer. *Eur. J. Cancer,* 8:387–389.
27. Heuson, J. C., Engelsman, E., Blonk-Van Der Wijst, J., Maass, H., Drochmans, A., Michel, J., Nowakowski, H., and Gorins, A. (1975): Comparative trial of nafoxidine and ethinyloestradiol in advanced breast cancer: An E.O.R.T.C. study. *Br. Med. J.,* 2:711–713.
28. Engelsman, E., Heuson, J. C., Blonk-Van Der Wijst, J., Drochmans, A., Maass, H., Cheix, F., Sobrinho, L. G., and Nowakowski, H. (1975): Controlled clinical trial of L-dopa and nafoxidine in advanced breast cancer: An E.O.R.T.C. study. *Br. Med. J.,* 2:714–715.
29. Cole, M. P., Jones, C. T. A., and Todd, I. D. H. (1971): A new antioestrogenic agent in late breast cancer: An early clinical appraisal of ICI 46,474. *Br. J. Cancer,* 25:270–275.
30. Ward, H. W. C. (1973): Anti-oestrogen therapy for breast cancer: A trial of tamoxifen at two dose levels. *Br. Med. J.,* 1:13–14.
31. Rippel, R. H., Moyer, R. H., Johnson, E. S., and Mauer, R. E. (1974): Response of the ewe to synthetic gonadotropin releasing hormone. *J. Anim. Sci.,* 38:605–612.
32. Jensen, E. V., and DeSombre, E. R. (1972): Mechanism of action of the female sex hormones. *Annu. Rev. Biochem.,* 41:203–230.

Breast Cancer: Trends in Research and Treatment, edited by J. C. Heuson,
W. H. Mattheiem, and M. Rozencweig. Raven Press, New York © 1976.

Predictive Mammary Tumor Test Systems for Experimental Chemotherapy

Arthur E. Bogden and D. Jane Taylor

*Department of Immunobiology, Mason Research Institute,
Worcester, Massachusetts 01608; and Breast Cancer Program Coordinating Branch,
Division of Cancer Biology and Diagnosis, National Cancer Institute, NIH,
Bethesda, Maryland 20014*

It is becoming increasingly apparent that the future of cancer treatment lies in the greater application of combined therapy. Combined therapy can mean either "combination chemotherapy" employing two or more drugs, or it may involve "combinations of therapeutic modalities" in which single-drug or combination chemotherapy is used as an adjuvant to surgery and/or radiotherapy. With increasing emphasis on the use of combined therapy, and the resultant logistical and ethical problems of empirically determining "optimal combinations" clinically, there is a correspondingly greater need for animal model tumor systems that could predict the clinical success of combinations of new and existing chemotherapeutic agents and modalities.

In the United States leukemia L1210 has been the major screening tool of the National Cancer Institute's Drug Development Program for many years (1). A close second has been the leukemia P-388, used for testing natural products because of its greater sensitivity for crude fractions (2). There is little question that the preoccupation of the experimental chemotherapists with the leukemia test systems has played a significant role in the overall progress of chemotherapy against the hematologic malignancies, especially acute lymphocytic leukemia and advanced Hodgkin's disease. However, by the same token, one wonders whether this same preoccupation with the leukemia test systems may not be partially responsible for the paucity of antineoplastic drugs really effective against the so-called solid tumors in man.

Although experimental tumor systems such as the L1210 and P-388 leukemias have proved to be and still are extremely useful and logistically practical in screening programs, there is growing evidence that the solid tumors as well as the *natural* metastases from such tumors present unique drug sensitivities and treatment problems and must be added to the armamentarium of refined test systems for preclinical drug and therapy evaluation. Ideally, animal tumor models should not only be representative of human malignancies histologically but should also

95

originate in the organ or tissues and have the growth and metastasizing characteristics of the particular neoplastic disease for which they serve as a model.

In this context, therefore, we might define breast cancer as a disease of the mammary gland characterized by neoplasms, and identify the variations in tumor growth and invasiveness, as well as variations in histopathology and in responsiveness to chemotherapy, that are encountered clinically, as manifestations of the individual neoplasms found within a disease. Although more of a statement than a definition, this points to the obvious—that no one animal tumor can completely represent and be predictive for breast cancer disease. Although animal tumors can be found that reproducibly mimic certain responses to therapy observed clinically, and can be manipulated to serve as a test system, at best a single animal tumor can only serve as a model and be predictive for a certain class of tumors found within a disease.

Realistically, therefore, for a model test system to be predictive for human breast cancer it should be made up of a *block* of animal tumors that reflect a spectrum of growth patterns and reactivities. Providing that all other criteria are met, in such a test system the role of the tumor that is unresponsive or resistant to chemotherapy is as important as that of the responsive tumor. One should not lose sight of the fact, however, that animal tumor models are assay systems and as such must have well-defined and reproducible growth patterns and reactivities so that modifications in such parameters resulting from experimental manipulations can be correctly interpreted. To be practical as a model, the model itself must be predictable, its use logistically feasible, and the time frame for its use as a test system reasonable. A rationale for the development of experimental systems compatible with clinical needs was recently discussed by Carter (2), and a rationale of combination chemotherapy based on preclinical experiments was presented by Goldin (3).

The purpose of this chapter is to present both a potential model for the whole disease of breast cancer as well as an experimental animal tumor that mimics the chemotherapy responsiveness and acquired drug resistance of those clinical breast cancers sensitive to the alkylating agents.

MATERIALS AND METHODS

Rat Mammary Tumor Systems

The following tumors were randomly selected from the tumor bank at the Mason Research Institute.

DMBA 1—a dimethylbenzanthracene-induced, papillary cyst mammary adenocarcinoma; metastasizes only rarely to regional lymph nodes and lungs; originally received from Dr. Wilhemina F. Dunning.

DMBA 14—a dimethylbenzanthracene-induced mammary adenocarcinoma with very-well-defined acini; metastasizes occasionally to regional lymph nodes and lungs; originally received from Dr. Wilhemina F. Dunning.

R3230AC—a well-differentiated mammary adenocarcinoma of spontaneous origin; metastasizes occasionally to regional lymph nodes and lungs, and responds to exogenous estrogens by milk secretion; originally received from Dr. Russell Hilf.

3M2N—a mammary squamous cell carcinoma which shows some keratinization and pearl formation; metastasizes only occasionally; induced by 3-methyl-2-naphthylamine at the Mason Research Institute.

SMT-2A—a poorly differentiated mammary carcinoma characterized by sheets of anaplastic epithelial cells having pleomorphic, hyperchromatic nuclei and abundant cytoplasm; has a high incidence of metastases to regional lymph nodes and lungs; induced by methylcholanthrene and *in vivo* immunoselection by Dr. Untae Kim.

13762—a dimethylbenzanthracene-induced mammary adenocarcinoma with typical histologic structures; metastasizes regularly to regional lymph nodes, lungs, abdominal organs, and occasionally to the brain and spinal column; originally received from Dr. Albert Segaloff.

Tumor Transplantations

All mammary tumors were routinely carried in syngeneic females. The 13762, R3230AC, DMBA 1, and DMBA 14 tumors were transplanted with 1- to 2-mm^3 pieces injected subcutaneously (s.c.) on the right side, via trocar, and the 3M2N tumor by injecting one-fourth of a 2-inch, 13-gauge trocar subcutaneously on the right side. All grafts were placed approximately midway between the axillary and inguinal areas. The SMT-2A mammary tumor was prepared as a mince in a 1:1 ratio of tumor tissue/tissue culture medium 199 (containing no serum), of which 0.1 ml was inoculated directly into the right inguinal mammary fat pad. Experimental groups within studies were made up of 10–20 tumor-bearing animals.

Chemotherapeutic Agents, Dose Levels, and Treatment Regimens

For comparing the chemotherapy responsiveness of the six transplantable mammary tumors as a potential predictive test system for general clinical activity, L-phenylalanine mustard (PAM) was administered at 1.6 mg/kg orally (p.o.); 5-fluorouracil (5FU) at 20 mg/kg s.c.; and methotrexate (MTX) at 0.8 mg/kg p.o. All agents were prepared in a 0.9% solution of sodium chloride containing 0.3% hydroxypropyl cellulose (Klucel) and administered three times weekly.

In assay 1871, PAM, 5FU, and MTX were administered in a Klucel vehicle at the same dose levels and in the same regimen as above. In assay 1872, PAM was administered at 1.6 mg/kg, p.o. three times weekly; 5FU at 25 mg/kg, s.c. five times weekly; and adriamycin (ADR) at 0.8 mg/kg intraperitoneally (i.p.) five times weekly. ADR was prepared in saline, and PAM and 5FU in the Klucel vehicle.

RESULTS AND DISCUSSION

A "Block" of Mammary Tumors as a Test System Predictive for General Clinical Activity

To determine the spectrum of reactivities that could be obtained with a block of animal mammary tumor systems, six transplantable rat mammary tumors were selected at random from the tumor bank of the Mason Research Institute (Table 1). These tumors have been well established in serial transplantation, have stable growth characteristics in the syngeneic strain of origin, and show a range in maximum growth rate (at mid-log phase of measurable growth) of 1.06–2.57 mm/day, a range in mean survival time of 45.4–84.7 days, and incidences of metastases ranging from 0% to 93%. The growth curves of these tumors, as approximated by the Gompertz function and plotted on an arithmetic scale, are illustrated in Fig. 1. The plots, obtained by simple caliper measurements of the longest and shortest diameters, show that these tumors represent a range of growth patterns.

The six mammary tumors were tested for their responsiveness to PAM as a single agent and in a three-drug combination with MTX and 5FU. The spectrum of responses illustrated by the tumor growth and/or regression curves in Fig. 2 were obtained by tumor size measurements taken three times weekly. All tumor systems are plotted on the same scale, and dose levels and treatment regimens were identical. Significantly, although these mammary tumors were chosen at random, they show gradations of responses with 13762 tumor being most responsive to both PAM and the three-drug combination, and R3230AC being unresponsive to PAM and the three-drug combination.

The responses of the six tumors to the three clinically active chemotherapeutic agents (PAM, 5FU, and MTX) administered singly and in combination have been graded in Table 2. The most striking response was the inactivity of MTX at the dose levels and regimens used; 5FU, on the other hand, inhibited growth slightly to moderately in all tumor systems. Administered alone, PAM showed some activity in all tumor systems and was oncolytic, producing remissions in two tumor systems. The three-drug combination of PAM, 5FU, and MTX was oncolytic in three tumor systems, showed moderate to marked activity in two, and showed no activity in only one. Significantly, drug synergism with marked tumor growth inhibition or oncolysis was evident in three tumor systems, when the same agents administered singly showed only slight to moderate inhibitory activity. This type of synergism was evident in the SMT-2A and 3M2N tumor systems. Although studies with PAM and 5FU are still underway, it is evident that the two-drug combination had an overall activity similar to that of the three-drug combination.

A further summary of these activities shows that when tested against this "block" of six mammary tumor systems PAM had a response rate of 67%, response being defined as a significant inhibition of tumor growth, inducing a few

TABLE 1. Syngeneic transplantable mammary tumor systems: A potential animal mammary tumor model predictive for general clinical activity

Tumor designation	Histologic type	Rat strain of origin and transplantability	Maximum growth rate (mm/day)	Survival time (days)[a]	Metastases (% incidence)[b]
DMBA 14	Adenocarcinoma	Fischer 344	1.06	84.7 ± 15	15
SMT-2A	Poorly differentiated carcinoma	Wistar-Furth	1.06	61.1 ± 7	80
DMBA 1	Adenocarcinoma	Fischer 344	1.39	58.9 ± 11	0
R3230AC	Adenocarcinoma	Fischer 344	1.35	49.8 ± 16	10
13762	Adenocarcinoma	Fischer 344	1.85	48.7 ± 8	93
3M2N	Squamous cell carcinoma	Fischer 344	2.57	45.4 ± 8	10

[a] Means ± standard deviation.
[b] Detected macroscopically at necropsy. Therefore incidences reflect early rather than late metastases, since only early metastases have sufficient time to develop into macroscopically discernible masses before cachexia and death.

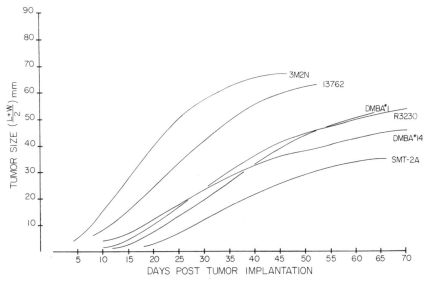

FIG. 1. Tumor growth curves of transplantable rat mammary tumors approximated by the Gompertz function mammary tumor systems. Tumor sizes were determined three times weekly by averaging the caliper measurements of the longest and shortest diameters.

complete remissions in 33% of the tumor systems. The three-drug combination (PAM, MTX, 5FU) had a response rate of 83%, inducing many complete remissions in 50% of the tumor systems treated. Although these transplantable rodent tumors were chosen at random, the activities demonstrated with them are not that different from activities reported for the same compounds in clinical studies. The inference is made, therefore, that such a "block" of tumors may

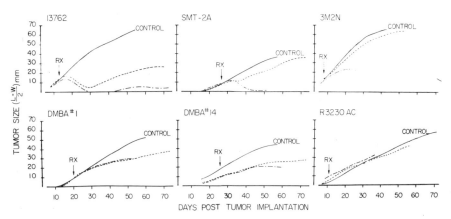

FIG. 2. Tumor growth and regression curves illustrating the response of transplantable rat mammary tumors to chemotherapy: (——) vehicle-treated controls; (- - - -) treated with PAM; and (— · —) treated with the combination of PAM + MTX + 5FU.

TABLE 2. *Responsiveness of transplantable rat mammary tumors to three clinically active chemotherapeutic agents administered singly and in combination*

Tumor designation	Histologic type	Effect of chemotherapeutic agents[a]				
		PAM	5FU	MTX	PAM + 5FU + MTX	PAM + 5FU
13762	Adenocarcinoma	+++	+	0	++++ (S)	++++ (S)
DMBA 14	Adenocarcinoma	+++	+	0	+++	+++ (S)
SMT-2A	Poorly differentiated carcinoma	+	+	0	+++ (S)	
3M2N	Squamous cell carcinoma	±	±	0	++ (S)	
DMBA 1	Adenocarcinoma	++	±	±	+	+
R3230AC	Adenocarcinoma	±	±	0	0	±

[a]Key:
++++ oncolytic with many complete remissions.
+++ oncolytic with a few complete remissions.
++ markedly growth inhibitory.
+ moderately growth inhibitory.
± slightly growth inhibitory.
0 no effect.
(S) Combination induces a synergistic effect.

serve as a more realistic predictive test system for general clinical activity. There is little question that PAM is predicted to be an effective agent for clinical use, and that combining PAM with MTX and/or 5FU significantly enhances its activity.

A Predictive Mammary Tumor Test System That Mimics Certain Clinical Responses

Of the six tumor systems just reviewed, the 13762 mammary adenocarcinoma best mimics the chemotherapy responsiveness and acquired drug resistance of those human breast cancers that are sensitive to alkylating agents (4,5). Its potential as a preclinical test system for drug and therapy evaluation is further underscored by the fact that when tested against 14 chemotherapeutic agents that show clinical activity against human breast cancer it responded significantly to 13, a positive response of 93%, compared to a 54% response to those compounds having clinical activity against a variety of "solid" tumors *(unpublished data)*. Thus the 13762 mammary tumor system appears to have a degree of selectivity for those agents active against breast cancer.

Tumor cell suspensions as small as 1,000 cells produce lethal tumors, and routine grafts (1–2 mm^3) implanted subcutaneously into a 35- to 45-day-old Fischer strain females kill their hosts within approximately 42 ± 6 days (S.D.). "Natural" metastases from the subcutaneous grafts to regional lymph nodes, lungs, abdominal organs, and occasionally to the brain and spinal column occur in almost 100% of the implanted animals by day 20 postimplantation. Progressive growth of this tumor in young, sexually maturing females causes measurable antiuterotrophic (6) and antimammotrophic (7) effects. This is due to competition between the tumor and the normal uterus for endogenous estrogens and with normal mammae for endogenous prolactin. Similar to human breast cancer, this experimental animal tumor induces hypercalcemia and splenomegaly. It also reverses lymphocyte/polymorphonuclear leukocyte ratios and is immunosuppressive. Ovariectomy and hypophysectomy produce a slight growth-retarding effect, whereas increasing endogenous prolactin levels stimulates tumor growth. This tumor is minimally affected by food deprivation. The rat has 42 chromosomes, and the normal chromosomal mode for this tumor is 45.

In the studies which follow, the experimental design provided a rigorous test of therapeutic activity. Tumor grafts were implanted subcutaneously on day 0, and chemotherapy was initiated only when tumors were well established in early log phase of measurable growth. Simple caliper measurements of tumor size made three times weekly permitted the establishment of tumor growth and regression curves for following therapy response.

The objective of the studies was to induce oncolysis with prolonged remission, with special attention paid to: (a) evidence of drug synergism; (b) duration of remissions; (c) induction of drug resistance; and (d) toxicity resulting from prolonged therapy. Figure 3 illustrates the results obtained with PAM, MTX, and 5FU tested alone and in a three-drug combination. Treatment was initiated on day

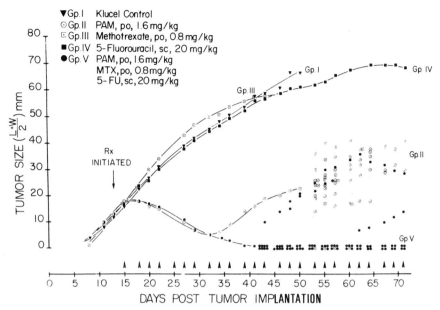

FIG. 3. Response of the 13762 mammary adenocarcinoma to PAM, MTX, and 5FU administered alone, and in a three-drug combination (assay No. I1838). Rx indicates day treatments were initiated, and *arrows* along abscissa the actual treatment days. Individual tumor sizes are shown for group II after day 50 and for group V after day 40.

13, and compounds were administered three times weekly. Treatment days are indicated by the arrowheads along the abscissa.

A typical growth curve for this tumor system is indicated by group I. The average survival for this vehicle-treated group was 52 days. The MTX-treated group III exhibited a slightly faster growth rate and had an average survival of only 44 days. This evidence of a stimulatory effect by MTX is peculiar to the treatment regimen and is reproducible. Group IV, treated with 5FU, showed no inhibitory effects on the solid subcutaneous growth. However, survival was significantly prolonged to an average of 62 days. 5FU appears to be more effective against metastases than against the primary subcutaneous growth, permitting prolonged survival with large subcutaneous tumor masses.

The oncolytic effect of PAM is illustrated by group II. After therapy was initiated on day 13 tumors regressed to barely measurable nodes by day 32. Tumor regrowth occurred, however, and was progressive despite continuing therapy. Individual tumor sizes for this now drug-resistant group are plotted after day 50 to illustrate individual variability. Most interesting was the effect of the three-drug combination indicated by group V. Oncolysis was progressive after day 13, and all but one animal was in complete remission by day 38. Individual tumor sizes were plotted after day 40 to show the relative number of tumors that remained in complete remission in this group as well as the number of tumors that regrew as drug-resistant entities. Four animals were alive and in complete remission on day 92. Duration of remission in the two animals whose tumors regrew was 9 and 33 days, respectively. Since both MTX and 5FU were used at dose levels having no significant oncolytic effects, the marked enhancement of anti-tumor activity when combined with PAM indicates a synergism of drug activities.

To determine whether the synergistic effect obtained with PAM was due to MTX or 5FU, or whether a three-drug combination was required, a second study was initiated. Table 3 summarizes the results obtained when the three agents were tested separately, as well as in two- and three-drug combinations, at the same dose levels used in the previous assay.

PAM given alone induced complete remission in 40% of the animals treated; neither MTX nor 5FU when administered alone induced remissions. PAM plus MTX was about as effective as PAM alone in remission induction. PAM plus 5FU, on the other hand, induced complete remissions in 90% of the animals treated, and the three-drug combination (PAM + MTX + 5FU) induced complete remission in every animal treated. However, regrowth of drug-resistant tumors during prolonged chemotherapy was evident in all PAM-treated groups.

Prolonged remissions were induced in 20% of the animals treated with PAM alone. PAM + MTX induced 30% prolonged remissions; PAM + 5FU induced remissions in 40%; and the three-drug combination induced prolonged remissions in 50%. The relative toxicity resulting from prolonged administration of MTX is evidenced by the shorter survival of group III animals and by the number of animals still alive in groups V, VI, and VII on day 100. Twenty to thirty percent of the animals in remission in groups V and VII died while in remission.

It is evident that PAM is a very effective oncolytic agent in this mammary tumor model. Combining MTX and 5FU with PAM produced a synergistic effect, inducing not only a greater number of complete tumor remissions but earlier remissions, as well as a greater number of possible "cures." Of the two-drug combinations, PAM + 5FU was most effective, showed less toxicity, and evidenced synergism, although it was not as marked as the three-drug combination.

TABLE 3. *Response of the 13762 mammary adenocarcinoma to treatment with two- and three-drug combinations of PAM, MTX, and 5FU*

Group no.	Treatment	Complete remissions (%)	Prolonged remissions (%)	Toxicity (% alive on day 100)	Increased survival (% T/C)
I	Klucel control	0	0	0	—
II	PAM	40	20	30	151
III	MTX	0	0	0	0
IV	5FU	0	0	0	102
V	PAM + MTX	40	30[a]	10	124
VI	PAM + 5FU	90	40	90	161
VII	PAM + MTX + 5FU	100	50[b]	40	131

[a] Group V, 20% died while in complete and prolonged remission.
[b] Group VII, 30% died while in complete and prolonged remission.

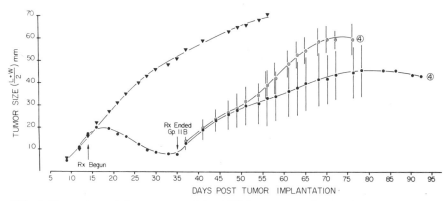

FIG. 4. Comparison of the response of the 13762 mammary adenocarcinoma to continuous treatment with PAM (group IIA; ●) and after discontinuation of treatment following the induction of maximum remission (group IIB; ⊙) (study No. P1871). Vehicle-treated control tumor growth is represented by (▼). Rx with *arrow* indicates when treatment was begun or ended; points with vertical lines indicate means and standard deviations; and numbers within circles indicate the number of animals alive within each group at a particular time.

The 13762 mammary tumor lends itself easily to experiments designed to answer specific clinical questions. As an example, the following study was initiated to determine whether continuing treatment with PAM, after the induction of maximum remission, would continue to produce any therapeutic effects.

In this study (Fig. 4) treatment with PAM was initiated on day 14 and continued three times weekly. Group I illustrates the vehicle-treated control tumor growth curve. Group IIA represents the tumors under continuing PAM therapy, and group IIB those tumors treated with PAM only from days 14 to 35, when all tumors were in maximum remission. In this latter group treatment was discontinued after day 35. Maximum remission was induced in groups IIA and IIB at about day 35 when drug-resistant tumors began to regrow despite continuing drug therapy. Of particular interest is the growth pattern of group IIB tumors in which therapy had been discontinued. During a period of 14 days following cessation of therapy, the regrowth of untreated tumors paralleled that of the drug-resistant tumors undergoing continuing treatment. It appears either that prolonged treatment with PAM imparted a "residual" inhibitory effect on tumor growth or that the emerging drug-resistant tumor cells had a slower growth rate, suggesting that after the induction of maximum remission treatment with PAM may be discontinued for a short period allowing recovery from drug toxicity without jeopardizing survival. The results also suggest that although maximum remission had been induced and drug-resistant tumors were beginning to emerge, continuing PAM treatment was better than no treatment. Such information will aid in estimating parameters for determining true biochemical resistance versus kinetic resistance to PAM.

The following study (Table 4) is based on the classic design of a clinical crossover. Animals were implanted with the 13762 mammary tumor on day 0 and

TABLE 4. *Experimental design for crossover studies*

	Therapy A		Therapy B	
Group no.	First compound	Treatment period	Second compound	Treatment period
I	Vehicle control			
IIA	5FU	Continuous		
IIB	5FU	Days 10–22	ADR	Day 24–ST
IIC	5FU	Days 10–22	PAM	Day 24–ST
IIIA	ADR	Continuous		
IIIB	ADR	Days 10–27	5FU	Day 29–ST
IIIC	ADR	Days 10–27	PAM	Day 29–ST
IVA	PAM	Continuous		
IVB	PAM	Day 10 to remission	ADR	Day 24–ST
IVC	PAM	Day 10 to remission	5FU	Day 24–ST

then randomly allocated to receive as therapy A either 5FU, ADR, or PAM at the onset of treatment on day 10. Those animals progressing over the ensuing 2–3 weeks were then automatically crossed over to an alternate therapy B. Animals initially treated with 5FU were crossed over to ADR or PAM, and those treated initially with ADR were crossed over to 5FU or PAM. The animals treated only with PAM to remission were continued on therapy until relapse, at which point they were crossed over to the alternate treatment with ADR or 5FU.

Figure 5 illustrates the results obtained with PAM as the initial therapeutic agent. The oncolytic activity of PAM with typical regrowth of PAM-resistant tumors despite continuing therapy is represented by group IVA. Eight of 30

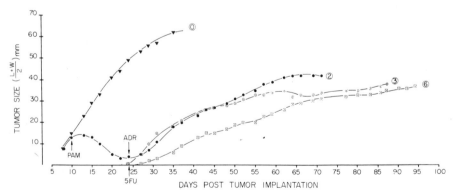

FIG. 5. Response of the 13762 mammary adenocarcinoma in a chemotherapy crossover study (assay No. 1872). Group IVA was treated continuously with PAM (●). Group IVB was treated initially with PAM and crossed over to ADR (⊙); Group IVC was treated initially with PAM and crossed over to 5FU (▫). Group I comprised the vehicle-treated controls (▼). Numbers within the circles indicate the number of animals alive within a group.

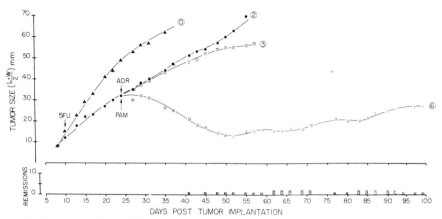

FIG 6. Response of the 13762 mammary adenocarcinoma in a chemotherapy crossover study (assay No. 1872). Group IIA was treated continuously with 5FU (●). Group IIB was treated initially with 5FU and crossed over to PAM (⊙,▨). Group IIC was treated initially with 5FU and crossed over to ADR (▣). Group I comprised the vehicle-treated controls (▼). Numbers within circles indicate the numbers of animals alive within a group.

animals (27%) experienced complete remission with PAM. Substitution of 5FU for PAM on day 24 had an inhibitory effect on tumor regrowth, while the inhibitory effect of ADR appears to have been delayed until after day 50.

Figure 6 illustrates the results obtained with those experimental groups in which treatment was initiated with 5FU. Substitution of ADR for 5FU on day 24 had a measurable though only nominal tumor-inhibitory effect. The marked oncolytic activity by PAM is a typical response of this tumor system, but it appears that pretreatment with 5FU slightly enhanced the maintenance of PAM-induced remissions. This effect is indicated by the delayed regrowth of PAM-resistant tumors and is best visualized by comparing the tumor regrowth curves of group IIB in Fig. 6 with that of group IVA in Fig. 5.

In the experimental grouping illustrated in Fig. 7, treatment was initiated with ADR. Substituting 5FU for ADR on day 29 had a measurable, although minimal, effect on tumor growth. The oncolytic effects of PAM, substituted for ADR on day 29, as usual, was striking. Most unexpectedly, however, were the number of complete remissions induced (80%) and the duration of remissions in the PAM-treated group. As of day 110 only two animals developed drug-resistant tumors, and both had been in partial remission; one died on day 77 and the tumor in the other is growing progressively.

Table 5 summarizes the effects of 5FU or ADR pretreatment of mammary tumors on the oncolytic activity of PAM. There is little question that initial treatment with ADR significantly enhanced the remission-induction activity of PAM and either markedly prolonged the duration of remissions or produced "cures." One might postulate that the propensity of ADR to bind to tumor DNA may have enhanced the "cell kill" activity of PAM, which is also a DNA reacting agent, or in some way may have interfered with the mechanism by which

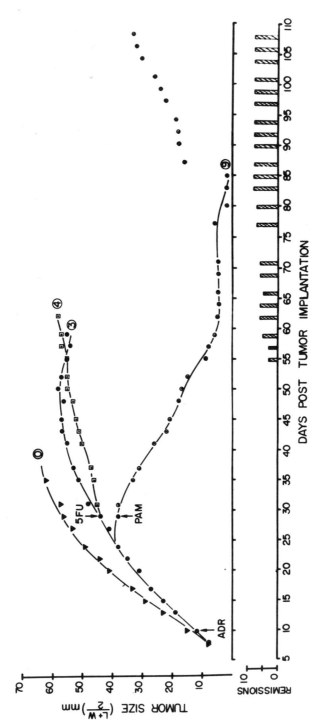

FIG. 7. Response of the 13762 mammary adenocarcinoma in a chemotherapy crossover study (assay No. 1872). Group IIIA was treated continuously with ADR (●). Group IIIB was treated initially with ADR and crossed over to 5FU (□). Group IIIC was treated initially with ADR and crossed over to PAM (⊙, ▨). Group I comprised the vehicle-treated controls (▼). There was a single regrowing tumor in group IIIC (⊙ without connecting lines). ▨ indicates number of remissions. Numbers within circles indicate the number of animals alive within a group.

TABLE 5. *Effects of pretreatment with 5FU or ADR on the oncolytic activity of PAM*

Treatment[a]		Complete remissions (%)	Average duration of remissions (days)	"Cures"[b] (%)
First compound	Second compound			
PAM (continuous)		10	—	10
5FU	PAM	30	13	10
ADR	PAM	80	—	80

[a]Chemotherapy crossover study.
[b]"Cures" defined as negative for tumor regrowth at implant site on day 115 after tumor implantation.

resistance to PAM is induced. It is obvious that, in this test system at least, ADR therapy followed by PAM is an effective sequence for crossover studies.

SUMMARY

It has been our objective to demonstrate that transplantable, syngeneic rat mammary tumors can be used effectively as test systems for preclinical evaluation of existing, as well as new, chemotherapeutic agents and modalities. However, we stress that no one animal tumor can represent all of the variations in growth potential or in endocrine and chemotherapy responsiveness encountered in human breast cancer. Caution must be exercised therefore in extrapolating the chemotherapeutic results obtained in a *single* tumor test system to the whole of breast cancer disease. To be realistically predictive of general clinical activity, a "block" of mammary tumor systems reflecting a spectrum of growth characteristics and chemotherapy responsiveness must be used as the evaluating test system. On the other hand, specific tumors (e.g., the 13762 mammary adenocarcinoma) that reproducibly mimic the chemotherapy responsiveness and acquired drug resistance of certain breast cancers encountered clinically can be manipulated and used effectively in experiments designed to answer specific clinical questions.

We sincerely hope—for it is necessary if experimental animal systems are to be used most effectively—that if a Breast Cancer Task Force is created by the EORTC, the liaison between the clinical chemotherapist and the animal experimentalist will be close enough to permit the use of animal model tumor systems in a predictive mode and in direct support of the clinician.

ACKNOWLEDGMENTS

These studies were supported by Contract NO1-CB-43914 from the Division of Cancer and Biology and Diagnosis, National Cancer Institute, NIH.

The authors gratefully acknowledge the excellent technical assistance of Anastasia Speropoulos, and thank Wendy Grant for preparing the many figures.

REFERENCES

1. Zubrod, C. G., Schepartz, S., Leiter, J., Endicott, K. M., Carrese, L. M., and Baker, C. G. (1966): The chemotherapy program of the National Cancer Institute: History, analysis and plans. *Cancer Chemother. Rep.,* 50:349–396.
2. Carter, S. K. (1973): Some thoughts on experimental models and their clinical correlations. *Eur. J. Cancer,* 9:833–841.
3. Goldin, A. (1973): Rationale of combination chemotherapy based on preclinical experiments. *Cancer Chemother. Rep.,* 4:189–198.
4. Bogden, A. E., Taylor, D. J., Esber, H. J., and Menninger, F. F., Jr. (1974): Effect of surgery, chemotherapy and immunotherapy, alone and in combination, on metastases of the 13762 mammary adenocarcinoma. *Cancer Res.* 34:1627–1631.
5. Taylor, D. J., and Bogden, A. E. (1970): Antitumor activity of some steroidal alkylating agents on a rat mammary tumor. In: *Tenth International Cancer Congress; Abstracts,* p. 408. University of Texas Press, Austin.
6. Bogden, A. E., Taylor, D. J., Esber, H. J., and Menninger, F. F., Jr. (1971): Anti-uterotrophic effect of mammary tumor growth. *Proc. Am. Assoc. Cancer Res.,* 12:55.
7. Bogden, A. E., Taylor, D. J., Kuo, E. Y. H., Mason, M. M., and Speropoulos, A. (1974): The effect of perphenazine induced serum prolactin response on estrogen-primed mammary tumor-host systems, 13762 and R-35 mammary adenocarcinomas. *Cancer Res.,* 34:3018–3025.

Breast Cancer: Trends in Research and Treatment, edited by J. C. Heuson, W. H. Mattheiem, and M. Rozencweig. Raven Press, New York © 1976.

Hormone-Responsive Human Breast Cancer in Continuous Tissue Culture

Marc Lippman

Medicine Branch, National Cancer Institute, Bethesda, Maryland 20014

Despite nearly a century of awareness of the efficacy of various kinds of endocrine therapies in the management of patients with metastatic breast cancer, many facets of the mechanisms whereby hormones influence the growth of neoplastic tissue remain incompletely understood. Recently significant progress has been made in the field of steroid hormone action (1) highlighted by the identification of specific receptors for estrogen in some tumor samples accompanied by an appreciation of their potential usefulness in therapeutic decision making (2). This progress notwithstanding, many aspects of the relationship between hormones and the responses they evoke in human breast tumors remain to be elucidated. Particularly vexing problems have included: the role of prolactin in human breast cancer (3); the mechanisms by which pharmacologic concentrations of estrogens, androgens, and progestins exert their inhibitory effects (4); the mechanisms of tumor escape from hormone dependency (5); if human breast cancer is androgen-dependent (6); and how glucocorticoids inhibit the growth of some human mammary tumors.

Reasons for the failure to come to grips with these problems effectively are manifold, but one of the most notable has surely been the lack of adequate long-term *in vitro* tissue culture systems for mammary tissue in which the effects of various hormonal stimuli could be studied independently of the actions of other trophic hormones. Such systems would have many additional potential advantages, including the opportunity to develop variant hormone-independent cell lines that could be used as reagents for complementation and somatic cell hybridization studies, thus allowing more complete characterization of the steps in hormone action.

In this chapter we review some of our studies concerning the establishment of two, and the characterization of five additional, human breast cancer cell lines in continuous tissue culture. Each of these cell lines displays varying responses to glucocorticoids, androgens, and estrogens, ranging from complete hormone unresponsiveness to significant sensitivity to all three. We hope that these model systems may be used in experiments that help to clarify some of the perplexing issues alluded to above.

TABLE 1. *Characteristics of human breast cells in long-term tissue culture*

Morphology
  Acinar structures and ducts
  Microvilli
  Golgi and rough endoplasmic reticulum
  Domes

Synthesis and/or secretion
  α-Lactalbumin
  Casein
  Carcinoembryonic antigen (CEA)
  β-glucuronidase, lysozyme

Chromosomal studies
  Human chromosomes
  Similar numbers and markers compared with fresh malignant material

Receptors: hormonal receptors and/or responsiveness to
  Glucocorticoids
  Estrogens
  Androgens
  Progestins
  Insulin

CHARACTERISTICS OF CELL LINES

Two of the cell lines described below were established by us, using methods previously described (7), from a malignant ascitic effusion from a postmenopausal patient with metastatic breast cancer. The MCF-7 cell line was generously provided by Dr. Marvin Rich (Michigan Cancer Foundation). HT-39, MDA 231, 496, and G-11 were supplied by Dr. Ronald Herberman (NIH, Bethesda) and Ms. Grace Cannon (Litton Bionetics, Rockville, Md.). These cell lines are mycoplasma-free, noncontact-inhibited, cloned cell lines that have been propagated for a minimum of a year in tissue culture as previously described (7). Some of the characteristics of the cell lines are summarized in Table 1; all appear epithelioid by both light and electron microscopy, manifesting varying amounts of rough endoplasmic reticulum and golgi. They have other characteristics of breast cells in that they have desmosomes and microvilli, and tend to arrange themselves in gland-like acinar structures. These cell lines synthesize and secrete certain protein products characteristic of breast cells. All contain α-lactalbumin, confirmed by specific enzymatic assay (kindly performed by Dr. Barbara Vonderhaar, NIAMDD, Bethesda, Md.) and sensitive radioimmunoassay (measured by Dr. David Kleinberg, New York University). At least one line and in some cases several synthesize carcinoembryonic antigen, casein, lysozyme (muramidase), and β-glucuronidase. In addition, the EVSA lines after 6 months in culture contain both identical telocentric marker chromosomes as well as a median chromosomal number (84 versus 76) nearly identical with the fresh malignant material from which the cell lines were begun. Russo and co-workers (8) demonstrated glandular structures using light and scanning electron microscopy of MCF-7 cells grown on collagen-coated sponges using the Leighton technique (9). In collaboration with Dr. R. Knazek (NCI, Bethesda, Md.), we observed the arrangement of these cells into glandular arrays and ducts using a unique capillary support system. A typical section is shown in Fig. 1. This striking degree of morphologic differentiation is paralleled by the hormone responsiveness described below.

EFFECTS OF ESTROGENS

One cell line, MCF-7, shows marked responsiveness to estrogen. As shown in Fig. 2, 10^{-8} M 17β-estradiol or 10^{-8} M diethylstibestrol (DES) both stimulate ^{3}H-thymidine incorporation. This stimulation of precursor incorporation is demonstrable whether cells are grown in totally serum-free medium or in medium containing 2% charcoal-treated serum from which more than 99% of the endogenous steroid has been removed (7). Untreated commercial sera contain physiologic quantities of 17β-estradiol as well as other steroids (10), and this may in part explain our failure to demonstrate stimulation by exogenously added estradiol unless serum-free or hormone-depleted conditions are employed. If, instead of estrogen, antiestrogens such as tamoxifen (ICI 46474) are added to the medium, marked inhibition of ^{3}H-thymidine incorporation is observed. If the cells are left in either tamoxifen, nafoxidine (Upjohn U11, 100A), or Parke Davis CI-628 for

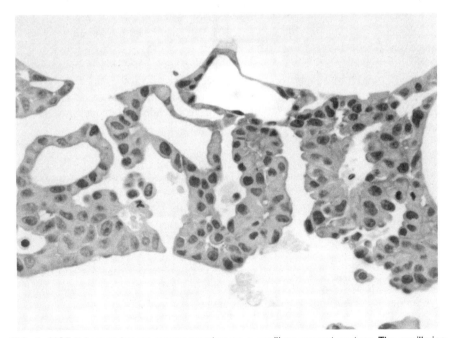

FIG. 1. MCF-7 human breast cancer growing on a capillary support system. The capillaries themselves are not present in the section. Note the glandular array of the cells and the formation of ducts. H&E section. ×200.

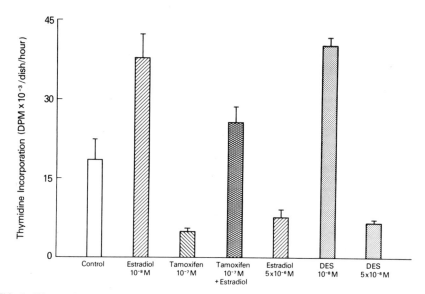

FIG. 2. Effects of estrogen and antiestrogen on ^{3}H-thymidine incorporation into DNA in MCF-7 human breast cancer. Experiments are performed in media free of endogenous steroids. Cells are treated with hormones for 48 hr and then pulsed for 1 hr with ^{3}H-thymidine. Cells are harvested with trypsin-EDTA solution, washed, and precipitated with 10% trichloracetic acid; the precipitates are collected and washed on 0.45-μm Millipore filters. Results are averages of triplicate determinations and are shown $\pm$1 S.D.

longer than approximately 48 hr, virtually all cells are killed. A rare cell (occurring with a frequency of approximately 10^{-6} to 10^{-7}) is resistant to antiestrogen, grows, and eventually forms colonies on the surface of the dish despite the continued presence of antiestrogen. The mechanism(s) of resistance in these cells is currently under investigation. This inhibition is largely obviated if, as shown, as little as 10-fold less estradiol is added to the medium simultaneously with the antiestrogen. Also shown in Fig. 2 are the effects of higher concentrations of estrogen. Both DES and estradiol at concentrations of 5×10^{-6} M inhibit thymidine incorporation below control levels. If the cells are left in these concentrations of steroid for periods exceeding approximately 48 hr, the cells begin to round up from the bottom of the dish, detach, and die. Evidence that killing by higher concentrations of estrogen is not a specific response under the conditions we employ receives further attention later.

A similar although somewhat less striking stimulation of amino acid incorporation into protein by estrogen is shown in Fig. 3. In this experiment ^{14}C-leucine incorporation into acid-precipitable material is measured for 1 hr after a 48-hr incubation in hormones at the concentrations indicated. Once again, 10^{-8} M estradiol stimulates and antiestrogen inhibits precursor incorporation. Tamoxifen inhibition is largely overcome by the simultaneous administration of 10-fold less 17β-estradiol.

The kinetics of the response of these cells to estrogen and antiestrogen are shown in Fig. 4. In this experiment cells are incubated in medium to which

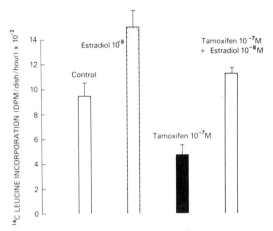

FIG. 3. Effects of 17β-estradiol and antiestrogen on ^{14}C-leucine incorporation into acid-precipitable material. Cells are incubated in media free of endogenous steroid. Hormones are added at the concentrations shown; after 48 hr ^{14}C-leucine is added for 1 hr, cells are harvested, and acid-precipitable counts are collected on 0.45-μm Millipore filters. Results are averages of triplicate determinations and are shown ±1 S.D.

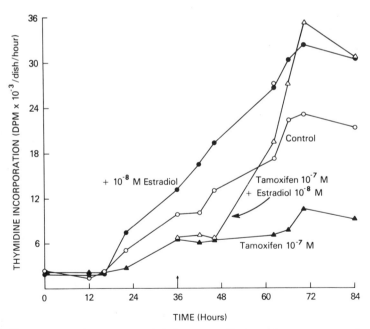

FIG. 4. Time course of estrogen and antiestrogen effects on hormone-responsive MCF-7 human breast cancer. Cells are replicately plated in hormone-depleted medium 24 hr prior to the start of the experiment. At zero time, hormones are added as indicated. ^{3}H-Thymidine is added to dishes 1 hr before harvesting. At 36 hr (*arrow*) 10^{-8} M 17β-estradiol is added to some of the cells continuously maintained in 10^{-7} M tamoxifen. Values shown are means of triplicate determinations; standard deviations rarely exceed 10% of the average value shown.

hormones at the concentrations shown have been added. After approximately a 12-hr lag, estradiol stimulates and antiestrogen inhibits ^{3}H-thymidine incorporation into DNA. After 36 hr, 10^{-8} M estradiol is added to some of the dishes containing 10^{-7} M tamoxifen. After an additional 12-hr lag, there is an abrupt rise in ^{3}H-thymidine incorporation to values that exceed even estradiol-treated cells, while cells incubated in antiestrogen alone continue to be markedly inhibited. We interpret this highly reproducible "rescue" phenomenon as consistent with the hypothesis that the antiestrogen tamoxifen, as part of its inhibitory effect, causes the cells to arrest at a uniform stage of the cell cycle. Then, when the antiestrogen "block" is removed by the addition of estradiol, a larger cohort of cells enters the DNA synthetic phase of the cell cycle. The possibility that antiestrogens may partially synchronize estrogen-responsive cells has obvious clinical ramifications, particularly when the combination of hormone- and cell cycle-specific cytotoxic chemotherapy are entertained. The reversal of antiestrogen effect by delayed addition of estradiol even at lower concentrations, combined with prevention of most antiestrogen effects by the simultaneous addition of estrogen, strongly suggests that these compounds are not nonspecifically toxic, but rather interfere with a pathway(s) that can be stimulated by estrogen.

The effects on precursor incorporation described above are accompanied by an overall effect on cell multiplication (Fig. 5). In this experiment cells are replicately plated into dishes, and 24 hr prior to the start of the experiment the medium is changed to serum-free medium. At zero time 17β-estradiol, tamoxifen, or nothing is added to each dish; the cell numbers are assessed daily. Clear-cut stimulation by estradiol and inhibition by antiestrogen is apparent. These effects are somewhat less striking than the effects on precursor incorporation previously shown. This is probably due to a general slowing of cell division under the totally serum-free conditions employed in this experiment. A contributory possibility is that estrogen may induce significant changes in intracellular thymidine pool size or transport, which may exaggerate incorporation rates as compared to net effects on macromolecular synthesis.

Estrogen receptor was previously described in the MCF-7 cell line by Brooks and co-workers (11). In Fig. 6 we confirm by the presence of a high-affinity ($Kd = 6.89 \times 10^{-10}$; $r = .986$) estrogen receptor in these cells. This binding is of limited capacity, usually approximately 75 femtomoles (fmoles) of ^{3}H-17β-estradiol bound per milligram of cytoplasmic protein (Table 2), a value that essentially remained constant for these cells during a year in culture. Further characterization of the steroid-binding specificities of this receptor is shown in Fig. 24 (below) as part of the discussion distinguishing the estrogen from the androgen receptor also found in these cells. If this putative estrogen receptor is a mediator of estrogen action in these cells, one might predict a reasonable correlation between concentrations of estrogen that bind to receptor and concentrations that evoke characteristic effects. Results of a comparison of binding and inductive effects are shown in Fig. 7. Two points are particularly noteworthy. First, the sensitivity of these cells to estrogen is apparent. As little as 2–3 $\times$ 10^{-11} M

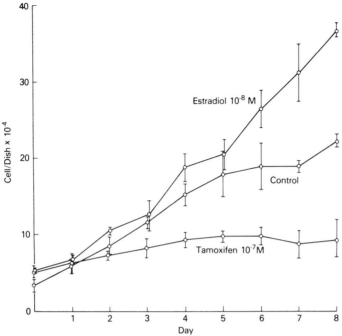

FIG. 5. Effects of 17β-estradiol (10^{-8} M) or tamoxifen (10^{-7} M) on cell devision in MCF-7 human breast cancer. At 36 hr prior to the start of the experiment, cells were plated into 60-mm plastic petri dishes in complete medium; 12 hr later this medium was exchanged and serum-free medium substituted. At zero time hormones were added, and at the times shown the dishes were harvested and cells counted. Values shown are averages of triplicate determinations ± 1 S.D.

estradiol is reproducibly stimulatory of precursor incorporation. Thus it may be that some previous studies have failed to note stimulation of cell lines by the addition of exogenous estrogen since the experiments are frequently performed in media supplemented with commercially available sera, which may already contain physiologic concentrations of estradiol as well as other steroids (10). Second, it should be noted that the curve for ^{3}H-thymidine incorporation shows near-maximal stimulation at concentrations of estradiol that occupy only a small percentage of the receptor sites. This raises the possibility that only a few receptor sites may need to be occupied to induce maximal effects; however, it should be recalled that precursor incorporation experiments are performed on intact cells incubated with hormone at 37°C, while the dextran-coated charcoal receptor assays were performed on cytosol extracts incubated at 0°C. Thus it seemed worthwhile to examine the binding of ^{3}H-estradiol to intact cells at both 0° and 37°C. Results are shown in Fig. 8. Not only are there more apparent receptor sites at 37°C as compared to 0°C, but the affinity of the receptor appears to be approximately threefold higher at 37°C. The net result of this decrease in the affinity constant at 37°C would be to shift the binding curve shown in Fig. 7 to

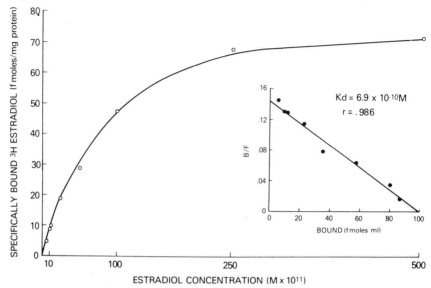

FIG. 6. Demonstration of high-affinity, limited-capacity estrogen receptor in cytoplasm of MCF-7 human breast cancer. The assay was performed using a dextran-coated charcoal competitive protein-binding assay at 0°C (41). The binding data are replotted in the inset using the Scatchard technique (20).

the left, i.e., toward the dose-response curve of these cells to estrogen. Thus there appears to be generally good agreement between concentrations of estrogen that bind to receptor and those that stimulate the cells.

Many studies suggested that antiestrogens inhibit cells by competing with estrogen for specific receptor sites (1). If this is true, it could be predicted that there would be good agreement between concentrations of estrogen that inhibit macromolecular synthesis and concentrations that displace estradiol from receptor. Results are shown in Fig. 9. In this experiment the ability of increasing concentrations of tamoxifen to displace 10^{-9} M ^{3}H-estradiol from receptor is compared with the effect of increasing concentrations of tamoxifen on ^{3}H-thymidine incorporation. As shown, these concentrations agree closely. It should also be noted

TABLE 2. *Quantity of estradiol receptor in various human breast cancer cell lines as determined by dextran-coated charcoal assay*

Cell line	Estrogen receptor (fmoles/mg protein)
MCF-7	71.6 ± 12.9
MDA 231	6.6
HT-39	4.2
G-11	5.0

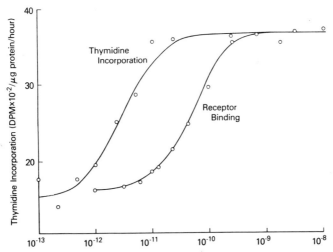

FIG. 7. Comparison of binding of ³H-17β-estradiol to receptor and stimulation of thymidine incorporation in MCF-7 human breast cancer. Binding studies were performed exactly as described in Fig. 6; precursor incorporation studies followed using the methodology described in Fig. 2 with concentrations of estradiol noted on the abscissa of this figure.

that one-half maximally effective concentrations for tamoxifen as both a competitor for receptor and as an inhibitor of precursor incorporation are 100- to 1,000-fold higher than half maximally effective concentrations of estradiol for the same effects. This result may explain the ability of less estradiol to reverse the effects of tamoxifen, as shown in Figs. 2 through 4.

One puzzling feature of these studies is the fact that although estrogen clearly stimulates the cells above control levels, estrogen-deficient cells do grow, albeit more slowly. Antiestrogen treatment, on the other hand, is lethal, although not nonspecifically so, since estrogen reverses the effects and (as is shown in Fig. 11, below) does not inhibit breast cancer cell lines that lack receptor. The implication is that antiestrogen may inhibit cells by a mechanism which requires receptor but does not merely reset the cells at the estrogen-depleted level. One might hypothesize that estrogen-receptor complexes bind to chromatin, leading to the enhanced synthesis of mRNA segments, which directly or indirectly have an important regulatory role. Unstimulated cells may have a slower but finite rate of transcription of these same segments. Recently Clark (12) and Katzenellenbogen (13) and their associates suggested that antiestrogen may be transported to the nucleus bound to estrogen receptor; perhaps these "abnormal" antiestrogen-estrogen receptor complexes translocate to the nucleus to block even constitutive transcription of some segments of DNA which code for proteins having a regulatory effect on cell proliferation, thus leading to inhibition below control levels.

It has long been appreciated that pharmacologic administration of estrogens to postmenopausal females with breast cancer leads to objective tumor regressions in approximately a third of cases (14). The mechanism of this effect is unknown. It

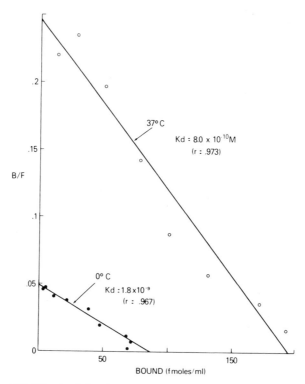

FIG. 8. Binding of ³H-17β-estradiol to intact MCF-7 human breast cancer cells. Cells growing logarithmically were changed to serum-free medium without hormones. Cells were harvested 24 hr later in trypsin-EDTA solution, centrifuged gently, and suspended in Dulbecco's phosphate-buffered saline (pH 7.4) supplemented with 5 mM glucose (PBSG) at 0°C at a density of 10⁻⁶ cells per milliliter. An 0.8-ml aliquot of this cell suspension was added to glass tubes, and varying concentrations of ³H-estradiol with or without unlabeled competitor were added. Tubes were incubated at either 0° or 37°C for 3 or 1 hr, respectively. Cells were collected and washed twice in ice cold PBSG at the end of the incubation and cell-associated radioactivity assessed. The results are shown plotted after the Scatchard technique (20).

has, however, been shown that the presence of cytoplasmic estrogen receptor in human tumor samples can be correlated with response to such pharmacologic hormone administration (2). Because the MCF-7 cell line is stimulated by physiologic concentrations of 17β-estradiol and also contains estrogen receptor, it seemed reasonable to examine the effects of higher concentrations on the MCF-7 cell line. Results are shown in Fig. 10. Thymidine incorporation is enhanced by approximately 2.5-fold in this experiment by adding physiologic concentrations of 17β-estradiol. As concentrations are increased above 10^{-7} M, stimulation is less effective; concentrations exceeding 10^{-6} M are strongly inhibitory. If the cells are left in these concentrations longer than 72 hr, the cells round up from the bottom of the dish and die. Some evidence that this may not be a specific response is suggested by the effects of 17α-estradiol, also shown in Fig. 10. 17α-Estradiol is not stimulatory at any concentration employed, and yet virtually equivalent con-

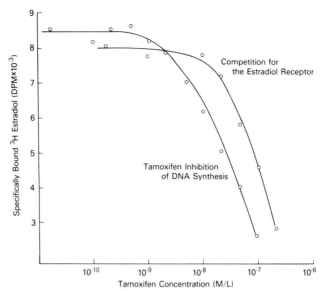

FIG. 9. Tamoxifen displacement of ³H-estradiol binding to estrogen receptor compared with tamoxifen inhibition of ³H-thymidine incorporation in MCF-7 human breast cancer. For binding displacement studies, cytosols were incubated with 5 × 10⁻⁹ M ³H-estradiol with or without increasing concentrations of unlabeled tamoxifen. After 18 hr of incubation at 0°C, bound and free steroid were separated by centrifugation with dextran-coated charcoal (41). Thymidine incorporation was measured as described in the legend of Fig. 2.

centrations of the 17α-compound are inhibitory of thymidine concentration. 17α-Estradiol has a much lower affinity for the estradiol receptor (Fig. 24, below) than the 17β compound. 3-Methylether estradiol induces effects parallel to those shown for 17α-estradiol.

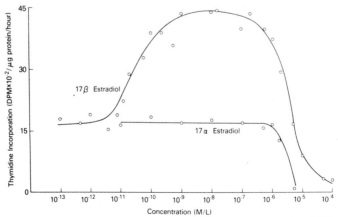

FIG. 10. Effects of 17α- and 17β-estradiol on ³H-thymidine incorporation into DNA. Conditions were as described in Fig. 2.

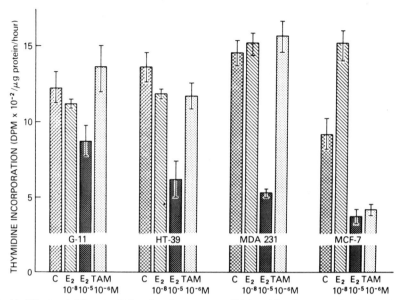

FIG. 11. Effects of 17β-estradiol and antiestrogen on ^{3}H-thymidine incorporation in four human breast cancer cell lines maintained in long-term tissue culture. Results are the averages of triplicate determinations and are shown ± 1 S.D. Conditions were as described in Fig. 2.

Further evidence that the effects of high concentrations of estradiol are nonspecific in this cell system is shown in Fig. 11. The effects of low and high concentrations of estradiol as well as the effects of tamoxifen on three other human breast cell lines are compared with the MCF-7 cell line. While physiologic concentrations of 17β-estradiol (10^{-8} M) do not stimulate and 10^{-6} M tamoxifen does not inhibit these other cell lines, high concentrations of steroid (10^{-5} M) inhibits all of the cell lines significantly. These other three cell lines contain virtually no receptor activity (Table 2). Clearly, high concentrations of estradiol inhibit otherwise unresponsive cells that lack demonstrable receptor activity, strongly suggesting that the effect is nonspecific. Thus conditions we employ do not seem to suggest a mechanism for the efficacy of high concentrations of estrogen in the management of human breast cancer *in vivo*, or an answer as to why this effect should appear to be linked to estrogen receptor.

This characterization of a human cell system in long-term culture that is responsive to physiologic concentrations of estrogen in terms of both macromolecular synthesis and the induction of specific protein products characteristic of mammary tissue should provide a valuable resource for the study of the mechanism whereby estrogens regulate the growth of target tissues in general and mammary cancer in particular.

EFFECTS OF GLUCOCORTICOIDS

Many studies have suggested that glucocorticoids can interact significantly with mammary tissue. For example, glucocorticoids are required for the growth and

TABLE 3. *Effects of dexamethasone or cortisol on* ^{14}*C-leucine incorporation into acid-insoluble radioactivity*

Conc. of steroid (M)	Dexamethasone[a]	Cortisol[a]
0	39.6 ± 0.68	
10^{-9}	39.1 ± 2.3	35.4 ± 2.8
10^{-8}	46.6 ± 6.8	43 ± 3.4
10^{-7}	37.3 ± 2.9	40.7 ± 2.0
10^{-6}	37.3 ± 3.3	38.6 ± 1.2

[a]Values are disintegrations per minute (dpm) ^{14}C-leucine × 10^{-2} per milligram of protein per hour ± 1 S.D.

differentiation of murine mammary gland in short-term organ culture (15). Similar effects have been noted in normal human mammary gland in primary tissue culture (16). Glucocorticoid receptors have been demonstrated in mouse mammary carcinoma (17), and recent reports suggest that the addition of glucocorticoids to mouse mammary tumor may enhance the release of viral particles (18). Finally, approximately 10% of patients with breast cancer have objective tumor regression when treated with glucocorticoids (19). The mechanism of this response has never been clarified. Clearly, glucocorticoids may act directly on the tumor to inhibit growth in some way. Alternatively, exogenous glucocorticoids may suppress adrenal function by inhibiting ACTH release, leading to a "medical adrenalectomy." Suppression of normal adrenal steroidogenesis would be accompanied by a decreased production of dehydroepiandrosterone and androstenedione. These weak androgens may stimulate tumors by being converted by either breast or other tissues to more potent androgens and estrogen. Thus it would obviously be of value to study the effects of glucocorticoids directly on human breast cancer under conditions that preclude the influence of other trophic hormones. We therefore tested five human breast cancer cell lines in long-term tissue culture for their response to glucocorticoids. Three contain glucocorticoid receptors and are directly inhibited by glucocorticoids.

The effects of 10^{-7} M dexamethasone on cell division in the MCF-7 cell line are shown in Fig. 12. After approximately 24 hr of incubation in glucocorticoid, cell division is significantly slowed. Unlike the effects of antiestrogen, however, the cells eventually grow to confluence and do not appear to be killed by glucocorticoid.

Slowing of cell division is accompanied by approximately a 50% decrease in ^{3}H-thymidine incorporation into DNA (Fig. 13). Interestingly, when ^{14}C-leucine incorporation into protein is measured at 48 hr (Table 3), it is apparent that glucocorticoids do not significantly alter amino acid incorporation at a time when thymidine is inhibited approximately 50% and cell growth has already been slowed.

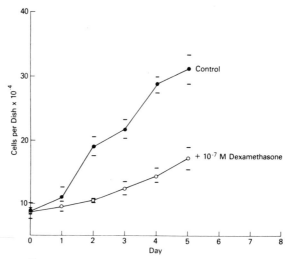

FIG. 12. Effects of 10⁻⁷ M dexamethasone on cell division in MCF-7 human breast cancer. Conditions for this experiment are identical to those employed in Fig. 5 with the exception that dexamethasone was the steroid added.

Demonstration of a specific glucocorticoid effect suggests that these cells might have specific receptors for this class of steroid hormones. Verification of this is provided by the binding data shown in Fig. 14. A high-affinity, limited capacity cytoplasmic receptor for dexamethasone is shown. Replotting the binding data

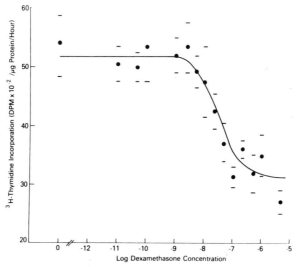

FIG. 13. Effects of dexamethasone on ³H-thymidine incorporation in MCF-7 human breast cancer. Conditions for this experiment are identical to those described in Fig. 2 with the exception of the different steroids employed.

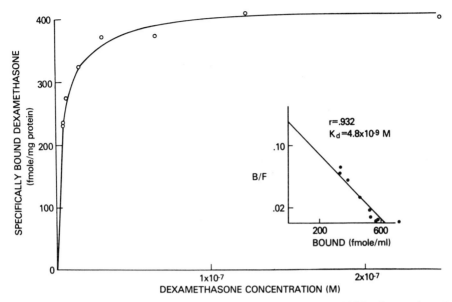

FIG. 14. Binding of ³H-dexamethasone to cytoplasmic receptor in MCF-7 human breast cancer. ³H-Dexamethasone (22 Ci/mM Amersham-Searle) was used in binding studies performed in a manner identical to that outlined in Fig. 6.

according to the Scatchard technique (20) reveals a straight line (r = .932). From the slope and intercept we estimate the equilibrium dissociation constant of this receptor to be 4.8×10^{-9} and the cells to contain 280 fmoles of receptor per milligram of cytoplasmic protein. This quantity of receptor is in the range reported for receptors in many other glucocorticoid target tissues (21).

This receptor was further characterized on sucrose density gradients (Fig. 15). A single peak of ³H-dexamethasone sedimenting at approximately 8S is apparent. This peak is lost if the extract is incubated with either an excess of unlabeled dexamethasone or R50-20 ($\Delta^{1,4}$-pregnadiene-17,21-dimethyl-19-nor-3,20-dione) a progestational agent. The 24-hr preincubation in serum-free medium before harvesting the cells for receptor studies, the fact that ³H-dexamethasone binds to this receptor, and the 8S position on gradients all suggest that this is true glucocorticoid receptor and not contaminating serum corticosteroid-binding globulin, which does not bind dexamethasone significantly (22) and sediments at 4S on sucrose gradients (23).

Further support for the direct relation between this receptor and glucocorticoid effect is provided by the data in Table 4. The effects of glucocorticoids on five human breast cancer cell lines in long-term tissue culture are contrasted with receptor analyses of these cell lines. Three lines (G-11, MCF-7, and MDA 231) have significant amounts of glucocorticoid receptor and show a hormonally provoked decrease in thymidine incorporation. Two other cell lines (496 and Evsa T) neither contain receptor nor are inhibited by glucocorticoids. For comparison, 11α-OH-cortisol fails to inhibit any cell line tested; and as discussed below, this

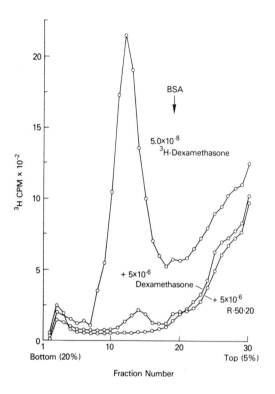

FIG. 15. Sucrose density gradients of glucocorticoid receptor in MCF-7 human breast cancer. Cells growing in log phase were switched to serum-free medium. Cells were harvested the next day in trypsin-EDTA solution, washed, and 100,000 G supernates prepared (7). Cytosol extracts were incubated with 10^{-7} M ^{3}H-dexamethasone with or without competitor as noted in the figure and layered on top of 5 – 20% sucrose density gradients in 10% glycerol, 10 mM tris HCl pH 7.4, 1 mM EDTA, 1 mM dithiothreitol buffer, and developed and counted as described elsewhere (42). The *arrow* refers to a ^{14}C-labeled bovine serum albumin marker run for each gradient.

compound is able to displace ^{3}H-dexamethasone competitively from receptor at any concentration tested.

Binding specificities of this receptor were further delineated by the competition studies summarized in Fig. 16. As shown, glucocorticoids such as dexamethasone and cortisol completely displace the labeled hormone from receptor sites while the

TABLE 4. *Comparison of maximal inhibition of DNA synthesis and quantity of glucocorticoid receptor*

	Maximal inhibition of thymidine incorporation (%)[a]		Glucocorticoid binding[b]
Inhibitor	Dexamethasone	11α-Cortisol	
G-11	76 ± 4	0 ± 6	146
MCF-7	46 ± 7	0 ± 7	199
MDA 231	23 ± 6	0.6 ± 6	77
496	4 ± 6	4 ± 8	5.3
Evsa-T	0 ± 6	0 ± 8	0

[a]Values are ± 1 S.D.
[b]Values are in femtomoles ^{3}H-dexamethasone bound per milligram of cytoplasmic protein.

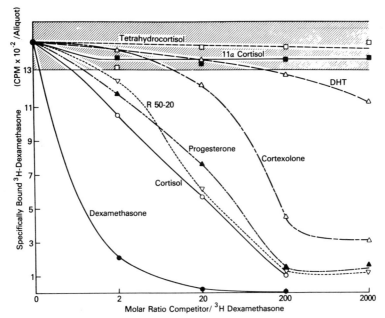

FIG. 16. Ability of various steroids to displace ³H-dexamethasone from receptor in MCF-7 human breast cancer. Cytosol extracts were prepared (Fig. 15) and incubated with 10⁻⁸ M ³H-dexamethasone with or without the addition of unlabeled steroids as shown in the figure. After 18 hr, bound and free steroid were separated, and the specifically bound steroid assessed as described in Fig. 6.

metabolite tetrahydrocortisol and a stereoisomer of cortisol, 11α-OH-cortisol, fail to compete at any concentration tested. Both progesterone and R50-20 can displace dexamethasone from its binding sites. This result is not unexpected when the known proclivity of progesterone for glucocorticoid receptor is recalled (24).

A comparison of apparent binding affinities and biologic effect is provided by the data presented in Fig. 17. Inhibitory effects are shown by dexamethasone, cortisol, and R50-20. The latter compound (which has been shown to have progestational activity and to bind to progesterone receptor but not to corticosteroid-binding globulin) appears in our own study to have significant glucocorticoid activity, which the results of Figs. 15 and 16 suggest are mediated through an interaction with glucocorticoid. Of interest is the fact that steroids which did not displace ³H-dexamethasone from receptor fail to show biologic activity. The only steroid whose apparent binding to glucocorticoid receptor does not parallel its biologic effect is progesterone, which is essentially devoid of inhibitory effect. Further exploration of this situation led us to the conclusion that the MCF-7 cell line contains a progesterone receptor in addition to the glucocorticoid receptor described above. These studies suggest that glucocorticoid receptor in MCF-7 cells has some binding affinity for glucocorticoid, whereas the progesterone receptor has affinity for progestational agents and to a lesser extent androgens only.

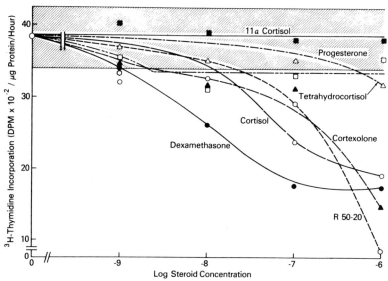

FIG. 17. Effects of various steroids on ³H-thymidine incorporation in MCF-7 human breast cancer. The experiment was performed using the methods outlined in Fig. 2.

Careful comparison of the binding curve of ³H-dexamethasone to receptor (Fig. 14) with its induction curve (Figs. 13 and 17) reveals a discrepancy between optimal concentrations for cell inhibition and concentrations that saturate receptor. It appears that most receptor sites must be occupied before inhibition is seen. It should be recalled, however, that thymidine incorporation studies are done at 37°C with intact cells, whereas binding studies employ cytosols incubated at 0°C. Thus it seemed important to see what alterations in binding affinity might occur with intact cells at 37°C. These studies are summarized in Fig. 18. Using intact cells, at 37°C the equilibrium dissociation constant is approximately equal to that obtained on cytosols. This dissociation constant suggests that the percent of receptor sites occupied correlates only moderately with the percent of maximal inhibition of thymidine incorporation seen in these cells.

Thus some human breast cancer, at least *in vitro*, can be shown to contain glucocorticoid receptor and to be directly inhibited by glucocorticoid interaction with these receptors. In addition, we recently noted that some fresh human breast tumor samples may also contain glucocorticoid receptors (25). The responses of these tumors to hormonal manipulations is as yet unknown. One may hope that analysis of tumor samples for glucocorticoid receptor may allow identification of a subset of patients in whom therapy with glucocorticoids would be of clinical value much as the study of estrogen receptor has aided in therapeutic decision-making processes in patients with breast cancer (26). Our previous work with glucocorticoid receptor in leukemia states also supports this hypothesis (25,27).

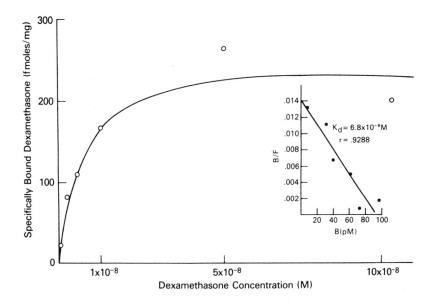

FIG. 18. Binding ^{3}H-dexamethasone to intact MCF-7 human breast cancer. Scatchard plots generated from the binding data obtained using the method described in Fig. 8 are shown.

EFFECTS OF ANDROGENS

The mechanism(s) of androgen interaction with mammary cancer are poorly understood. At least three lines of evidence suggest some breast cancer may be androgen-dependent. First, a mouse mammary cancer (Shionogi 115) both *in vivo* and in long-term tissue culture is moderately androgen-responsive (28). This cell line contains androgen receptor. Second, the response of some human breast cancer to adrenalectomy (29) has frequently been interpreted as a response to the ablation of weak adrenal androgens, dehydroepiandrosterone, and androstene-dione, which can be peripherally converted to more potent androgens. Perhaps in conflict with this interpretation is the recent finding that objective responses to adrenalectomy in patients with metastatic breast cancer are correlated with the presence of estradiol receptor, suggesting peripheral or tumor aromatization of androgen to estrogen. Third, approximately two out of three males with metastatic breast cancer have regression of tumor deposits following orchiectomy (30). On the other hand, approximately 20% of females with breast cancer show objective responses to the administration of androgens (31). For these reasons, it seemed important to examine our cell lines for the effects of various androgens. Some of these results were recently published (32).

The effects of 5α-dihydrotestosterone (DHT) on precursor incorporation into macromolecules are shown in Fig. 19. DHT stimulates thymidine incorporation approximately fourfold in the experiment shown; stimulation of leucine incorporation is approximately 2.5-fold. With a 48-hr incubation, some stimulation is apparent at 5×10^{-9} M DHT, reaching a maximum of 5×10^{-7} M. The androgen

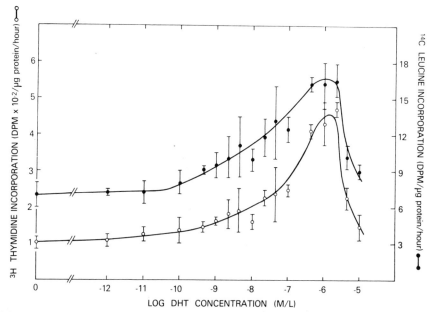

FIG. 19. Effects of 5α-dihydrotestosterone on ³H-thymidine and ¹⁴C-leucine incorporation into macromolecules in MCF-7 human breast cancer. Experiments are done using totally serum-free conditions as outlined in Fig. 2.

responsiveness shown clearly demonstrates that, at least *in vitro*, some human breast cancer may be responsive to androgen. Stimulation rapidly declines at concentrations greater than 10^{-6} M, and 10^{-5} M DHT is lethal to cells after 72 hr of incubation. This latter effect is probably nonspecific in that 5β-dihydrotestosterone (5β-DHT), which is not stimulatory at any concentration, also inhibits the cells at concentrations greater than 10^{-6} M. As shown in Fig. 25 (below), 5β-DHT does not bind to receptor. Thus killing by high concentrations of androgen, at least under the *in vitro* conditions we employ, is probably lethal to the cells by a nonspecific mechanism analogous to the effects of estradiol (Fig. 10).

Stimulation of precursor incorporation is accompanied by enhanced protein accumulation and cell proliferation. Results are shown in Fig. 20. At zero time cells preincubated for 24 hr in serum-free medium are treated with either 10^{-6} M DHT or R2956 (17β-hydroxy-2,2,17α-trimethyl-estra-4,9,11-trien-3-one), a potent antiandrogen provided by J. P. Raynaud of the Roussell Corporation. DHT stimulates and the antiandrogen inhibits net protein synthesis. Maximal effects are less impressive than those on precursor incorporation (Fig. 18). This is probably due to the fact that under serum-free conditions the cells grow considerably more slowly than in complete medium.

The presence of androgen responsiveness suggests that these cells might contain androgen receptor. Demonstration of such binding molecules on sucrose density gradients is shown in Fig. 21. A peak sedimenting at approximately 8S is

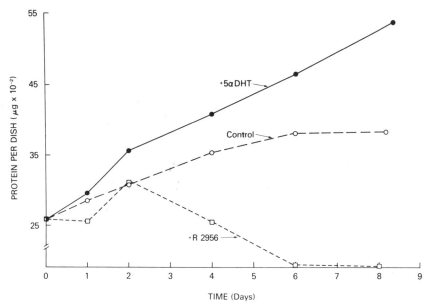

FIG. 20. Effects of 5α-dihydrotestosterone and R2956 on net protein synthesis in MCF-7 human breast cancer. At 48 hr prior to the start of the experiment, cells growing in log phase were harvested in trypsin-EDTA solution, collected by centrifugation, and replicately plated in 60-mm plastic petri dishes in complete medium. The medium was changed 24 hr later to serum-free medium. After another 24 hr (zero time) hormones (10^{-6} M DHT or 10^{-6} M R2956) were each added to one-third of the dishes. At the times shown, dishes were harvested in triplicate and the cell protein assessed.

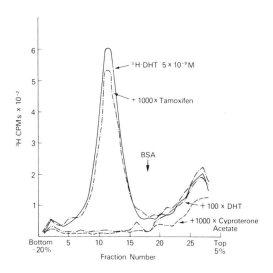

FIG. 21. Sucrose density gradients of androgen receptor in MCF-7 human breast cancer. Conditions are the same as in Fig. 15 except all extracts were incubated with 5×10^{-9} M ^{3}H-DHT with or without a 100-fold excess of unlabeled DHT or a 1,000-fold excess of cyproterone acetate of tamoxifen.

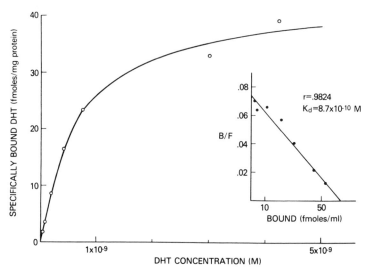

FIG. 22. Binding of ^{3}H-DHT to a cytoplasmic androgen receptor in MCF-7 human breast cancer. Methods are described in Fig. 6.

apparent in the gradient prepared from an extract incubated with 5×10^{-9} M ^{3}H-DHT. Excess unlabeled DHT or the antiandrogen cyproterone acetate incubated together with 5×10^{-9} M ^{3}H-DHT obliterates this peak of binding, whereas even a thousand-fold excess of the antiestrogen tamoxifen has little effect on the peak of androgen binding. These results suggest a receptor of limited capacity and some specificity for substances with androgenic or antiandrogenic properties.

This was examined further in competitive binding studies using dextran-coated charcoal to separate bound from free hormone (Fig. 22). ^{3}H-DHT is bound to a limited-capacity binder to the extent of 56 fmoles/mg cytoplasmic protein in the experiment shown. When the data are plotted according to the Scatchard technique (20) shown in the inset of Fig. 22, the straight line obtained ($r = .982$) suggests that the ^{3}H-DHT is bound to a single class of receptor molecules of uniform affinity ($Kd = 8.7 \times 10^{-10}$ M).

In many androgen-responsive tissues 5α-DHT rather than gonadally synthesized testosterone (T) is the "effector" androgen (33); in some tissues (e.g., levator ani muscle of the rat) testosterone appears to be the "effector" androgen (34). In order to determine whether DHT or T is the active androgen, affinity of the androgen receptor for T was measured directly and compared with DHT. Results are shown in Fig. 23. The dissociation constant for T, estimated from the Scatchard plot ($Kd = 1.5 \times 10^{-9}$; $r = .958$), is approximately twice that of DHT, suggesting that DHT is the more avidly bound and possibly the more potent steroid. In an experiment in which DHT and T binding were assessed on the same cytoplasmic extract, they were specifically bound to within 5% of each other, suggesting that they were associated with the same receptor protein.

Further characterization of the androgen and receptors in these cells were obtained by cross-competition studies shown in Figs. 24 and 25. In Fig. 24 the

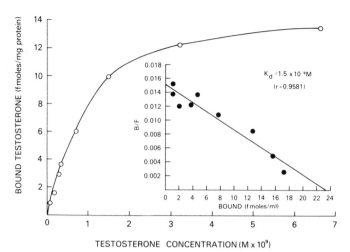

FIG. 23. Binding of ³H-testosterone to a high-affinity limited-capacity androgen receptor in MCF-7 human breast cancer. Methods are presented in Fig. 6.

ability of various steroids to displace ³H-17β-estradiol from receptor is shown. Note that estrogens and antiestrogens can completely displace the label from the receptor. Androgens, progesterone, and antiandrogens have essentially no ability to displace estradiol from receptor. This suggests a limited binding specificity for estrogen and closely related compounds.

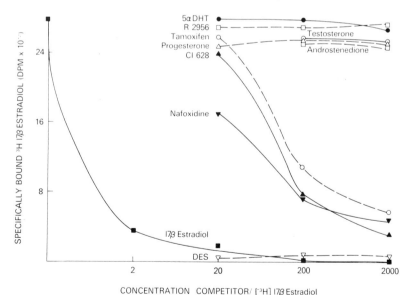

FIG. 24. Binding specificity of the estrogen receptor in MCF-7 human breast cancer. Cytoplasmic extracts were incubated for 18 hr at 0°C with 5 × 10⁻⁹ M ³H-estradiol with or without added unlabeled steroids at the concentrations noted. At the end of the incubation, specifically bound steroid was determined using a competitive protein-binding assay as before (41).

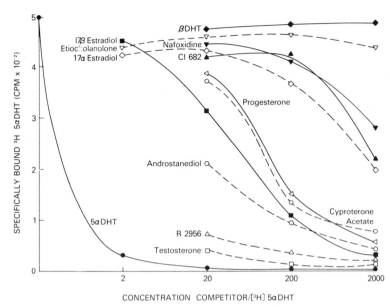

FIG. 25. Binding specificity of the androgen receptor in MCF-7 human breast cancer. Methods are described in Fig. 27. ³H- 5α-DHT (5 × 10⁻⁹ M) was used as the labeled steroid.

On the other hand, if ^{3}H-5α-DHT (5 × 10⁻⁹ M) is used as the trace (Fig. 25), a very different result is obtained. Androgens readily displace labeled DHT from the receptor; estradiol can also compete for binding sites but far less effectively than androgens. Antiestrogens have little ability to displace labeled androgen, whereas the antiandrogens do compete for binding sites. Note also that progesterone, which showed no ability to displace estradiol, displaces ^{3}H-DHT significantly. This is consistent with the known weak androgenic action of progesterone. These specificity studies suggest that androgen receptor has high affinity for androgens but some binding affinity for estrogen and progesterone. Taken together, Figs. 24 and 25 clearly distinguish between the androgen and estrogen receptor in the MCF-7 cell line. This is an important conclusion since one could imagine androgen stimulation being mediated by a weak interaction with the estrogen receptor or by conversion of testosterone to estradiol by breast cancer, a process known to occur in some tumors (35). The latter possibility appears extremely unlikely in the present case because DHT cannot be aromatized to estrogen or converted back to testosterone (36).

If the binding data of ^{3}H-DHT to receptor (Fig. 22) are compared with the dose-response curve of these cells to DHT (Fig. 19), it appears that because of the high affinity of the androgen receptor in these cells essentially every receptor site would be occupied before any effect on precursor incorporation was noted. Although this is certainly a conceivable result, there are other possibilities to be considered, including decreased uptake of DHT by intact cells, decreased binding affinity of receptor at 37°C (since binding studies were performed at 0°C on cytosols and incorporation experiments at 37°C on intact cells), and metabolism of the steroid to less active metabolites. The first two possibilities were examined directly in the whole cell binding experiments shown in Fig. 26. As shown, binding affinity at 37°C is even higher than at 0°C in intact cells. Essentially the same number of binding sites are identified at both temperatures. The *Kd* at 37°C is still 100- to 1,000-fold higher than the half maximally effective concentration of DHT.

Having ruled out any significant androgen transport effects or altered affinity for androgens as a function of physiologic temperature, we next examined androgen metabolism. Results are shown in Fig. 27. The control medium, as expected, contains counts migrating in the position of the DHT standard. At various times thereafter, the appearance of a new peak of radioactivity migrating in the position of androstanediol is noted. By 8 hr more than 60% of the ^{3}H-DHT has been converted to androstanediol, with the appearance of more polar metabolites not migrating from the origin. In addition, during the course of the incubation an increasing amount of radioactivity is unextractable by methylene chloride, quite possibly representing water-soluble conjugated steroids. As early as 1 min following the addition of ^{3}H-DHT to the cells, there is a small peak of radioactivity migrating in the position of androstanediol in the cytoplasmic extract.

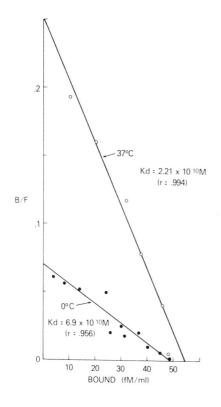

FIG. 26. Binding of ^{3}H-5α-dihydrotestosterone to intact MCF-7 human breast cancer cells. Scatchard plots of the binding data obtained at 0° and 37°C are shown. Methods are described in Fig. 8.

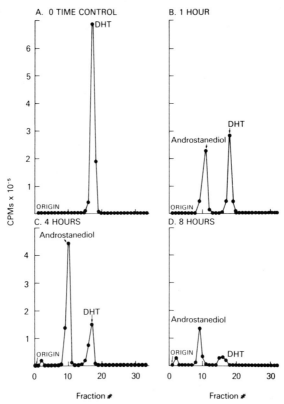

FIG. 27. Metabolism of ^{3}H-DHT by MCF-7 human breast cancer. ^{3}H-DHT was added to cells preincubated (or not) for 24 hr in serum-free medium. Unlabeled carrier steroids were added at various times; the medium was removed; and the cells harvested, homogenized, and separated into crude nuclear and cytoplasmic fractions by 800 G centrifugation for 10 min. The medium, cytosol, and nuclear fractions were extracted with methylene chloride, evaporated to dryness, redissolved in methylene chloride, and run on Silacagel TLC plates in chloroform:methanol 98:2 (v/v). Spots were identified with concentrated sulfuric acid:methanol 50:50 (v/v), scraped, and counted. The results shown are for the extracted supernatant medium.

Thus the most likely explanation for the large discrepancy between optimal androgen binding and inductive concentrations is the very significant metabolism of ^{3}H-DHT to less active and inactive metabolites. Possibly experiments conducted at earlier time points, when less metabolism had occurred, might permit a better approximation between optimal inductive and binding concentrations of androgen.

The studies of relative binding affinities of ^{3}H-DHT and ^{3}H-testosterone to receptor already discussed suggested that DHT may be the biologically active androgen in this cell system. For this to be true it would be necessary for the cells to contain 5α-reductase activity to convert testosterone to DHT. This was examined by incubating cells with ^{3}H-testosterone for varying periods of time,

TABLE 5. *Comparison of androgen binding and androgen effects on precursor incorporation in human breast cancer cell lines*

Cell line	Leucine incorporation[a]			Quantity androgen receptor[b]
	Control	5α-DHT 10^{-6} M	5β-DHT 10^{-6} M	
MCF-7	32.8 ± 35	63.4 ± 0.95	35.0 ± 1.0	12.0
G-11	32.6 ± 8.6	32.3 ± 2.1	29.8 ± 3.4	7.2
HT-39	24.9 ± 3.4	20.7 ± 5.6	27.6 ± 7.0	0
MDA 231	49.5 ± 0.38	45.4 ± 1.1	46.7 ± 4.0	0
EVSA-T	31.0 ± 0.78	35.8 ± 2.8	28.0 ± 6.8	15.3

[a]Values are in disintegrations per minute (dpm) ^{14}C-leucine incorporated × 10^{-3} per microgram of protein per hour.
[b]Values are in femtomoles ^{3}H-5α-dihydrotestosterone bound per milligram of cytoplasmic protein.

harvesting the medium and crude cytoplasmic and nuclear fractions, and identifying the steroid products in the various fractions. The methods employed are outlined in the legend to Fig. 27. Conversion of testosterone to DHT was assessed semiquantitatively by summing the appearance of radioactivity migrating in the positions of authentic DHT and androstanediol since the latter compound can be formed only by the action of 3-hydroxysteroid dehydrogenase on DHT. Using this method, 13.7% of the radioactivity added as ^{3}H-testosterone had been converted to 5α-reduced products by 4 hr. While essentially no ^{3}H-DHT was detectable in the medium, a significant ^{3}H-DHT peak was apparent in the nuclear and cytoplasmic fraction. We conclude that a significant proportion of testosterone can be converted to DHT by MCF-7 human breast cancer. Furthermore, since binding of DHT to receptor occurs with approximately twofold higher affinity, it seems likely that DHT is the major effector androgen in these cells.

Binding and androgen action were compared in four other human breast cancer cell lines. Results are given in Table 5. Three cell lines (G-11, HT-39, and MDA 231) contain little or no receptor activity and are essentially unresponsive to androgen additions. One cell line already discussed (MCF-7) contains androgen receptor and shows marked stimulation of precursor incorporation. Finally, the EVSA-T line contains androgen receptor but under the conditions we employ does not show enhanced precursor incorporation by any concentration of DHT employed. Explanations for the failure of a receptor-containing cell line to respond to steroid are manifold and have been discussed extensively elsewhere (1,31,37,38). Thus although our own studies with estrogen-, glucocorticoid-, and androgen-responsive cell lines strongly support the notion that a lack of receptor is uniformly associated with the absence of physiologically relevant responses to steroid hormone, the converse (i.e., a receptor guarantees a hormone-responsive cell) cannot be considered true.

CONCLUSION AND PROSPECTS

We described our work in characterizing the hormonal responses of several human breast cancer cell lines in long-term tissue culture. These lines exhibit a panoply of hormone receptors and responses—ranging from no receptors and no responses to three classes of steroid receptors and responses to all three shown by the MCF-7 cell. We are currently preparing variant cell lines resistant to the inhibitory effects of glucocorticoids, antiestrogens, and antiandrogens. These variant cell lines together with their parents should provide extremely useful reagents for the biochemical and genetic analysis of steroid hormone action in mammalian cells. We (39) and others (40) have used somatic cell hybridization to combine genetic information from cells with differing hormonal responses to analyze further the steps in hormone action. Such studies in the future may suggest methods for increasing the effectiveness of hormonal therapy in human malignancy.

ACKNOWLEDGMENT

I thank Ms. Gail Bolan and Karen Huff for devoted technical assistance; Dr. R. Herberman for providing the MDA 231, HT-39, and G-11 cell lines and Dr. M. Rich for the MCF-7 cell line employed in these studies; Drs. B. Vonderhaar and D. Kleinberg for enzymatic and immunoassays of α-lactalbumin; Dr. R. Knazek for performing the capillary culture experiments; Ms. Lois Trench of ICI America for tamoxifen; Dr. R. Wheelock of Parke Davis for CI 628; and Dr. J. P. Raynaud of the Roussel Corporation for R50-20 and R2956.

REFERENCES

1. King, R. J. B., and Mainwaring, W. I. P. (1974): *Steroid Cell Interactions*, pp. 1–430. University Park Press, Baltimore.
2. McGuire, W. L., Carbone, P. P., Sears, M. E., and Escher, G. C. (1975): In: *Estrogen Receptors in Human Breast Cancer*, edited by W. L. McGuire, P. P. Carbone, and E. P. Vollmer. pp. 1–8. Raven Press, New York.
3. Smithline, F., Sherman, L., and Kolodny, H. D. (1975): *N. Engl. J. Med.*, 292:784–792.
4. Williams, D. C. (1974): *Adv. Steroid Biochem. Pharmacol.*, 4:9–31.
5. McGuire, W. L., and Chamness, G. C. (1973): In: *Receptors for Reproductive Hormones*, edited by B. W. O'Malley and A. R. Means, pp. 113–136. Plenum Press, New York.
6. Bruchovsky, N., and Meakin, J. W. (1973): *Cancer Res.*, 33:1689–1695.
7. Lippman, M. E., and Bolan, G. (1975): *Nature (Lond.)*, 256:592–593.
8. Soule, H. D., Vazquez, J., Long, A., Albert, S., and Brennan, M. (1973): *J. Natl. Cancer Inst.*, 51:1409–1416.
9. Leighton, J. (1951): *J. Natl. Cancer Inst.*, 12:545–561.
10. Esber, H., Payner, I., and Bogden, A. (1973): *J. Natl. Cancer Inst.*, 50:559–562.
11. Brooks, S. C., Locke, E. R., and Soule, H. (1973): *J. Biol. Chem.*, 248:6251–6253.
12. Clark, J. H., Peck, E. J., and Anderson, J. N. (1974): *Nature (Lond.)*, 251:466.
13. Katzenellenbogen, B. S., and Ferguson, E. R. (1975): *Endocrinology*, 97:1–12.
14. Heuson, J. C. (1974): In: *The Treatment of Breast Cancer*, edited by H. Atkins, pp. 113–164. University Park Press, Baltimore.
15. Vonderhaar, B. K., and Topper, Y. J. (1973): *Enzyme*, 15:340–350.
16. Flaxman, B. A. (1973): *J. Invest. Dermatol.*, 61:67–71.

17. Shymala, G. (1974): *J. Biol. Chem.,* 249:2160–2163.
18. Parks, W. L., Scolnick, E., and Kuzihowski, E. (1974): *Science,* 184:158–160.
19. Stoll, B. A. (1972): In: *Endocrine Therapy of Malignant Disease,* edited by B. A. Stoll, pp. 176–182. Saunders, Philadelphia.
20. Scatchard, G. (1949): *Ann. N.Y. Acad. Sci.,* 51:660–672.
21. Thompson, E. B., and Lippman, M. E. (1974): *Metabolism,* 23:159–202.
22. Lippman, M. E., and Thompson, E. B. (1974): *J. Steroid Biochem.,* 5:461–465.
23. Toft, D. O., and Sherman, M. R. (1975): *Methods Enzymol.,* 36:156–166.
24. Rousseau, G. G., Baxter, J. D., and Tomkins, G. M. (1972): *J. Mol. Biol.,* 67:99–116.
25. Lippman, M. E., and Bolan, G. *(In preparation.)*
26. Lippman, M. E., Halterman, R., Leventhal, B. G., Perry, S., and Thompson, E. B. (1973): *J. Clin. Invest.,* 52:1715–1725.
27. Lippman, M. E., Perry, S., and Thompson, E. B. (1974): *Cancer Res.,* 34:1572–1576.
28. Smith, J. A., and King, R. J. B. (1972): *Exp. Cell Res.,* 73:351–359.
29. Fracchia, A. A., Randall, H. T., and Farrow, J. H. (1967): *Surg. Gynecol. Obstet.,* 125:747–756.
30. Treves, N. (1957): *Cancer,* 12:821.
31. AMA Committee on Research (1960): *J.A.M.A.,* 172:1271–1274.
32. Lippman, M. E., Bolan, G., and Huff, K. (1975): *Nature (Lond.),* 258:339–341.
33. Wilson, J. D. (1972): *N. Engl. J. Med.,* 287:1284–1287.
34. Jung, I., and Baulieu, E. E. (1972): *Nature [New Biol.],* 237:24–26.
35. Miller, W. R., McDonald, D., Forrest, A. P. M., and Shivas, A. A. (1973): *Lancet* 1:912–914.
36. Gual, C., Morato, T., Hayano, M., Gut, M., and Dorfman, R. J. (1962): *Endocrinology,* 71:920–925.
37. Lippman, M. E. (1976): *Life Sci.* 18:143–152.
38. Sibley, C. H., and Tomkins, G. M. (1974): *Cell,* 2:213–220.
39. Lippman, M. E., and Thompson, E. B. (1974): *J. Biol. Chem.,* 249:2483–2488.
40. Rosenau, W., Baxter, J. D., Rousseau, G. G., and Tomkins, G. M. (1972): *Nature [New Biol.],* 237:20–24.
41. McGuire, W. L., and DeLaGarza, V. I. (1973): *J. Clin. Endocrinol. Metab.,* 36:548–552.
42. Stancel, G. M., and Gorski, J. (1975): *Methods Enzymol.,* 36:166–175.

Breast Cancer: Trends in Research and Treatment, edited by J. C. Heuson,
W. H. Mattheiem, and M. Rozencweig. Raven Press, New York © 1976.

Organ Culture of Human Breast Cancer

J. L. Pasteels,* J. A. Heuson-Stiennon,* N. Legros,† G. Leclercq,† and J. C. Heuson†

*Laboratoire d'Histologie, Faculté de Médecine, Université
Libre de Bruxelles, Brussels; and †Service de Médecine et
Laboratoire d'Investigation Clinique, Institut J. Bordet, Brussels, Belgium*

Ablation of the ovaries, adrenal glands, or hypophysis and/or additive hormonal therapy constitute effective palliative treatment for 30–40% of patients with advanced carcinoma of the breast. The endocrine mechanisms by which tumor regression occurs in such patients have not been well defined. Moreover, it is impossible to forecast which patients may benefit from hormonal therapy because no specific histologic correlation was ever found with hormonal responsiveness.

Several authors tried to develop techniques for determining the hormone responsiveness of a given cancer, and various culture systems were proposed for this purpose. They are unique tools for investigating interactions of hormones on individual tumors, without interference of secondary actions through the hypothalamus and the pituitary. They proved efficient on animal models. The well-known 7,12-dimethylbenz(a)anthracene (DMBA)-induced mammary tumor in the rat was successfully maintained in organ culture and subjected to various combinations of several hormones. The data on hormonal responsiveness *in vitro* correlated satisfactorily with experimental results on living animals. Unfortunately, when the same organ culture procedures were tried on human breast cancers, they failed in some experiments and led to controversial results in others. We also made several attempts along this line. Finally, by trial and error we were able to devise a suitable method. It yielded interesting observations that are relevant to the mechanisms of hormone dependence.

ANIMAL MODELS

As discussed in another chapter in this section (Heuson et al.: "Hormone Dependency of Rat Mammary Tumors"), mammary tumors of rats can be maintained for several days as organ cultures in a chemically defined medium. No significant cell loss occurs, provided the explants are small enough to prevent central infarction. Thymidine-^{3}H incorporation and counts of mitoses after exposure of the cultures to colchicine were used as an index of tumor growth.

Mammary tumors induced by DMBA in the rat, when tested for hormone sensitivity in this organ culture system, proved responsive to insulin, prolactin, estradiol, and progesterone. Striking differences were found between individual tumors. There are excellent reasons to believe that their hormone responsivity is the same *in vivo* as it is *in vitro*. It is clear that if the performance of organ culture of breast cancer was as easy in the human as it is in the rat the method would be widely used at the present time.

CULTURE OF HUMAN BREAST CANCER

Early Attempts

In contrast to mammary carcinoma of mice and rats, human breast cancers were shown to be extremely difficult to maintain for several days in organ culture (1–6). This was related to their scirrhous character. Indeed, normal or dysplastic mammary tissue, fibroadenoma, and intraductal, colloid, and medullary carcinoma were successfully maintained under such culture conditions (3,4,7). This explains the discrepancy between results of culture of animal versus human material: The mammary cancers of rats and mice are not scirrhous. With the culture conditions tried, there remained a serious hindrance for the *in vitro* study of hormonal sensitivity of human breast cancers, for approximately 75% of them belong to the scirrhous type.

Because of the lack of adequate means to preserve organ cultures for several days, some authors (8–11) tried a "tissue survival test" (9) of 24 hr. They claimed that specific hormone supplementation could improve the maintenance of some tumors, while similar cultures in control medium died. Interestingly enough, some tumors were claimed to require estrogens for survival *in vitro* (8,10). This is in agreement with our own findings. However, the survival procedure has been strongly criticized. Testing the action of hormones on dying tissue might be hazardous (12). Using similar culture techniques, but of slightly longer duration, other workers failed to confirm the reported influence of estrogens (2,4,6).

Tissue cultures that allowed epithelial and fibroblastic outgrowth (13,14), or cell cultures using cell suspensions obtained by enzymic action (15,16), were apparently much more successful in preserving human breast cancer *in vitro*. A method using thymidine-^{3}H incorporation by cell suspensions has been proposed to demonstrate specific hormone influences on human breast cancers (16). Provided there is no doubt as to the epithelial (and tumoral) nature of the cells grown under such conditions, the technique could bring valuable information. However, the conditions of cell growth are highly artificial; and even if a specific hormone action is shown on a cell suspension, it is only speculation that it would be the same *in vivo*. The tumor cells might not be expected to behave the same way when free in liquid nutrient medium as they are when surrounded by a dense, scirrhous, collagen stroma. For this reason we preferred the organ culture procedure. As described in the next paragraph, giving support to the rationale of this choice, hormone-dependent interactions were found between tumor and stroma that may be instrumental in the spreading of the cancer.

Recent Results

The recent findings reported here were presented at another meeting (17) and are described in detail elsewhere (18). They may be summarized as follows: Starting with the organ culture method that proved efficient for rat mammary tumors, we tried to develop a technique suitable for human material. Ninety-four breast cancer tissue samples were collected from 88 women and one man. Seventy-five were from primary breast cancers and 19 from metastases in lymph nodes or skin. Twenty-three female patients were premenopausal, eight within 1 year of their last menstrual period, 56 were postmenopausal, and one was of undetermined status.

The sterile samples were placed in Earle's base at 0°C immediately after excision and transferred to the laboratory within 15 min. Tumor tissue was dissected free from adhering fat, connective tissue strands, and necrotic areas, and was cut into 1- to 2-mm explants. Culture units were comprised of five explants deposited on a Millipore filter or a small block of agar gel and transferred on stainless steel grids in Falcon disposable petri dishes containing 2.5 ml of liquid culture medium. The height of the grids was such that the explants were at the interphase of liquid medium and gas (95% O_2/5% CO_2). Medium 199 Earle's base supplemented with glucose (250 mg%) was used as the basal medium. It was changed every 2 days.

Two to three culture units (i.e., 10–15 explants) were fixed for histological examination at the end of each culture period of 4, 6, 7, or 14 days. After serial sectioning, eight regularly spaced sections were stained with hematoxylin and eosin (H & E). Specific staining of collagen was carried out with Masson's trichrome, van Gieson staining, and periodic acid-Schiff in selected experiments. Histological typing of the tumors was performed on samples collected at the start of the culture according to Stewart (19) and Kuzma (20). We further subclassified them into "soft" tumors with scanty or loose stroma, and "scirrhous" (collagen-rich) tumors.

Estrogen receptors in the tumor samples were assayed before culture, as described by Leclercq et al. (21). Tumors of the various histological types, including the soft and scirrhous types, were equally represented with regard to age and menopausal status of the patients. Of the 94 breast cancers studied, 32 were soft and 62 scirrhous.

A first observation in the present experiments was that as a general rule survival was excellent throughout the explants from soft tumors. Such tumors comprised 12 infiltrating ductal carcinomas, 5 medullary carcinomas, 4 colloid carcinomas, 4 comedocarcinomas, 3 papillary infiltrating carcinomas, 3 infiltrating lobular carcinomas, and 1 Paget's disease. No hormone supplementation of the medium (or collagenase treatment) was required. The only exceptions were the five medullary carcinomas. These tumors, characterized by a heavy lymphocyte infiltration, failed to survive under all culture conditions tried.

In contrast to the soft tumors, the scirrhous cancers showed very poor survival in basal medium. After 2 days of culture only the very peripheral tumor cells, exposed to the medium either directly or at least without interposition of dense collagen, were found to be viable. The more central tumor cords underwent pyknosis and karyorrhexis. Apparently such necrosis was not due to unspecific central infarction. Indeed, the fibroblasts surrounding the necrotic tumor cords in central areas were generally well preserved. Moreover, pyknosis of the tumor was observed very close to the edge of the explants (less than 0.05 mm from the periphery), whereas in cultures of soft tumors central infarction never occurred when the diameter of the explants was less than 1 mm.

In the first 23 experiments the explants were prepared for culture by cutting the tissue samples with opposed surgical scalpel blades on a porcelain plate. Histological controls performed on explants fixed immediately after cutting demonstrated crushed cancer cells, especially in the case of scirrhous tumors. Therefore the cutting method was improved. By trial and error we found that a suitable technique was to mince the tumor by means of opposed razor blades on a solidified paraffin surface. This greatly improved the condition of the explants at the start of culture. Even with the scirrhous tumors, significant destruction of cancer cells could no longer be ascribed to the cutting procedure. The improved method was therefore used for all subsequent experiments. Nevertheless, it did not allow survival of scirrhous explants during culture.

At this stage it was supposed that poor survival of the scirrhous tumors could be related to the presence of dense collagen. We therefore subjected explants from 35 tumors (27 scirrhous and 8 soft) to collagenase. Bacterial collagenase (Calbiochem, San Diego, Calif., 100 C units/mg) was added to basal medium at a concentration of 1 mg/ml. The explants were cultured in this medium for 24 to 48 hr. Afterward, collagenase was washed out and the explants were further cultured on agar gel under the usual conditions for periods ranging from 5 to 13 days.

At the end of the 1- or 2-day period of culture with collagenase, histological examination disclosed complete disappearance of the collagen. Tumor cells and fibroblasts appeared intact and settled on the support, forming flattened explants of very high cellular density. The same pattern was maintained when the explants were further cultured in fresh medium with or without hormone supplementation. In cultures from soft tumors, cell survival, already excellent in the controls, was not affected by collagenase pretreatment. In sharp contrast, the scirrhous tumors cultured after initial treatment with collagenase were considerably improved over their controls. In each case, pyknosis became very infrequent. The entire explants were composed of viable tumor cells and connective tissue cells. The tumor cells arranged themselves as epithelial cords, allowing clear distinction between tumor and fibroblasts. Maintenance of such explants did not seem grossly influenced by added hormones.

In parallel with the collagenase experiments, hormone supplementation of the medium was tried in various combinations at the following concentrations: insulin, 10 μg/ml; prolactin (ovine, NIH-P-S-10) 5 μg/ml; hydrocortisone 1 μg/ml; 17β-estradiol 0.01 ng to 10 μg/ml. No clear-cut differences were observed between controls and the explants cultured in medium supplemented with insulin, prolactin, and hydrocortisone, either alone or in combination. The survival of soft tumors or of scirrhous explants pretreated with collagenase remained excellent. The poor condition of scirrhous tumors not subjected to collagenase was essentially the same, although it is possible that in some cases insulin alone or in combination with prolactin induced discrete enlargement of peripherally located viable cancer cells and moderate lossening of the stroma.

In 23 experiments the medium was further supplemented with 17β-estradiol in combination with insulin alone or with insulin and prolactin. This was tried on three soft tumors (one carcinoma simplex, one comedocarcinoma, and one papillary carcinoma) and on 20 collagen-rich cancers (1 comedocarcinoma with very dense stroma and 19 scirrhous infiltrating ductal carcinomas). In none of the soft tumors did estradiol effect detectable changes. In contrast, dramatic changes occurred in 18 of the 20 scirrhous tumors. Culture in the presence of estradiol resulted in marked loosening and dissolution of the collagen and in survival of clusters of cancer cells throughout the explants, even in their central areas. In a few experiments collagen dissolution was nearly complete. In most instances, however, collagen lysis was restricted to the stromal areas immediately surrounding viable cancer cells (Figs. 1 and 2).

Dissolution of the collagen never occurred in the explants that were, by the hazards of sampling, devoid of tumor cells. The minimum concentration of estrogen effecting these changes was usually 1 ng/ml (ca. 3.7×10^{-9} M), but it differed slightly from one tumor to another, ranging from 0.1 to 10 ng/ml. Once the stroma was loosened through the action of estradiol, estrogen was no longer required to ensure cell survival. This was demonstrated in five experiments where explants from scirrhous tumors were cultured for 7 days in medium containing insulin, prolactin, and 17β-estradiol (1 ng/ml), then washed free of estradiol and further cultured for 7 days with insulin and prolactin only. At the end of both 7-day periods, we found excellent survival of cancer cells in cords surrounded by a loosened stroma.

Specific estrogen receptors were found in 26 of the 32 soft tumors and in 47 of 61 scirrhous tumors. In the experiment where 20 collagen-rich tumors were cultured with 17β-estradiol, 14 of the 18 improved tumors contained receptors. Both tumors found unaffected by estradiol in culture were receptor-positive.

DISCUSSION

From the results reported here, it becomes clear that previous failures in performing organ cultures of human breast cancers were due to the presence of large amounts of dense collagen in most tumors studied. Indeed, we confirmed that failures were restricted to the scirrhous tumors and that soft tumors were

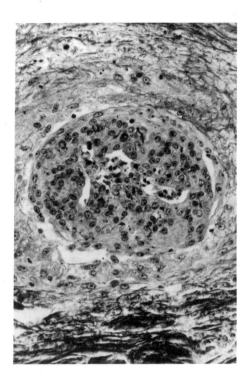

FIG. 1. Detail of a 7-day organ culture of a scirrhous carcinoma, carried out in the presence of insulin (10 μg/ml), prolactin (5 μg/ml), and 17β-estradiol (0.1 ng/ml). Van Gieson stain demonstrates the dark collagen fibrils. Disappearance of collagen is observed in the immediate surroundings of the cancer cells, while intact collagen is found in remote areas. $\times$225.

cultured easily, even in hormone-free medium. The same was observed for the scirrhous cancers when they were made soft by collagenase pretreatment. In such instances human breast cancers were cultured as readily as the mammary tumors of rats and mice (which are not scirrhous) and were then successfully maintained without any hormone supplementation of the medium. This does not necessarily mean that they were not hormone-sensitive. In organ cultures of DMBA-induced rat mammary tumors, we found that histological criteria of survival as were used in the study of human material are inadequate to assess hormone sensitivity. Thymidine-^{3}H incorporation provided more precise evidence. Unfortunately this method could not be applied as such to our organ cultures of human material because, in contrast to the mammary tumors of rats, they usually contained very few tumor cells compared to stromal cells. As a consequence, incorporation of thymidine-^{3}H was very small and variable. Furthermore, the contribution of incorporation of the isotope into stromal cells was to be expected. Assessment of such contribution would thus have required radioautographic studies, hardly practical for screening a large number of mammary tumors.

Although a complete picture of the hormone sensitivity of human breast cancer could not be drawn, the present organ culture experiment brought unexpected findings that might be of great significance *in vivo*. They are proof of hormone sensitivity in some tumors, and, perhaps more important, they throw some light on the mechanisms involved. The evidence may be summarized as follows:

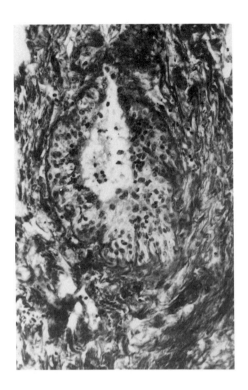

FIG. 2. Detail of a 7-day organ culture of the same tumor but cultured in hormone-free medium. Shrunken but viable cancer cells are present in this very peripheral area of an explant. No dissolution of collagen is observed. Compare the basement membrane to that in Fig. 1. Van Gieson stain. ×225.

1. When collagen is absent or destroyed by pretreatment with collagenase, the cultures are successfully maintained in hormone-free medium.

2. Scirrhous tumors can be maintained without collagenase pretreatment, provided they are exposed to estradiol.

3. In such cultures exposed to estradiol, collagenolysis invariably occurs in the immediate surroundings of cancer cells.

4. Once collagen digestion is achieved by means of exposure to estradiol, the cultures are successfully maintained in estrogen-free medium.

From this, we conclude that some human breast cancers display estrogen-dependent collagenolytic activity. Collagenolytic enzyme activity was reported in other neoplasms, either in homogenates (22) or in culture experiments (23–26).

A few of these experiments were conducted on breast cancers with negative results (23,26), but no hormone supplementation was tried. On the other hand, specific neutral collagenase activity was shown to be hormone-dependent in nontumoral tissue, such as the uterus (27,28). The correlation between our findings on *in vitro* hormone sensitivity and the assays of estrogen receptors was poor. This supports our previous view that, with the technique used, negative assays for estrogen receptors may be due to methodological artifacts (29).

The question arises whether the hypothesis of an estrogen-dependent collagenolytic enzyme system may apply to the growth of breast cancer *in vivo*. In a study of parenchymal growth in the normal mammary gland, Elliot and

Turner (30) described a spreading factor that had the properties of an enzyme, was distinct from hyaluronidase, and possibly was acting on collagen. Their hypothesis was that "the spreading factor is either elaborated or activated in the growing mammary gland cells by hormones (especially estrogens) which initiate both duct and lobule-alveolar growth of the mammary glands. The spreading factor may then break down the connective tissue in some manner allowing the rapid forward growth of the mammary ducts and lobes." In breast cancer patients subjected to treatment with large doses of estrogen, Emerson et al. (31) described loosening of connective tissue stroma surrounding the cancer cells. "This appeared to occur by partial solution of the collagen, for there was an over-all depletion of the amount of collagen." Quantitative methods should be devised to measure the collagenolytic activity of human breast cancers, and to investigate whether other hormones than estrogen are involved in its control. Regardless, the results of our organ culture studies strongly suggest that an estradiol-dependent collagenolytic enzyme system exists in human breast cancers, and that it could play an important role in the hormonal control of their growth and invasiveness.

SUMMARY

An organ culture method suitable for the maintenance of viable human breast cancer for up to 14 days has been described. Even in hormone-free medium, it allowed excellent survival of 27 of 32 "soft" tumors and all 27 scirrhous cancers, provided the latter were pretreated with collagenase. When not subjected to collagenase, the 62 scirrhous tumors cultured in hormone-free medium invariably showed survival of only clusters of cancer cells located at the very periphery of the explants—those cells in direct contact with the culture medium. Supplementation of the medium with various combinations of insulin, ovine prolactin, and hydrocortisone did not improve the viability of central tumor cords in scirrhous explants. Further supplementation of the medium with 17β-estradiol (minimum effective dose, 0.1–10 ng/ml) markedly improved survival of 18 of 20 of the scirrhous tumors tried. This occurred throughout the whole explant, with evidence of collagen dissolution around the cancer cells. It is concluded that when breast cancer cells are surrounded by dense collagen estradiol ensures their survival by inducing them to produce collagenolytic enzymes. It is suggested that this estrogen-dependent collagenolytic enzyme system could play an important role in the hormonal control of their growth and invasiveness.

ACKNOWLEDGMENTS

We are grateful to the surgeons and pathologists at the Institut J. Bordet for kindly providing the specimens. We are indebted to Mr. S. Verset and to Miss M. C. Deboel for skillful technical assistance. Our thanks are due to Mr. P. G. Condliffe from the National Institutes of Health who generously provided ovine prolactin.

This work was supported by grants from the "Fonds Cancérologique" de la Caisse Générale d'Epargne et de Retraite de Belgique and were performed in part under contract of the Ministère de la Politique Scientifique within the framework of the Association Euratom, University of Brussels, University of Pisa.

REFERENCES

1. Archer, F. L. (1968): Normal and neoplastic human tissue in organ culture: Reaction to environmental factors. *Arch. Pathol.*, 85:62–71.
2. Stoll, B. A. (1970): Investigation of organ culture as an aid to the hormonal management of breast cancer. *Cancer*, 25:1228–1233.
3. Wellings, S. R., and Jentoft, V. L. (1972): Organ cultures of normal, dysplastic, hyperplastic, and neoplastic human mammary tissues. *J. Natl. Cancer Inst.*, 49:329–338.
4. Willcox, P. A., and Thomas, G. H. (1972): Oestrogen metabolism in cultured human breast tumors. *Br. J. Cancer*, 26:453–460.
5. Lagios, M. D. (1974): Hormonally enhanced proliferation of human breast cancer in organ culture: An *in vitro* system for assessment of specific hormonal response. *Oncology*, 29:22–33.
6. Sellwood, R. A., and Castro, J. E. (1974): The effect of hormones on organ cultures of human mammary carcinoma. *J. Pathol.*, 113:223–225.
7. Elias, J. J., and Armstrong, R. C. (1973): Hyperplastic and metaplastic responses of human mammary fibroadenomas and dysplasias in organ culture. *J. Natl. Cancer Inst.*, 51:1341–1343.
8. Chayen, J., Altmann, F. P., Bitensky, L., and Daly, J. R. (1970): Reponse of human breast-cancer tissue to steroid hormones in vitro. *Lancet*, 1:868–870.
9. Hobbs, J. R., Salih, H., Flax, H., and Brander, W. (1973): Prolactin dependence among human breast cancers. In: *Human Prolactin*, edited by J. L. Pasteels and C. Robyn, pp. 249–265. Excerpta Medica, Amsterdam.
10. Salih, H., Flax, H., and Hobbs, J. R. (1972): In vitro oestrogen sensitivity of breast cancer tissue as a possible screening method for hormonal treatment. *Lancet*, 1:1198–1202.
11. Salih, H., Flax, H., Brander, W., and Hobbs, J. R. (1972): Prolactin dependence in human breast cancers. *Lancet*, 2:1103–1105.
12. Heuson, J. C., and Tagnon, H. J. (1973): Androgen dependence of breast cancers. *Lancet*, 2:203–204.
13. Dickson, J. A. (1966): Tissue-culture approach to the treatment of cancer. *Br. Med. J.*, 1:817–823.
14. Barker, J. R., and Richmond, C. (1971): Human breast carcinoma culture: The effect of hormones. *Br. J. Surg.*, 58:732–734.
15. Foley, J. F., and Aftonomos, B. T. (1965): Growth of human breast neoplasms in cell cultures. *J. Natl. Cancer Inst.*, 34:217–220.
16. Burstein, N. A., Kjellberg, R. N., Raker, J. W., and Schmidek, H. H. (1971): Human carcinoma of the breast *in vitro*; the effect of hormones: A preliminary report. *Cancer*, 27:1112–1116.
17. Heuson, J. C., Pasteels, J. L., Legros, N., Heuson-Stiennon, J. A., and Leclercq, G. (1975): Study of hormone dependence of human breast cancer in organ culture. In: *Proceedings of the International Symposium on Hormones and Breast Cancer*. Nice, May 23–24, INSERM, 55:129–138.
18. Heuson, J. C., Pasteels, J. L., Legros, N., Heuson-Stiennon, J. A., and Leclercq, G. (1975): Estradiol-dependent collagenolytic enzyme activity in long-term organ culture of human breast cancer. *Cancer Res.*, 35:2039–2048.
19. Stewart, F. W. (1950): Tumors of the breast. In: *Atlas of Tumor Pathology*, Sect. IX, Fasc. 34, pp. 5–114. Armed Forces Institute of Pathology, Washington, D. C.
20. Kuzma, J. F. (1953): The breast. In: *Pathology*, edited by W. A. D. Anderson, 2nd ed., pp. 1102–1129. Henry Kimpton, London.
21. Leclercq, G., Heuson, J. C., Schoenfeld, R., Mattheiem, W. H., and Tagnon, H. J. (1973): Estrogen receptor in human breast cancer. *Eur. J. Cancer*, 9:665–673.
22. Harris, E. D., Faulkner, C. S., and Wood, S. (1972): Collagenase in carcinoma cells. *Biochem. Biophys. Res. Commun.*, 48:1247–1253.

23. Riley, W. B., and Peacock, E. E., Jr. (1967): Identification, distribution and significance of a collagenolytic enzyme in human tissues. *Proc. Soc. Exp. Biol. Med.,* 124:207–210.
24. Robertson, D. M., and Williams, D. C. (1969): *In vitro* evidence of neutral collagenase activity in an invasive mammalian tumor. *Nature (Lond.),* 221:259–260.
25. Taylor, A. C., Levy, B. M., and Simpson, J. W. (1970): Collagenolytic activity of sarcoma tissues in culture. *Nature (Lond.),* 228:366–367.
26. Dresden, M. H., Heilman, S. A., and Schmidt, J. D. (1972): Collagenolytic enzymes in human neoplasms. *Cancer Res.,* 32:993–996.
27. Jeffrey, J. J., Coffey, R. J., and Eisen, A. (1971): Studies on uterine collagenase in tissue culture. II. Effect of steroid hormones on enzyme production. *Biochem. Biophys. Acta,* 252:143–149.
28. Ryan, J. N., and Woessner, J. F., Jr. (1974): Oestradiol inhibition of collagenase role in uterine involution. *Nature (Lond.),* 248:526–528.
29. Leclercq, G., Heuson, J. C., Deboel, M. C., and Matheiem, W. H. (1975): Oestrogen receptors in breast cancer. *Br. Med. J.,* 1:185–189.
30. Elliot, J. R., and Turner, C. W. (1953): The mammary gland spreading factor. *Res. Bull. Univ. Missouri Coll. Agric.,* 537:1-52.
31. Emerson, W. J., Kennedy, B. J., Graham, J. N., and Nathanson, I. T. (1953): Pathology of primary and recurrent carcinoma of the human breast after administration of steroid hormones. *Cancer,* 6:641–670.

Breast Cancer: Trends in Research and Treatment, edited by J. C. Heuson,
W. H. Mattheiem, and M. Rozencweig. Raven Press, New York © 1976.

Roundtable Discussion: Experimental Models

Chairman: L. M. van Putten

van Putten: Dr. Maass, would you summarize your experience on some of the drugs
mentioned at the end of Dr. Heuson's presentation, which are alkylating agents coupled to
steroids, and which could therefore be expected to concentrate in tumors.

Maass: We tested three substances of this group, phenesterine, estradiol mustard, and
dehydroepiandrosterone (DHA) mustard for their capacity to combine with estrogen and
androgen receptors. For measuring these receptors we used sucrose gradients, centrifugation, and agar gel electrophoresis. On agar gel electrophoresis there is competition only for
estradiol receptors with nafoxidine but no competition with estradiol mustard at two
concentrations. There is absolutely no competition, and it is the same with DHT receptors.
On agar gel electrophoresis, after incubation with cyproterone acetate, you find a competition but none with DHA mustard. If calf tissue slices are incubated in the presence of an
excess of cold estradiol, there is inhibition of the uptake of labeled estradiol; likewise
uptake of hot estradiol is inhibited by nafoxidine, estradiol mustard and phenesterine, but
there is no inhibition with DHA mustard. The same is true with DHT uptake; there is
inhibition with a high excess of cold DHT, and in this case there is also signficant
inhibition of DHT uptake with DHA mustard. So the effects of these substances are
obviously due to the splitting of the steroid alkylating molecule, and the binding or
inhibiting effect is found only in *in vivo* experiments; there is no competition *in vitro* at all.
So the sites of the molecules necessary for binding to the receptor are obviously blocked by
the alkylating agent.

van Putten: Dr. McGuire, will you discuss steroid binding in tissue culture?

McGuire: Our chairman mentioned at the beginning of the session that an ideal model
for studying breast cancer would be a tumor which is sensitive to insulin as well as to all
four steroid hormones. Dr. Lippman presented data on the MCF7 line in which he showed
evidence for three separate steroid receptors. I have data on the same tissue culture line
demonstrating receptors for four steroids: estradiol, progesterone (measured with R5020, a
Roussel compound), DHT, and dexamethasone. So perhaps at least in terms of a tissue
culture line, this meets one of the chairman's criteria for an ideal situation. I think the data
that Dr. Lippman presented, in terms of some of the biology of the steroids, supports this.

Lippman: I would like to confirm that finding. The MCF7 cell line has all four receptors
and, in addition, an extremely high-affinity receptor for insulin. It is, in fact, a model
system for studying the response to insulin in the physiological range, so it meets that
additional requirement of breast cancer that was putatively raised. To my knowledge,
several people have sought prolactin receptor in this line, uniformly without success, but
perhaps someone here is willing to change that.

Rochefort: Do you have any data or ideas concerning the mechanism of the toxic effect
of tamoxifen on MCF cells? Do you think that the prolonged nuclear retention of the
receptor-antiestrogen complex, which has been shown for nafoxidine, is involved?

Lippman: There is relatively incontrovertible evidence that the effect of the antiestrogen
on these cells is not a nonspecific toxic effect but interferes with the estrogen pathway for
these reasons. (1) The simultaneous addition of estradiol at a hundred-fold lower concen-

151

tration compared with the antiestrogen can prevent the action of the antiestrogen. (2) By adding estradiol to cultures incubated with the antiestrogen after the cells have been inhibited, the effects of the antiestrogen can be reversed. (3) Antiestrogen is inactive in breast cells and other cell lines which lack estrogen receptor. Finally, in studies we just completed, using three different lines of experiment we were able to show that the antiestrogen bound to the estrogen receptor can translocate to the nucleus. We feel there is good evidence to support the idea that the antiestrogen bound to the estrogen receptor is acting at a nuclear level. I do not have any information concerning retention of this abnormal receptor complex in the nucleus.

Baulieu: Is there any information on the karyotype or the virus genome content of DMBA-induced tumors? Secondly, concerning your very interesting progesterone effect, Dr. Heuson, could you decide whether part of this was due to transformation of progesterone into estrogen in the animal body?

Heuson: I do not have much of an answer for the first question. I do not know the karyotype of this tumor. As far as progesterone is concerned, I have no idea on the possible transformation of progesterone into estrogen, but it is a possibility.

Konyves: Have you some results with other hormones—for example, corticoids or gestogens—on the 13762 mammary adenocarcinoma?

Bogden: The 13762 mammary tumor is very slightly inhibited by cortisone or prednisone.

Konyves: You had a very high remission rate from combinations of 5-FU and PAM, perhaps 90%, but the toxicity was also very high.

Bogden: This has to do with the response of the tumors to the single drug and the three-drug combinations. A number of animals died while they were in complete remission. They showed no evidence of tumor at necropsy, but they did show evidence of gastrointestinal toxicity—typical degeneration of the small and large intestines—primarily, we feel, from the methotrexate.

There was a question on the chromosomes. This one tumor, the 13762, has a chromosomal mode of 45, and the normal rat has 42. We have observed that where the tumor was put into prolonged remission—for 50, 60, 70, and 100 days—the tumors that emerged had a changed mode, to 43, and were drug-resistant.

These animals were treated with phenesterine, interestingly enough, and only the tumors were checked for chromosomal mode changes. We were primarily interested that, histologically, the tumor that arose was an adenocarcinoma that very definitely had a mode of two fewer chromosomes and was drug-resistant. We established this in serial transplantation studies; furthermore, it maintained that mode and its drug resistance.

Labrie: Did you study long-term effects of high concentrations of estradiol to see if an escape phenomenon occurs?

Lippman: We are currently trying to make variants or mutants for all of the antisteroids and for the high concentrations of steroids. Trying to give cell lines the high concentrations so far has been a uniformly unrewarding experience for us; with 10^{-5} M concentrations of steroids, at least in our *in vitro* system, we have produced no resistant cell lines. I imagine that cells are being killed at these concentrations by nonspecific physical-chemical interaction of steroids with membranes, and so I do not know if we will be successful.

Vakil: Certain epidemiological factors, such as early age at first pregnancy, protect against breast cancer in rats, as they do in man; but in mice early pregnancy is a high-risk factor for breast cancer. Should more use be made of animal models other than mice to extrapolate the results to human breast cancer?

van Putten: This points out that there is no ideal model for man, and that in some aspects mice are better and in others rats are better. We might despair of ever getting the perfect model if we have also to take into account virology and so on, in addition to treatment, epidemiology, carcinogenesis.

Heuson: Several steroid hormones, given before DMBA administration to rats, inhibit tumor induction and formation, and I do not know if this has anything to do with pregnancy in humans, but at least it is hormone impregnation at the time of tumor induction.

Spittle: Could someone who described the effect of cytotoxic drugs and hormones on whole animal systems relate the dose levels achieved to those possible in the clinical situation?

Bogden: There is a formula based on body surface area which can be applied to extrapolate doses roughly from the rat or dog to man, or vice versa, but I do not have that information. I might add in reference to the last statement of Dr. Heuson that Dr. Firth recently performed a study in which the mammary tumor in genesis in the Sprague Dawley rat was related to hormone levels in the pituitary. He related this to the human, and there appears to be a period that could be related to the female between the ages of, say, 13 and 18. If hormones are administered and the maturation effect on the mammary gland is speeded up during this time, you match that critical period of 50–60 days in the maturation of the female rat when the mammary gland is most susceptible to carcinogens. Therefore being pregnant early appears to be indicated also in a rat.

Heuson: Dr. Leclercq and I, like many other workers, have been measuring estrogen receptors in breast cancer tissue for years now, and we have claimed that probably all human breast cancers contain some estrogen receptors. Of course it is impossible to state with certainty that these receptors are related to any estrogen action on the target tissue. However, if estrogen receptors are the mediators of estrogen actions, then it is striking to see that in the experiments reported by Pasteels 18 of 20 tumors seem to be estrogen-dependent or estrogen-sensitive to some degree, which is in agreement with our results on estrogen receptors.

Question: May I suggest that on the animal models there is one factor that has not arisen during this meeting so far. I am sure you are familiar with the fact that there are more mammary tumors in dogs than in people. Certainly in the United States, as in Europe, there are good veterinary schools that are equipped to study this problem.

Answer: That is a good point. One of the most exciting possibilities, of course, is the development whereby human tumors are transplanted into nude mice. There is a lot of work going on in that field in terms of their possibilities.

Breast Cancer: Trends in Research and Treatment, edited by J. C. Heuson,
W. H. Mattheiem, and M. Rozencweig. Raven Press, New York © 1976.

Steroid Receptors and the Control of Mammary Tumor Growth

R. J. B. King and J. A. Smith

*Hormone Biochemistry Department, Imperial Cancer Research Fund, Lincoln's Inn Fields,
London WC2A 3PX, England*

Clinical data emerging from studies on estrogen receptor (R_E) levels in human breast tumors indicate that R_E-negative tumors do not respond to endocrine therapy. Patients with R_E-positive tumors, on the other hand, exhibit a more heterogeneous behavior, partitioning approximately equally in the responsive and unresponsive groups (1,2). These studies were based on the general idea that responsive cells contain specific steroid receptors (R) which are absent or present only in small amounts in unresponsive cells. The human data just mentioned, together with those from several animal systems, show that this idea is too simple when applied to tumors; R-negative tumors are unresponsive, but many R-positive tumors are also unresponsive. It is important to delineate the biological reasons for the behavior of the latter category of so-called "false-positive" tumors. The present chapter discusses this topic. It is probable that several very different reasons can be advanced to explain the behavior of these false-positive tumors. Commonly quoted reasons are cellular heterogeneity (3), imprecise clinical assessment (1), and inadequate methodology for measuring the overall steroid-binding process (2). These are undoubtedly important factors and are mentioned later. The main purpose of this chapter is to discuss what factors affect proliferation of mammary tumor cells. This is important because we feel that steroid hormones are only one class of many factors that regulate overall tumor size. The thesis to be developed is summarized by the equation

$$(P_A + P_B + P_C + P_S) - (L_X + L_Y + L_Z) = G$$

where P represents the factors determining proliferation rate, P_S being steroids, and L the factors affecting cell loss. The difference between P and L gives an index of the overall growth (G) of the tumor. If $P_S > G$, steroid removal results in regression, but growth continues if $P_S < G$. It is thus possible that a steroid-responsive, receptor-positive neoplasm might not regress after steroid therapy, so that it behaves as a "false-positive" tumor.

FACTORS AFFECTING TUMOR CELL GROWTH

Experiments on endocrine-related tumors growing in animals have led to the idea that many such tumors are hormone-dependent and so regress on removal of the hormonal stimulus. The idea is also prevalent that one could get complete regression of such tumors by endocrinological means if tumors of a homogeneous cell type existed; partial regressions are usually ascribed to mixed populations of hormone-dependent and hormone-independent cells. However, as more studies are published on the effect of steroids on cells growing in culture, an anomaly is apparent between the animal and culture data. Provided attention is confined to culture systems in which steroids stimulate proliferation, it is apparent that steroids as a group are only one of many factors that can regulate proliferation. A specific example is illustrated in Fig. 1. The S115 mouse mammary tumor cells exhibit androgen responsiveness in culture as the androgen modulates an existing proliferation rate (Fig. 1A) (4,6). In the mouse the tumor is androgen-dependent because castrated male mice do not support tumor growth in the absence of exogenous dihydrotestosterone or testosterone (Fig. 1B) (5,7). We feel that the difference between the growth patterns seen in culture and in the mouse can be explained by considering what factors affect proliferation and tumor size.

Figure 1A illustrates three characteristics of these cells that relate to ways in which their proliferation might be regulated. They grow in the absence of steroid, their growth rate is approximately doubled by androgen, and proliferation is density regulated.

Growth in the absence of added steroid is not due to endogenous steroids present in the 2% fetal calf serum routinely added to such cultures. The cells do

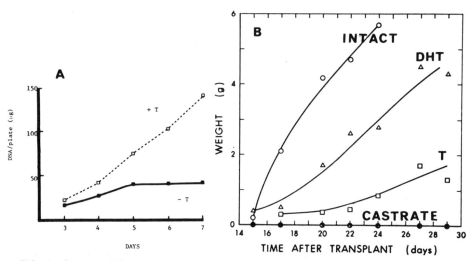

FIG. 1. Growth of S115 cells in culture (**A**) and in male mice (**B**). Data for **A** are from ref. 4, and for **B** from ref. 5. T, testosterone. DHT, 5α-dihydrotestosterone. In **B** the DHT and T were administered to castrated male mice.

TABLE 1. *Modulating effects of steroids on proliferation in culture*

Cells	Steroid	Ref.
Mouse fibroblasts	Corticoid	9
Mouse mammary tumor	Androgens	8
Human mammary tumor	Androgens	10
	Estrogens	11
Human fibroadenoma	Estrogens	12
	Corticoids	
Rat DMBA-induced mammary tumor	Estrogens	12
	Corticoids	

grow in the absence of serum (8), and insufficient endogenous dihydrotestosterone and testosterone are present in the serum to promote growth (6). The androgen-independent growth is not due to more than one cell type in the cultures as the effect is also seen with recently cloned cells.

The acceleration of an existing rate of proliferation by androgen as exhibited by the S115 cells seems to be a general phenomenon for other classes of steroid hormones (Table 1). How can this modulating effect of steroids work? In the absence of steroid, receptor protein might directly affect the proliferative machinery, the addition of steroid merely increasing the efficiency of the receptor (Fig. 2). This idea is based on our experience with S115 cells. If these cells are grown in the absence of androgen, they retain their androgen responsiveness for approximately 4 weeks, but this is then rapidly lost over the next 1–2 weeks. The loss of responsiveness is always accompanied by a fall in growth rate (4). Preliminary data suggest that androgen receptor is also lost when the cells become unresponsive. If substantiated, these results would indicate that proliferation in the absence of steroid is related to receptor levels. The loss of responsiveness just described cannot be explained by cell mutation because of the speed with which the cells

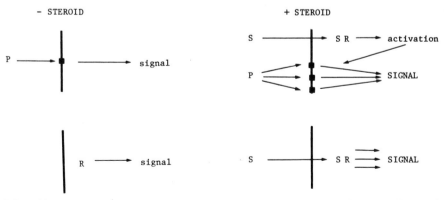

FIG. 2. Modulating effect of steroids on proliferation. P, protein stimulator. S, steroid. R, steroid receptor. ■, membrane receptor for P. Activation is the process leading to formation of the membrane receptor. The *vertical bar* represents the cell membrane.

become unresponsive, so one should not generalize that unresponsive cells produced by mutation grow more slowly than their counterparts.

The second model is one in which the steroid acts indirectly by making the cell more sensitive to other stimuli (Fig. 2). As shown here, the steroid increases the number of membrane receptors for an external agent (P). This mechanism has been used to explain the synergistic effect of glucocorticoids and fibroblast growth factor in the proliferation of 3T3 cells (9).

The growth pattern of S115 cells in culture both in the presence and absence of androgen depends on the retention of density regulation by these cells; as they become more dense, their proliferation rate declines (6,8). Density regulation is a common but ill-understood phenomenon (13) related to the proximity of other cells. It might therefore be anticipated that in solid tumors *in vivo* such contacts might provide an important regulatory mechanism. This would presumably be via inhibitory signals (13), but other forms of cell-cell contact might act in a stimulatory way (14). The general point to be made here is that proliferation of these mammary tumor cells can be regulated by contact with other cells; such contacts could be between homologous or heterologous cells.

In addition to S115 cell proliferation being regulated by androgens and cell density, these cells are markedly affected by serum. Proliferation, both in the presence and absence of androgen, is increased by serum (8). At very high serum levels the proliferation rate is so high in the absence of androgen that addition of androgen has no effect. The stimulatory factors in serum have not been fully identified but are undoubtedly of a complex nature (15).

For experiments in culture, conditions are usually imposed on the cells to maximize growth. The three regulatory components just mentioned for our cells may thus only partly represent the regulatory stimuli impinging on tumor cells growing in a host animal. Other stimuli that come to mind are immunological factors, the blood supply, and tumor encapsulation. Hence the *in vivo* situation could be represented by the model in Fig. 3. Tumor size represents a balance between cell death and proliferation, each of which can be regulated by several factors. The effect on tumor size of a change of any one of these factors depends on the importance of that factor relative to all the others. Figure 3 is thus a pictorial representation of the equation at the beginning of this chapter.

OTHER POTENTIAL CAUSES OF "FALSE-POSITIVE" TUMORS

Defects in the Receptor Mechanism

Studies with virtually every class of steroid suggest that the overall reaction sequence shown in Fig. 4 is operative (16). As depicted here, some of the steps are still debatable, but this does not affect the ensuing discussion. It is clear that with such a complex process the mere presence of receptors may not be sufficient to ensure responsiveness.

Defective nuclear transfer of a cytoplasmic receptor could explain some of the

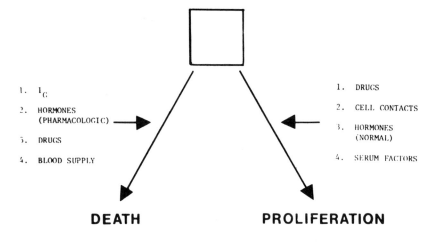

FIG. 3. Control of tumor size in animals. On the right side are listed some of the factors that might influence proliferation, and on the left are those affecting cell death. I_G, immunoglobulin.

false-positives. Suggestive evidence for such a defect existed with the estrogen-induced hamster kidney tumor (17) and spontaneous GRA mouse mammary tumor systems (18), but much more convincing data have now been published using the glucocorticoid-sensitive lymphoma tumor. Cells from this tumor can be grown in culture and retain their response (cell death) to glucocorticoids. A series of reports describe the isolation and characterization of a range of unresponsive cells from this tumor (19–21). Approximately 80% are R^+ and are subdivided into two approximately equal categories. One class contains R that does not transfer to the nucleus (nt^-) while the second group exhibits excessive nuclear transfer (nt^i). Both of these groups would be classified as false-positives by the criteria employed in the human breast tumor work.

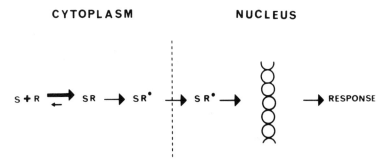

FIG. 4. Intracellular transport of steroids in responsive cells. S, steroid. R, specific receptor. SR•, activated steroid-recepter complex. ⦸ = chromatin.

A possible example in human breast tumors of R existing in a state that cannot be activated is the "4S"R_E. This is a soluble form of receptor that occurs in some human breast tumors (22,23) and other estrogen-sensitive cells (16). It does not bind to nuclei or subnuclear fractions (24,25) and therefore is presumed to be an inactive form of ER complex. Wittliff and Savlov (23) claim that the "4S" receptor is found predominantly in tumor cytosols from unresponsive patients. Such a receptor would not be distinguishable from other "active" receptors in any of the current assay procedures except the sucrose gradient analysis. However, the clinical evidence that "4S" receptor is associated with unresponsive tumors is not in accord with the data from Jensen's group (22) so this point needs further study.

Defect in the Postreceptor Sequence of Events

Some steroid-unresponsive cells may have a completely normal receptor binding and nuclear transfer mechanism, but subsequent expression of the steroid effect is blocked at a point distal to chromatin activation. Examples of such malfunctions are certain glucocorticoid-sensitive leukemias (26), androgen-responsive mouse mammary tumors (27), and glucocorticoid-sensitive hepatoma cells (28,29).

SHOULD R_E MEASUREMENTS BE PROGNOSTIC FOR ALL ENDOCRINE THERAPIES?

At first glance there is no reason to suppose that R_E measurements should indicate tumor response to a spectrum of treatments ranging from hypophysectomy to androgen therapy. However, the limited clinical data currently available suggest that this is the case (1). The biological background to this result is not known but might involve some sort of pleiotypic response (2). It is possible that measurement of receptors for other steroid and protein hormones will show that some unresponsive but R_E-positive tumors are deficient in some other class of receptor.

Another factor to be considered here is whether the presence of R_E in mammary tumor cells is always indicative of a proliferative rather than some other estrogenic response. Insufficient data are available for the human to provide an answer, but in the R_E-positive rat R3230AC mammary tumor estrogens do not affect tumor size but do induce a lactational response (30,31).

CELL HETEROGENEITY

Cellular heterogeneity of mammary tumors has already been mentioned in relation to density-regulated proliferation, but it is also important if any one tumor contains a mixture of responsive and unresponsive cells. Such a tumor could behave as a "false-positive." This was discussed by McGuire and Chamness (3).

CONCLUSIONS

This chapter has pointed out several ways in which a mammary tumor containing abundant cytoplasmic R_E might not respond to endocrine therapy. Whether these suggestions have any relevance to human breast tumors remains to be proved, but by describing the possible reasons for false positives it is also possible to suggest ways in which they may be rectified. From the points made in the section on tumor growth, it is evident that no refinement of steroid receptor methodology will be of use for these types of tumor. Rather it indicates that the range of clinical tests should be as broad as possible so that many tumor-related factors can be measured. The section dealing with defects in receptor mechanism beyond the cytoplasmic R can be resolved by better receptor methodology, while the problem of prognosis for different types of therapy may be overcome by extending the range of hormone receptors being measured.

REFERENCES

1. McGuire, W. L., Carbone, P. P., Sears, M. E., and Escher, G. C. (1975): Estrogen receptors in human breast cancer: an overview. In: *Estrogen Receptors in Human Breast Cancer,* edited by W. L. McGuire, P. P. Carbone, and E. P. Vollmer. Raven Press, New York.
2. King, R. J. B. (1976): Clinical relevance of steroid-receptor measurements in tumours. *Cancer Treatment Rev.,* 2:253–273.
3. McGuire, W. L., and Chamness, G. C. (1973): Studies on the estrogen receptor in breast cancer. In: *Receptors for Reproductive Hormones,* edited by B. W. O'Mally and A. R. Means, pp. 113–136. Plenum Press, New York.
4. Smith, J. A., Robinson, J. H., Jagus-Smith, R., and King, R. J. B. (1975): The stimulation of cell proliferation by steroids. In: *Regulation of Growth and Differentiated Function in Enkaryote Cells,* edited by G. P. Talwar, pp. 355–367. Raven Press, New York.
5. Bruchovsky, N., and Lesser, B. (1975): Control of proliferative growth in androgen responsive organs and neoplasms. *Adv. Sex Horm. Res. (in press).*
6. King, R. J. B., Jagus-Smith, R., Robinson, J. H., and Smith, J. A. (1976): Steroid hormones and the control of tumour growth: studies on androgen responsive tumour cells in culture. In: *Receptors and Steroid Hormone Action,* edited by J. Pasqualini. Marcel Dekker, New York. *(in press).*
7. Minesita, T., and Yamaguchi, K. (1965): An androgen-dependent mouse mammary tumour. *Cancer Res.,* 25:1168–1175.
8. Smith, J. A., and King, R. J. B. (1972): Effects of steroids on growth of an androgen-dependent mouse mammary carcinoma in cell culture. *Exp. Cell Res.,* 73:351–359.
9. Rudland, P. S., Seifert, W., and Gospodarowicz, D. (1974): Growth control in cultured mouse fibroblasts: Induction of the pleiotypic and mitogenic responses by a purified growth factor. *Proc. Natl. Acad. Sci. U.S.A.,* 71:2600–2604.
10. Lippmann, M. E. Personal communication.
11. Lippmann, M. E., and Bolan, G. (1975): Oestrogen-responsive human breast cancer in long term tissue culture. *Nature (Lond.),* 256:592.
12. Hallowes, R. C. Personal communication.
13. Wolstenholme, G. E. W., and Knight, J., editors (1971): *Growth Control in Cell Culture.* Churchill Livingstone, London.
14. Cox, R. P., Krauss, M. R., Balis, M. E., and Dancis, J. (1974): Metabolic cooperation in cell culture. In: *Cell Communication,* edited by R. P. Cox, pp. 67–95. Whiley, London.
15. Holly, R. W., and Kiernan, J. A. (1974): Control of the initiation of DNA synthesis in 3T3 cells: Serum factors. *Proc. Natl. Acad. Sci. U.S.A.,* 71:2908–2911.
16. King, R. J. B., and Mainwaring, W. I. P. (1974): *Steroid-Cell Interactions.* Butterworths, London.

17. King, R. J. B., Smith, J. A., and Steggles, A. W. (1970): Oestrogen binding and the hormone responsivensss of tumours. *Steroidologia,* 1:73–88.

18. Shyamala, G. (1972): Estradiol receptors in mouse mammary tumours: Absence of the transfer of bound estradiol from the cytoplasm to the nucleus. *Biochem. Biophys. Res. Commun.,* 46:1623–30.

19. Sibly, C. H., and Tomkins, G. M. (1974): Isolation of lymphoma cell variants resisant to killing by glucocorticoids. *Cell,* 2:213–220.

20. Sibly, C. H., and Tomkins, G. M. (1974): Mechanisms of steroid resistance. *Cell,* 2:221–227.

21. Yamomoto, K. R., Stampfer, M. R., and Tomkins, G. M. (1974): Receptors from gluco-corticoid-sensitive lymphoma cells and two classes of insensitive clones: Physical and DNA-binding properties. *Proc. Natl. Acad. Sci. U.S.A.,* 71:3901–3905.

22. Jensen, E. V., Polley, T. Z., Smith, S., Block, E., Ferguson, D. J., and De Sombre, E. R. (1975): Prediction of hormone dependency in human breast cancer. In: *Estrogen Receptors in Human Breast Cancer,* edited by W. L. McGuire, P. P. Carbone, and E. P. Vollmer, pp. 37–55. Raven Press, New York.

23. Wittliff, J. L., and Savlov, E. D. (1975): Estrogen-binding capacity of cytoplasmic forms of the estrogen receptors in human breast cancer. In: *Estrogen Receptors in Human Breast Cancer,* edited by W. L. McGuire, P. P. Carbone, and E. P. Vollmer, pp. 73–91. Raven Press, New York.

24. Salas-Trepat, J. M., and Vallet-Strouve, C. (1974): Binding of the estradiol receptor from calf uterus to the chromatin: Active forms. *Biochim. Biophys. Acta,* 371:186–202.

25. Toft, D. (1972): The interaction of uterine estrogen receptors with DNA. *J. Steroid Biochem.,* 3:512–515.

26. Lippman, M. E., Parry, S., and Thompson, E. B. (1974): Cytoplasmic glucocorticoid-binding proteins in glucocorticoid-unresponsive human and mouse leukemic cell lines. *Cancer Res.,* 34:1572–1576.

27. Bruchovsky, N., Sutherland, D. J. A., Meakin, J. W., and Minesita, T. (1975): Androgen receptors: Relationship to growth response and to intracellular androgen transport in nine variant lines of the Shionogi mouse mammary carcinoma. *Biochim. Biophys. Acta,* 381:61–71.

28. Thompson, E. B., and Geleherter, T. D.(1971): Expression of tyrosine amino transferase activity in somatic-cell heterokaryons: Evidence for negative control of enzyme expression. *Proc. Natl. Acad. Sci. U.S.A.,* 68:2589–2593.

29. Croce, C. M., Koprowksi, H., and Litwack, G. (1974): Regulation of the corticosteroid inducibility of tyrosine aminotransferase in interspecific hybrid cells. *Nature (Lond.),* 249:839–841.

30. Hilf, R., Michel, I., and Bell. C. (1967): Biochemical and morphological responses of normal and neoplastic mammary tissue to hormonal treatment. *Recent Prog. Horm. Res.,* 23:229–290.

31. McGuire, W. L., Julian, J. A., and Chamness, G. C. (1971): A dissociation between ovarian-dependent growth and estrogen sensitivity in mammary carcinoma. *Endocrinology,* 89:969–973.

DISCUSSION

Lippman: There are three additional mechanisms whereby tumors give these so-called false-positives. Firstly, everything may go according to plan, but the gene trial involved in the cell may be of itself defective, and so the cell cannot respond. Secondly, it is well known, and I think the cell line I have shown is a good example of it, that the cells may be able to metabolize the steroid hormone such that it has the receptor, but there is no particular response seen because it can do something to the steroid before an effect can be achieved. Thirdly, the question of positive and negative is based on a clinical trial in these patients, and very frequently one can imagine a situation in which the clinical trial is inadequate as compared with the receptor. For example, the ablation may be inadequate, and there is enough adrenal androgen production remaining to produce estrogen peripherally and so there is not an adequate response to castration. It was also recently shown that there is a dose response to DES such that the normal doses of 5 mg t.i.d. may be inadequate. Some patients may respond more, so that some responses we call "false-positives" may in fact reflect therapeutic inadequacy rather than a lack of responsiveness of the tumor.

McGuire: It sounds as though Drs. King and Lippman are trying to defend this theory of estrogen receptor and hormone dependence very vigorously. I object to the term false-positive; it somehow implies that there is something wrong with the assay—you get a positive result and you really should not. Or there is something wrong with the clinical evaluation—the patient really should have responded.

King: It is false-positive in the sense that it has receptor and that clinically it does not respond.

Hayward: Surely the fact that there are different response rates to different endocrine maneuvers means that there could not, by definition, ever be a complete association between hormone receptor sites and responders?

King: Agreed.

Tubiana: In vitro we know that there is the possibility of mutations, especially for lymphocytes, which might change from receptor to nonreceptor. Is the same possibility applicable in breast cancer, and does this happen *in vivo*?

King: Obviously it applies from the studies that have been done on mutation rates with eukaryotic cells. The data are not very grand, but they do suggest that it is approximately 1 in 10^6 to 10^7 cells, so the answer is that it is eminently possible.

Breast Cancer: Trends in Research and Treatment, edited by J. C. Heuson,
W. H. Mattheiem, and M. Rozencweig. Raven Press, New York © 1976.

Steroid Receptors and Hormone Receptivity: New Approaches in Pharmacology and Therapeutics

Etienne-Emile Baulieu

*Unité de Recherches sur le Métabolisme Moléculaire et la Physio-Pathologie des
Stéroides de l' Institut National de la Santé et de la Recherche Médicale,
Département de Chimie Biologique, Faculté de Médecine Paris-Sud,
78 Rue du Général Leclerc, 94270 Bicêtre, France*

Hormones are informational molecules. These chemical messengers must find, at the target cell level, specific recognition mechanism(s) for selecting them appropriately from all other components of the *milieu intérieur*. These recognition mechanisms, which involve binding sites (r in Fig. 1.) of very high affinity (dissociation constant, K_D, between 0.1 and 10 nM adjusted to the low concentration of hormones in the plasma) and strict (stereo) specificity, constitute the primary function of receptors. Parenthetically, one knows that the catalytic sites of enzymes also display specificity, but the affinity is 10^4 times lower than that of the hormone receptor binding sites, since substrates consumed mainly for energy purposes (e.g., sugars, amino acids, or lipids) are found in higher concentrations and transformed into products. In contrast, the interaction of hormones with their receptors does not alter their chemical composition *per se:* it is a purely "physical" phenomenon.

RECEPTORS: DEFINITION AND STUDIES

Specific binding, even of high affinity, does not define a receptor completely. There are other proteins, particularly in the plasma, which bind hormones rather tightly and specifically (e.g., in the human, transcortin for cortisol and progester-

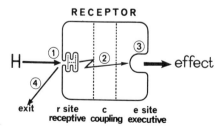

FIG. 1. Phenomenology of the steroid hormone receptor. H represents any steroid hormone. It binds to the "receptive" site (1) with high affinity, and there is transduction (2) coupling the hormone binding to the activation of the "executive" site (3). The latter may, for instance, interact with another macromolecule or catalyze some reaction. When this effect is switched on, the hormone can do nothing but leave (4).

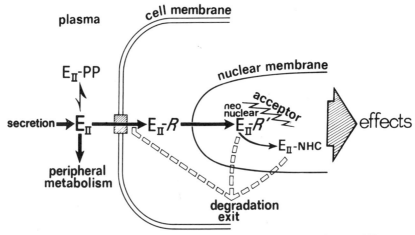

FIG. 2. Natural history of estradiol. Estradiol (E_{II}), taken as a representative steroid hormone, is secreted and circulates in the plasma, mostly bound to specific plasma protein (PP). It is subjected to degradative peripheral metabolism. It is currently believed that free E_{II} enters the cell, perhaps through a membrane-specific step indicated in the figure. Binding to the receptor (R) leads to its transconformation (R becomes R') and translocation of the complex to a neonuclear position, with binding to an "acceptor" still undefined. The possible role of high-affinity chromatin protein (NHC) is reported here and discussed elsewhere (1). At any moment of its cellular life, estradiol may be degraded and/or released from the cell.

one, and SBP-steroid binding plasma protein for estradiol and testosterone); and if these "transport" proteins are of still obscure *raison d'être*, they are certainly not receptors. Indeed, the full meaning of the word receptor implies responsibility for the interpretation of the received signal (hormone) in terms of cellular response. The binding of the hormone leads to activation of the "executive" site (e) of the receptor (r), interacting in turn with "acceptor" component(s) of the cellular machinery set up to initiate a cascade of effects known as the overall "hormonal response" (Fig. 2). At the molecular level there is transduction between the r and the e sites, indicating an allosteric transition of the receptor protein. At the organizational (cellular) level, the receptor is the last molecular entity with which the hormone has to interact in order to trigger the response; afterward it may and indeed does leave, as indicated by the permanent renewal of hormone in target cells, (justifying the continuous hormonal secretion in the intact organism) (1).

Early experiments of Jensen and Jacobson (2) and Glasscock (3) demonstrated the selective concentration and retention of radioactive estrogens in their target organs. Further studies during the mid-1960s performed by Jensen (4), Gorski (5,5a,6), Segal (7), and in our laboratory (8–10) established the proteinic nature and the intracellular localization of estrogen receptors, the first hormonal receptors to be demonstrated and characterized. Thereafter similar results were obtained with all steroid hormones—of both sexual (progesterone and androgens) and adrenal origin (for a decade of research see ref. 11). The entry of steroids into cells and then the intracellular presence of their receptors contrasts with the location of specific binding to plasma membranes found subsequently for most polypeptidic hormone receptors. A part of the "executive" activity of these membrane receptors is to activate the membrane-bound enzyme adenyl cyclase and to increase cAMP, a second messenger for the cell response according to E. Sutherland. cAMP does not play a role in triggering the cellular response to steroid hormones.

That the intracellular steroid binding proteins are "real" receptors is likely, but this has not been formally demonstrated since the acceptor to which the receptor executive site corresponds has not been defined in molecular terms. Three very strong but circumstantial arguments and a fourth that is more direct have been advanced: (a) There is satisfactory parallelism between the affinities of different steroids (or even of nonsteroidal derivatives) of a given series for the receptor and their biological activities (e.g., weak estrogens have low affinity). Such a correlation does not hold with transport plasma proteins. (b) Receptors are present in target organs, although they are undetectable in normal nontarget organs and in genetically nonresponsive tissues (androgen target organs in the testicular feminizing syndrome). (c) After entry into the cell by a process poorly understood (12), the hormone binds to the receptor, which is found in the cytoplasm and provokes a change in its properties (4,6) termed "acidophilic activation" (13). This makes the hormone-receptor complex capable of interacting with a variety of polyanions, notably DNA. The effect is probably related to the secondary location of the hormone-receptor complex in the cell nucleus (4,6,14), also designated "neonuclear" receptor (15). The final nuclear localization of the steroid hormone agrees well with different biochemical studies of the hormonal response, indicating the fundamental importance of gene transcription (again, molecular details are still unknown). (d) In a series of experiments initially developed in our laboratory (16,17), the nuclear gene-transcribing machinery of nonstimulated tissue has been exposed to preparations containing receptor-steroid complexes. There is a hormone-dependent, cytosol-dependent increase in RNA synthesis, a result which, whatever the limitations are from the molecular biological point of view (1,18), may indicate directly a function for the receptors.

These considerations are basic to the belief that the specific proteins binding selectively to the corresponding hormones of a given tissue are receptors, capable of recognition and operational in message execution. Therefore it is tempting to ask whether their qualitative and quantitative evaluation may be of practical value for a better understanding of hormone "receptivity," and consequently if their pharmacological manipulation can contribute to better control of cellular functioning in the intact living organism.

The technicalities of these studies involve: (a) The correct delineation of specific binding from nonspecific binding (albumin and many other proteins bind all steroids indistinctly with an affinity corresponding to $K_D \geqslant 10^{-5}M$). (b) Measurement of the binding affinity and determination of the number of sites per tissue unit (e.g., milligrams of protein or DNA). (c) A survey of binding characteristics with different hormonal derivatives and of molecular properties (e.g., sensitivity to SH blocking agents) not only in order to assess the proteinic nature of the binding but also to differentiate between receptors and plasma proteins (see also ref. 19). (d) An evaluation of the available binding sites (unoccupied by hormone at the time of the study and labeled directly by radioactive hormone added to the extract) and/or, often better, total binding sites taking into consideration the endogenous hormone occupying part of them and using an "exchange technique" for this purpose (20). (e) Eventually, an estimation of the receptor content of the soluble part (cytosol) and of the nuclear (KCl-extractable and "insoluble") fractions of tissue homogenates. All these requirements necessitate precise and rather complex analyses, and warn against "simplified" methods, which may indeed be very seriously misleading.

PHYSIOLOGICAL CHANGES OF RECEPTOR CONTENT AND RECEPTIVITY

Recent studies in the guinea pig demonstrate that the amount of progesterone receptor in the uterus varies during the estrous cycle, depending on complex hormonal control (21,22). Progesterone levels in the plasma and concentration of the progesterone receptor per uterine cell (whether it is free or occupied by the endogenous hormone) show cyclic variations that are not coincidental. Plasma progesterone exhibits an increase at ovulation and a prolonged high level during diestrus (luteal phase). On the other hand, a peak of uterine receptor is rapidly developed at proestrus. However, the maximum value is not maintained very long and a decrease follows, so that the receptor level is very low during the luteal phase, even though this is also the period when implantation eventually takes place. Incidentally, during pregnancy the receptor concentration is similar to that found in the absence of fertilization, up to the time of implantation.

These observations suggest that, if the progesterone receptors have an obligatory involvement in egg implantation, progesterone available when its receptors are high (around ovulation) may be physiologically "important." There is circumstantial evidence that this might be the case, since Deanesly (23) obtained a number of successful implantations in the guinea pig even after ovariectomy, provided the latter was performed after the third day following ovulation (implantation takes place on the seventh day after ovulation).

The increase of progesterone receptor during proestrus is probably attributable to estrogens, and in castrated animals estradiol provokes an important augmentation of binding sites. Such an increase of receptors—suppressible by protein and RNA synthesis inhibitors (Fig. 3)—may be the molecular mechanism of the classic priming of progesterone action by previously administered estradiol (24). The apparent decay of the progesterone receptor induced by estradiol in noncycled (castrated) animals corresponds to a half-life of at least 5 days and does not explain the rapid decrease during the cycle. However, in this model situation where hormonal manipulations are performed easily, progesterone can be injected when receptor is maximum; indeed it accelerates the decay of binding sites, only 20% remaining measurable after 1 day (22). Therefore during the guinea pig estrous cycle, there is a logical possibility to attribute the rapid decrease of the progesterone receptors after proestrus to the progesterone of the first and possibly of the early part of the second luteal peaks (Fig. 3). During the diestrous period, progesterone receptor level is even lower than that measured in castrated animals not treated by hormone, a fact still poorly understood that some "negative" effect of progesterone might explain. Such results suggest that the high level of progesterone receptor at midcycle might be a target for pharmacological inactivation in order to intercept processes leading to blastocyst implantation. None of the related preliminary observations in the human[1] to date discourage the possibility of midcycle contraception (25).

Other recent work shows that the uterine estrogen receptor undergoes changes during early pregnancy in the rat (26). The estradiol and progesterone levels are elevated in the plasma, and the concentrations of the cytosol estradiol receptor were different in the myometrium and the endometrium (Fig. 4). There are always more binding sites per DNA unit in the latter, and they increase markedly in the endometrium after the third day, reaching a maximum by 5–6 days, while the change is modest in myometrium. Implantation in the rat takes place on the fifth day and is not possible either before or after a narrowly defined critical period (27). On the basis of increased estradiol and progesterone concentrations in the blood during early pregnancy, hormones were given to castrated (at day 2 of pregnancy) rats after 3 weeks without treatment. The estrogen-induced increase of estradiol receptor in both endometrium and myometrium is not unexpected. However, it is remarkable that progesterone does increase the estrogen receptor in the endometrium (not significantly in the myometrium), whereas when given with estradiol it abolishes the receptor increase provoked by the latter in the myometrium. The relative concentrations of receptor in endometrium and myometrium are remarkably similar in both the physiological circumstances and the progesterone plus estrogen model. The antagonistic effect of progesterone on estradiol receptor induction in the myometrium may favor implantation by decreasing the estrogen-dependent sensitivity to catecholamines and prostaglandin F 2α (28).

In conclusion, physiological and hormone-induced changes of receptor concentrations have been demonstrated and will probably be further observed in a variety of tissues and circumstances, including development (29,30). Indeed recent work with insulin and growth hormone receptors (31) enlarges the concept to nonsteroid hormones. Detailed studies of the relationship between receptor concentration and hormone action are now necessary, as well as analyses of qualitative changes (e.g., modification of hormone specificity, difference in receptor-genome interactions) that may also occur and be of great importance.

---

[1]For instance, estrogen and progesterone receptors are found in the human endometrium; and whereas blood progesterone shows only a small increase at midcycle, there is a relatively high concentration of the hormone in the uterus (J. Ferin, *personal communication*).

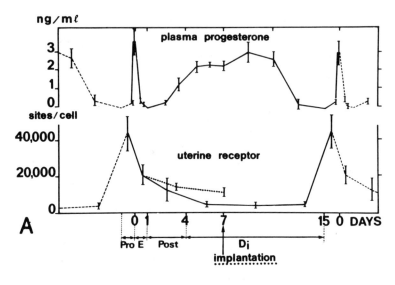

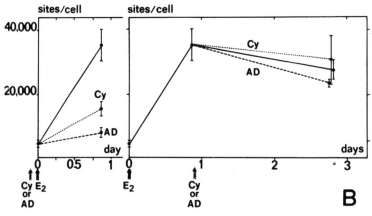

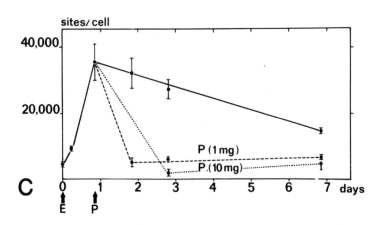

DIFFERENT RECEPTORS FOR THE SAME HORMONE IN DIFFERENT TARGET CELLS

It is not known whether receptors for a hormone are the same in different target tissues. For instance is estradiol receptor in the endometrium identical to that in cervical mucosa, normal and pathological mammary glands, or hypothalamus and anterior pituitary?

There is one example showing that a given hormone circulating in the blood may play its part in different target tissues through different receptors. The case is relatively easy to demonstrate since testosterone is active in target cells either as testosterone itself—in muscles, levator ani or skeletal (32,33), and in kidney (34) —or after transformation into metabolites such as androstanolone (dihydrotestosterone) in ventral prostate and seminal vesicles (35–37), or as estrogen(s) in hypothalamus (38). These results suggest a difference between tissues that respond to the same blood testosterone hormone; such a diversity may be of pharmacological interest since it may be possible to obtain dissociated activities for various androgens, and indeed empirical attempts to separate anabolic properties from virilizing effects of steroids are well known.

DIFFERENT RECEPTORS FOR DIFFERENT HORMONES IN THE SAME CELLS

The very fact that estradiol can induce the progesterone receptor (see above) suggests that uterine cells which synthesize it also contain an estradiol receptor. Formal evidence for two receptors per cell comes from the analysis of cloned cells (MI_1) from a mammary tumor SHI-115 in mice, the growth of which is androgen-dependent, an effect that estrogens antagonize. There are two different receptors in these (single type, hopefully) cells: E (estrogen) and A (androgen) receptors, binding estradiol and testosterone, respectively, with very high affinity (39). The E receptor does not bind testosterone, while the A receptor binds estradiol with relatively high affinity, although lower than that of the E receptor. Therefore, referring to the antiandrogenic effect of estradiol, the problem is to determine whether it "passes" through a competitive binding for the A receptor (which would not be "activated" as with testosterone) or if it implicates the E receptor (which would either carry an antagonistic order to a particular site of the genome or would compete with the A receptor for its acceptor site).

FIG. 3. Changes and hormonal control of progesterone receptor in guinea pig uterus. **A:** Plasma levels of progesterone during the cycle, and concentration per cell of its uterine receptor. Pro, proestrus. E, estrus. Post, postestrus. Di, diestrus. The case of pregnancy is indicated by (...). **B:** Estrogen induction of progesterone receptor in castrated guinea pig uterus. Maximum approximately 1 day after injection of estradiol (E_2). The negative effects of protein and RNA synthesis inhibitors (Cy and Ad) are shown. The prolonged apparent disappearance of the receptor (half-life 5 days) is shown on the right panel and would not account for the physiological decrease of the receptor observed during the cycle between days 0 and 4. **C:** Progesterone injected when R is maximum (as in **B**) accelerates the decay of the receptor and therefore may be implicated in its physiological control.

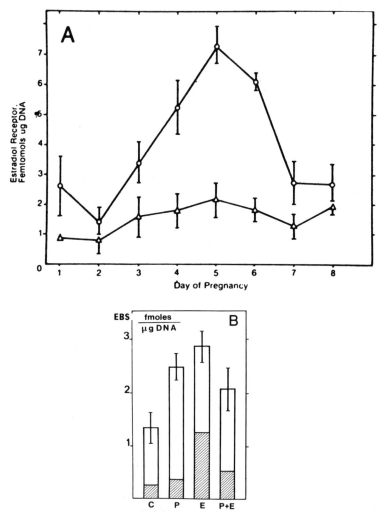

FIG. 4. Changes and hormonal control of estradiol receptor in rat uterus during early pregnancy. **A:** Concentration of endometrium (top line) and myometrium (bottom line) estradiol receptor during early pregnancy. **B:** Estradiol receptor in castrated rats' endometrium *(open bars)* and myometrium *(hatched bars)* in control animals and after various hormonal regimens. It can be observed that (a) estradiol (E) increases receptor in both endometrium and myometrium; (b) progesterone (P) increases estradiol in endometrium but not in myometrium; (c) progesterone abolishes the estradiol-induced increase of myometrium receptor. Therefore simultaneous administration of P and E gives a picture similar to that observed during early pregnancy (3–6 days) when both hormones are increased in the plasma.

DIFFERENT RECEPTORS FOR THE SAME HORMONE IN THE SAME CELL

Incidentally, since in the previous observations it is reported that estradiol binds to both the E and A receptors, this is evidence that two different receptors can bind the same steroid, depending on the concentration: When estradiol is low, the higher-affinity E receptor is first occupied, while at higher concentration the A receptor also begins to be saturated. If the effects promoted by the E receptor-estradiol and A receptor-estradiol complexes are opposite, we may observe a dose-response curve rising initially with increasing concentrations, until values at which the A receptor-estradiol complexes become operative and invert the slope, reproducing a well-known pattern of pharmacological response not well explained until now.

It was also remarked that diethylstilbestrol (DES), a nonsteroidal estrogen, binds to the E receptor in a similar fashion as to the estradiol itself, while its interaction with the A receptor is very weak. DES has been noted to be a perfect estrogen when its activity has been tested on the uterus; it is also a widely used compound in cancer therapy (40). Indeed the reported observation suggests that one can dissociate estradiol and DES effects: While the presence of the E and A receptors binding estradiol can explain a change of slope when estradiol concentration increases, the binding of DES by the E receptor alone leads to the prediction that this change of slope will not be seen with DES.

NEW THERAPEUTIC APPROACHES: RECEPTORS AND RECEPTIVITY, DISSOCIATION OF EFFECTS, AGONISM AND ANTAGONISM

From the above data, it follows that one can re-examine now, on biophysical grounds instead of on the basis of global observations, a series of pharmacological concepts of primary therapeutic importance. Receptivity to a given hormone may indeed depend on the amount of the corresponding receptor in target cells. The nonresponse of secondary sex organs to testosterone in the testicular feminizing syndrome (41), or in lymphoma cell mutants resistant to corticosteroids (42), are interesting examples, since no receptor is found in these tissues. There are also good correlations between the hormonal response of breast cancer and the estradiol receptor content (43) and of lymphoblastic leukemia and corticosteroid receptors (44), results which are of obvious theoretical and practical interest. Whether subtle pharmacological manipulations will be of therapeutic and practical interest, as proposed above in the case of contraception, remains to be demonstrated.

The induction of steroid receptor by steroid hormones is of great value for explaining "priming," a sort of synergism acquired over a well-defined time sequence. The negative influence of steroid on receptor induction (26) is one way to explain certain antagonisms between hormones, other possibilities being the simultaneous presence of different receptors (39) or their competition for the same receptor (45).

Finally, one can dissociate responses ordinarily (physiologically) linked by the very nature of a natural circulating hormone. We have seen that testosterone effects are mediated by different steroidal products in target cells, and that all estradiol effects may not be shared by the synthetic DES. These results may lead to new therapeutic advances.

Regulatory proteins, the steroid hormone receptors, provide some of the most advanced models for rational physicochemical and physiological approaches of pharmacological and therapeutic problems. Their purification and complete characterization will undoubtedly lead to even more progress in clinical medicine.

ACKNOWLEDGMENT

From many references, it is clear that I am indebted to my colleagues for their collaboration. The work has been supported partially by the Ford Foundation and the Délégation Générale à la Recherche Scientifique et Technique. I thank Dr. R. Sutherland for help in writing this manuscript.

REFERENCES

1. Baulieu, E. E. (1973): A 1972 survey of the mode of action of steroid hormones. In: *Proceedings of the 4th International Congress of Endocrinology*, edited by R. O. Scow, pp. 30–62. Excerpta Medica, Amsterdam.
2. Jensen, E. V., and Jacobson, H. I. (1962): Basic guides to the mechanism of estrogen action. *Recent Progr. Horm. Res.*, 18:387–314.
3. Glasscock, R. F., and Hoekstra, W. G. (1959): Selective accumulation of tritium-labelled hexoestrol by the reproductive organs of immature female goats and sheep. *Biochem. J.*, 72:673.
4. Jensen, E. V., Suzuki, T., Kawashima, T., Stumpf, W. E., Jungblut, P. W., and De Sombre, E. E. (1968): A two-step mechanism for the interaction of oestradiol with the rat uterus. *Proc. Natl. Acad. Sci. U.S.A.*, 59:632–638.
5. Toft, D., and Gorski, J. (1966): A receptor molecule for estrogens: Isolation from the rat uterus and preliminary characterization. *Proc. Natl. Acad. Sci. U.S.A.*, 55:1574–1581.
5a. Toft, D., Shyamala, G., and Gorski, J. (1967): A receptor molecule for estrogens: Studies using a cell free system. *Proc. Natl. Acad. Sci. U.S.A.*, 57:1740–1743.
6. Gorski, J., Toft, D., Shyamala, G., Smith, D., and Notides, A. (1968): Hormone receptors: Studies on the interaction of estrogen with the uterus. *Recent Progr. Horm. Res.*, 24:45–80.
7. Talwar, G. P., Segal, S. J., Evans, A., and Davidson, O. W. (1964): The binding of estradiol in the uterus: A mechanism for derepression of RNA synthesis. *Proc. Natl. Acad. Sci. U.S.A.*, 52:1059–1066.
8. Alberga, A., and Baulieu, E. E. (1965): Concentration élective de l'oestradiol dans l'endomètre chez la ratte. *C. R. Acad. Sci. Paris*, 261:5226–5228.
9. Baulieu, E. E., Alberga, A., and Jung, I. (1967): Récepteurs hormonaux: Liaison spécifique de l'oestradiol à des protéines utérines. *C. R. Acad. Sci. Paris*, 265:354–357.
10. Baulieu, E. E., Alberga, A., Jung, I., Lebeau, M. C., Mercier-Bodard, C., Milgrom, E., Raynaud, J. P., Raynaud-Jammet, C., Rochefort, H., Truong, H., and Robel, P. (1971): Metabolism and protein binding of sex steroids in target organs: An approach to the mechanism of hormone action. *Recent Prog. Horm. Res.*, 27:351–419.
11. Raspé, G., editor (1971): *Advances in the Biosciences*, Vol. 7. Pergamon Press-Vieweg, Oxford.
12. Milgrom, E., Atger, M., and Baulieu, E. E. (1973): Studies on estrogen entry into uterine cells and on estradiol-receptor complex attachment to the nucleus: Is the entry of estrogen into uterine cells a protein-mediated process? *Biochim. Biophys. Acta*, 320:267–283.
13. Milgrom, E., Atger, M., and Baulieu, E. E. (1973): Acidophilic activation of steroid hormone receptors. *Biochemistry*, 12:5198–5205.
14. Fanestil, D. D., and Edelman, I. S. (1966): Characteristics of the renal nuclear receptors for aldosterone. *Proc. Natl. Acad. Sci. U.S.A.*, 56:872–879.
15. Rochefort, H., and Baulieu, E. E. (1968): Récepteurs hormonaux: Relations entre les "récepteurs" utérins de l'oestradiol, "8 S" cytoplasmique et "4 S" cytoplasmique et nucléaire. *C. R. Acad. Sci. Paris*, 267:662–665.
16. Raynaud-Jammet, C., and Baulieu, E. E. (1969): Action de l'oestradiol in vitro: augmentation de la biosynthèse d'ARN dans les noyaux utérins. *C. R. Acad. Sci. Paris*, 268:3211–3214.
17. Mohla, S., DeSombre, E. R., and Jensen, E. V. (1972): Tissue-specific stimulation of RNA synthesis by transformed estradiol-receptor complex. *Biochem. Biophys. Res. Commun.*, 46:661–667.

18. Baulieu, E. E., Alberga, A., Raynaud-Jammet, C., and Wira, C. R. (1972): New look at the very early steps of oestrogen action in uterus. *Nature [New Biol.]*, 236:236–239.

19. Milgrom, E., and Baulieu, E. E. (1970): Progesterone in the uterus and the plasma. II. The role of hormone availability and metabolism on selective binding to uterus protein. *Biochem. Biophys. Res. Commun.*, 40:723–730.

20. Anderson, J., Clark, J. H., and Peck, E. J. (1972): Oestrogen and nuclear binding sites: Determination of specific sites by ³H-oestradiol exchanges. *Biochem. J.*, 126:561–567.

21. Milgrom, E., Atger, M., Perrot, M., and Baulieu, E. E. (1972): Progesterone in uterus and plasma. VI. Uterine progesterone receptors during the estrus cycle and implantation in the guinea pig. *Endocrinology*, 90:1071–1078.

22. Milgrom, E., Luu Thi, M., Atger, M., and Baulieu, E. E. (1973): Mechanisms regulating the concentration and the conformation of progesterone receptor(s) in the uterus. *J. Biol. Chem.*, 248:6366–6374.

23. Deanesly, R. (1960): Implantation and early pregnancy in ovariectomized guinea-pigs. *J. Reprod. Fertil.*, 1:242–248.

24. Courrier, R. (1950): Interactions between estradiol and progesterone. *Vitam. and Horm.*, 8:197.

25. Baulieu, E. E. (1976): Antiprogesterone effect and mid-cycle (periovulatory) contraception. *(In preparation.)*

26. Mester, J., Martel, D., Psychoyos, A., and Baulieu, E. E. (1974): Hormonal control of oestrogen receptor in uterus and receptivity for ovoimplantation in the rat. *Nature (Lond.)*, 250:776–778.

27. Psychoyos, A. (1973): Hormonal control of ovoimplantation. *Vitam. Horm.*, 31:201–256.

28. Baudouin-Legros, M., Meyer, P., and Worcel, M. (1974): Effects of prostaglandin inhibitors on angiotensin, oxytocin and prostaglandin F$_{2\alpha}$ contractile effects on the rat uterus during the oestrous cycle. *Br. J. Pharmacol.* (in press).

29. Clark, J. H., and Gorski, J. (1970): Ontogeny of the estrogen receptor during early uterine development. *Science*, 169:76–78.

30. Michel, G., Jung, I., and Baulieu, E. E., Aussel, C., and Uriél, J. (1974): Two high affinity estrogen binding proteins of different specificity in the immature rat uterus cytosol. *Steroids*, 24:437–449.

31. Gavin, J. R., Roth, J., Neville, D. M., De Meyts, P., and Buell, D. N. (1974): Insulin-dependent regulation of insulin receptor concentrations: A direct demonstration in cell culture. *Proc. Natl. Acad. Sci. U.S.A.*, 71:84–88.

32. Jung, I., and Baulieu, E. E. (1972): Testosterone cytosol receptor in the rat levator ani muscle. *Nature [New Biol.]*, 237:24–26.

33. Michel, G., and Baulieu, E. E. (1974): Récepteur cytosoluble des androgènes dans un muscle strié squelettique. *C. R. Acad. Sci. Paris*, 279:421–424.

34. Bullock, L. P., and Bardin, C. W. (1974): Androgen receptors in mouse kidney: A study of male, female and androgen-insensitive (tfm/y) mice. *Endocrinology*, 94:746–756.

35. Bruchovsky, N., and Wilson, J. D. (1968): The conversion of testosterone to 5α-androstan-17β-ol-3-one by rat prostate in vivo and in vitro. *J. Biol. Chem.*, 243:2012–2021.

36. Anderson, K. M., and Liao, S. (1968): Selective retention of dihydrotestosterone by prostatic nuclei. *Nature (Lond.)*, 219:277–279.

37. Baulieu, E. E., Lasnitzki, I., and Robel, P. (1968): Metabolism of testosterone and action of metabolites on prostate glands grown in organ culture. *Nature (Lond.)*, 219:1155–1156.

38. Naftolin, F., Ryan, K. J., Davies, I. J., Reddy, V. V., Flores, F., Petro, Z., Kuhn, M., White, R. J., Takaoka, Y., and Wolin, L. (1975): The formation of estrogens by central neuroendocrine tissues. *Recent Prog. Horm. Res.*, 31:295–319.

39. Jung-Testas, I., and Baulieu, E. E. (1974): Plusieurs récepteurs par cellule pour la même et pour différentes hormones stéroides: Conséquences pharmacologiques possibles. *C. R. Acad. Sci. Paris*, 279:671–674.

40. Huggins, C., (1967): Endocrine-induced regression of cancers. *Science*, 156:1050–1054.

41. Bullock, L. P., and Bardin, C. W. (1972): Androgen receptors in testicular feminization. *J. Clin. Endocrinol. Metab.*, 35:935–937.

42. Sibley, C. H., and Tomkins, G. M. (1974): Mechanisms of steroid resistance. *Cell*, 2:221–227.

43. Jensen, E. V., Block, G. E., Smith, S., Kyser, K., and De Sombre, E. R. (1971): Estrogen receptors and breast cancer response to adrenalectomy: Prediction of response in cancer therapy. *Natl. Cancer Inst. Monogr.*, 34:55–70.

44. Lippman, M. E., Halterman, R. H., Leventhal, B. G., Perry, S., and Thompson, E. B. (1973):

Glucocorticoid binding proteins in human acute lymphoblastic leukemic blast cells. *J. Clin. Invest.*, 52:1715–1725.

45. Geynet, C., Millet, C., Truong, H., and Baulieu, E. E. (1972): Estrogens and antiestrogens. *Gynecol. Invest.*, 3:2–29.

Breast Cancer: Trends in Research and Treatment, edited by J. C. Heuson,
W. H. Mattheiem, and M. Rozencweig. Raven Press, New York © 1976.

A Biochemical Basis for Selecting Endocrine Therapy in Human Breast Cancer

W. L. McGuire, K. B. Horwitz, and M. De La Garza

University of Texas Health Science Center, San Antonio, Texas 78284

The human mammary gland is exquisitely sensitive to a number of hormones, and one would predict that tumors arising by malignant transformation of mammary gland cells retain these hormone controls. Indeed regression of metastatic breast cancer in response to ovariectomy was first demonstrated 78 years ago (1). Unfortunately only 30% of such metastatic tumors are responsive, and they usually respond equally well to adrenalectomy or hypophysectomy (2). Since little is known of the complex hormonal interrelationships involved in tumor growth, tumors are classified simply as "hormone-dependent."

Target tissues for any hormone contain specific receptors for that hormone—cytoplasmic proteins for the steroids and surface membrane molecules for polypeptides and some others. Hormone-dependent tumors also contain receptors, but it now appears that independent, or autonomous, tumors often may not (3). These findings, which are discussed in detail, have led to the following hypothesis:

1. Normal mammary cells contain cytoplasmic or membrane receptor sites for each of the hormones known to influence the growth and function of the mammary gland. These receptor sites are responsible for the initial interaction between the hormone and the cell, and trigger the biochemical events characteristic for the particular hormone.

2. When malignant transformation occurs, the cell may retain all or part of the normal population of receptor sites. If the malignant cell retains receptors, its growth and function are potentially capable of being regulated by the hormonal environment, as in a normal cell, and such tumors would be responsive to endocrine therapy.

3. If specific receptors are lost from the tumor, this may indicate that the tumor is endocrine-resistant and so would be unresponsive to endocrine manipulation.

Only estrogen receptors have thus far been studied with respect to this hypothesis. The preferential uptake of radioactive estrogen by target tissues and endocrine-responsive tumors was demonstrated *in vivo* and *in vitro* during the years following 1959; endocrine-resistant tumors were less active (4–10). The discovery of the specific receptor for estrogen in these responsive tissues explained the preferential uptake of the hormone and also suggested that tumors could be assayed for receptor to predict hormone dependence.

ESTROGEN RECEPTOR IN HUMAN BREAST TUMORS

The properties of the estrogen receptor (ER), as determined in induced hormone-dependent rat tumors, have now been found in human mammary tumor cytosols as well (11). Two of these properties are employed in our laboratory to quantitate ER in human breast cancer specimens obtained at surgery (12,13). The first is the high-affinity binding of ^{3}H-estradiol, evaluated by equilibrating cytosol with various low concentrations of labeled hormone and then removing the unbound hormone with dextran-coated charcoal. Scatchard plots of the binding data show that the receptor, if present, has a very-high-affinity binding component ($Kd < 1 \times 10^{-10}$M). The amount of this component can be determined by direct extrapolation. The second property—sedimentation of receptor primarily at 8S in low-salt sucrose gradients—is employed to confirm the results of the charcoal assay by an independent method. Because part of the 4S binding peak may also be due to specific receptor, a parallel gradient is always run with a 100-fold excess of unlabeled diethylstilbestrol to measure any nonspecific binding components.

With these techniques we are in a position to explore Jensen's original suggestion that the presence of ER in a human breast tumor might indicate that the tumor was hormone-dependent and could be made to regress by appropriate endocrine manipulation (6). To date our laboratory has assayed ER in 700 human breast tumors for eventual correlation with response to endocrine therapy (14).

We find that the values in primary tumors range from 0 to approximately 1,000 femtomoles (fmoles)/mg cytosol protein. (The level of sensitivity in the two methods is such that a value of less than 3 fmoles/mg is essentially equivalent to 0 and is considered a negative assay.) Positive ER values ($\geq$ 3 fmoles) are found in 70% of primary specimens and 58% of metastatic specimens. We previously speculated that the wide range of values apparent in our results are due to a combination of factors, including: (a) variations in epithelial versus stromal content of the tumors; (b) the degree of dedifferentiation of the tumor; and (c) the patient's endogenous estrogen levels (since endogenous estradiol would occupy ER sites and make them unavailable for assay). This last point may at least partially explain why the highest values for tumor ER are seen in postmenopausal patients.

CLINICAL CORRELATION

A number of other laboratories (using a variety of techniques) have also assayed ER in breast tumor specimens. Data on clinical response to endocrine therapy is now available in many of these cases. To correlate these data, an international workshop sponsored by the Breast Cancer Task Force of the National Cancer Institute was held in Bethesda, Maryland, on July 18–19, 1974. Details of both ER assay procedures and clinical evaluation criteria were examined, and 436 treatment trials in 380 patients were ultimately accepted. We provide here a brief overview of the data presented at that meeting, indicating the current status of ER assays in predicting response to endocrine therapies in patients with metastatic breast cancer. For details the reader should consult the specific manuscripts and summary chapter published in the conference proceedings (15).

Response to Endocrine Therapy

1. *Extramural review*—Since the organizing committee for this conference felt that clinical response data were as critical as the ER assay data, it was arranged that participating institutions could request an extramural review of their case material. Prior to the conference, eight institutions were visited by two oncologists (Mary E. Sears and George C. Escher), and a total of 531 treatment trials in 453 patients were reviewed by the following criteria.

Objective remission was defined as a decrease in size of at least 50% of the measurable lesions by more than 50% while other lesions remained unchanged and no new lesions appeared. As the standard basis for determining the size of a lesion, the product of the two longest perpendicular diameters of the lesion was used. In osteolytic metastasis evidence of healing on roentgenography was necessary, again without increase in size or number of destructive lesions. Osteoblastic metastasis as the only measurable lesion was not an acceptable criterion for the study. In cases with multiple skin lesions, which often are impossible to measure accurately, photographs served as the means for evaluation of response. Neither the healing of an ulcerating lesion nor the clearing of pleural effusion was accepted as objective evidence of remission. Complete agreement between the investigators' and the reviewers' evaluations was attained in 442 of the 531 reviewed treatment trials. There were only 17 instances of total disagreement, but in a relatively large number (72) the intramural evaluation could not be supported because of inadequate documentation.

2. *Clinical correlation of ER and response to endocrine therapy*—The 436 treatment trials in 380 patients evaluated by the extramural review team are summarized in Table 1.

Surgical Ablation (Castration, Adrenalectomy, Hypophysectomy)

Thirty-three percent of 211 treatment trials resulted in objective tumor regressions. Only 8 (8%) of the 94 trials in patients with negative tumor ER values were successful, whereas 59 (55%) of the 107 trials in patients with positive tumor ER values succeeded. Patients with borderline tumor ER values had a 30% response rate.

TABLE 1. *Objective breast tumor regressions according to ER assay and type of therapy as judged by extramural review*

Therapy	ER+	ER–	ER±
Adrenalectomy	32/66	4/33	3/8
Castration	25/33	4/53	0/2
Hypophysectomy	2/8	0/8	—
Total	59/107 (55%)	8/94 (8%)	3/10 (30%)
Androgen	12/26	2/24	0/1
Estrogen	37/57	5/58	0/2
Glucocorticoid	2/2	—	—
Total	51/85 (60%)	7/82 (8%)	0/3 (0%)
Antiestrogens	8/20	5/27	—
Other	2/3	0/5	—
Total	10/23 (43%)	5/32 (16%)	—

Adapted from McGuire et al., ref. 15.

Additive Therapy (Pharmacological Doses of Estrogens, Androgens, and Glucocorticoids)

Thirty-four percent of 170 trials resulted in objective tumor regressions. Seven (8%) of the 82 trials in patients with negative tumor ER values were successful, whereas 51 (60%) of the 85 trials in patients with positive tumor ER values succeeded.

Miscellaneous Therapy

Twenty-seven percent of 55 trials resulted in responses to a variety of endocrine therapies, including antiestrogens, aminoglutethimide, etc. Five (16%) of 32 trials in patients with negative tumor ER values were successful, whereas 10 (43%) of 23 trials in patients with positive ER values succeeded.

Comment

There remains little doubt that estrogen receptor values can be helpful in predicting the results of endocrine therapy for metastatic breast cancer. It is clear that if a patient has a negative tumor ER value the chances of tumor regression in response to endocrine therapy are minimal. A large number of patients can thus be spared unrewarding major endocrine ablative therapy if ER assays are performed routinely. When the tumor ER value is positive, the response to endocrine therapy is 55-60%. This single piece of evidence—coupled with available clinical prognostic factors such as menopausal status, disease-free interval, site of dominant lesion, and especially response to previous hormonal therapies—should permit the practicing oncologist to select or reject endocrine therapy with relative confidence. Our concern now is to identify the 40% of ER-positive tumors that have lost their hormone dependence, so that these patients can be spared unrewarding therapies.

Progesterone Receptors in Human Breast Cancer

The presence of ER in malignant cells is evidence that at least part of the normal control system remains intact. However, since binding to receptors is only an early step in hormone action, it is possible that in ER-positive tumors where endocrine manipulations fail the lesion is at a later stage. An ideal marker of an endocrine-responsive tumor would therefore be a measurable product of hormone action rather than the initial binding step. Because in estrogen target tissues the synthesis of progesterone receptor (PgR) depends on the action of estrogen, we investigated the possibility that PgR might be such a marker (16). If so, PgR would be rare in tumors that lack ER. The presence of PgR in tumors containing ER indicate that the tumors are capable of synthesizing at least one endproduct under estrogen regulation, and that the tumors remain endocrine-responsive. Tumors with ER but no PgR would be resistant to endocrine therapy.

We used 8S binding of the synthetic progestin ^{3}H-R5020 (Roussel UCLAF) in sucrose gradients to identify PgR in human breast cancer tissue, rather than resort to indirect differential competition studies. Excess nonradioactive progesterone or R5020 completely inhibits the 8S ^{3}H-R5020 binding, whereas hydrocortisone, dexamethasone, or estradiol do not compete effectively (17). We have now determined the presence or absence of PgR and ER in more than 200 human mammary tumors. PgR is present in only 8% of the tumors lacking ER. Of the ER-positive tumors, 62% had PgR. This distribution is similar to the response rate to endocrine therapies for ER-positive and ER-negative tumors and is consistent with the hypothesis that PgR may be a marker for hormone dependence. Of course confirmation of this hypothesis requires direct correlation of the presence of PgR with objectively defined clinical remission. Our preliminary clinical data are encouraging (18). If further clinical correlations support our hypothesis, the presence of PgR will show that at least part of the hormone response system is functional, thus providing a more accurate marker of hormone dependence.

SUMMARY

In estrogen target tissues and hormone-dependent tumors, the steroid enters the cells and binds to a cytoplasmic protein called the estrogen receptor. The steroid-receptor complex then migrates to the nuclei, where it initiates the biochemical events characteristic of estrogen stimulation. Since ER is absent in tissues not responsive to estrogen, studies have been designed to show whether ER in human breast cancer tissue might be used to identify those patients likely to respond to endocrine therapy.

Data on 436 clinical trials contributed from a dozen centers around the world now clearly indicate that if a patient's tumor does not contain ER there is virtually no chance of tumor regression following endocrine therapy. When their tumors have ER, 55–60% of patients respond to endocrine therapy, so that this single piece of data—coupled with available clinical prognostic factors such as menopausal status, disease-free interval, site of the dominant lesion, and especially response to previous hormonal therapies—should permit the practicing oncologist to select or reject endocrine therapy with confidence. If our hypothesis involving the use of PgR as a marker of endocrine responsive tumors is supported, then the 40% of ER-positive tumors that are endocrine-resistant will also be identifiable, and a large number of patients will be spared unrewarding therapies.

ACKNOWLEDGMENTS

These studies were supported in part by the U. S. Public Health Service (CA-11378 and CB-23862) and the American Cancer Society (BC-23D). We thank Dr. J. P. Raynaud and Roussel UCLAF for the generous gift of R5020, and Dennis Perotta for his expert technical assistance.

REFERENCES

1. Beatson, G. T. (1896): On the treatment of inoperable cases of carcinoma of the mamma—suggestions for a new method of treatment, with illustrative cases. *Lancet,* 2:104–107, 162–165.
2. Dao, T. L. (1972): Ablation therapy for hormone dependent tumors. *Annu. Rev. Med.,* 23:1–18.
3. McGuire, W. L., Chamness, G. C., Costlow, M. E., and Shepherd, R. E. (1974). Hormone dependence in breast cancer. *Metabolism,* 23:75–100.
4. Folca, P. J., Glascock, R. F., and Irvine, W. T. (1961): Studies with tritium-labelled hexoestrol in advanced breast cancer. *Lancet,* 2:796–798.
5. Glascock, R. F., and Hoekstra, W. G. (1959): Selective accumulation of tritium-labelled hexoestrol by the reproductive organs of immature female goats and sheep. *Biochem. J.,* 72:673–682.
6. Jensen, E. V., DeSombre, E. R., and Jungblut, P. W. (1967): Estrogen receptors in hormone responsive tissues and tumors. In: *Endogenous Factors Influencing Host-Tumor Balance,* edited by R. W. Wissler, T. L. Dao, and S. Wood, Jr., pp. 15–30. University of Chicago Press, Chicago.
7. Jensen, E. V., and Jacobson, H. I. (1960): Fate of steroid estrogens in target tissues. In: *Biological Activities of Steroids in Relation to Cancer,* edited by G. Pincus and E. P. Vollmer, pp. 161–174. Academic Press, New York.
8. King, R. J. B., Gordon, J., Cowan, D. M., and Inman, D. R. (1966): The intranuclear localization of $(6,7,^3H)$-oestradiol-17 β in dimethylbenzanthracene induced rat mammary adenocarcinoma and other tissues. *J. Endocrinol.,* 36:139–150.
9. Mobbs, B. G. (1966): The uptake of tritiated oestradiol by dimethylbenzanthracene induced mammary tumours of the rat. *J. Endocrinol.,* 36:409–414.
10. Terenius, L. (1968): Selective retention of estrogen isomers in estrogen-dependent breast tumours of rats demonstrated by in vitro methods. *Cancer Res.,* 28:328–337.
11. McGuire, W. L., and De La Garza, M. (1973): Similarity of the estrogen receptor in human and rat mammary carcinoma. *J. Clin. Endocrinol. Metab.,* 36:548–552.
12. McGuire, W. L. (1973): Estrogen receptors in human breast cancer. *J. Clin. Invest.,* 52:73–77.
13. McGuire, W. L., and De La Garza, M. (1973): Improved sensitivity in the measurement of estrogen receptor in human breast cancer. *J. Clin. Endocrinol. Metab.,* 37:986–989.
14. McGuire, W. L., Pearson, O. H., and Segaloff, A. (1975): Predicting hormone responsiveness in human breast cancer. In: *Estrogen Receptor in Human Breast Cancer,* edited by W. L. McGuire, P. P. Carbone, and E. P. Vollmer, pp. 17–30. Raven Press, New York.
15. McGuire, W. L., Carbone, P. P., Sears, M. E., and Escher, G. C. (1975): Estrogen receptors in human breast cancer: an overview. In: *Estrogen Receptor in Human Breast Cancer,* edited by W. L. McGuire, P. P. Carbone, and E. P. Vollmer, pp. 1–7. Raven Press, New York.
16. McGuire, W. L., Chamness, G. C., Costlow, M. E., and Horwitz, K. B. (1976): Hormone receptors in breast cancer. In: *Modern Pharmacology,* edited by G. S. Levey. Marcel Dekker, New York (*in press*).
17. Horwitz, K. B., and McGuire, W. L. (1975): Specific progesterone receptors in human breast cancer. *Steroids,* 25:497.
18. Horwitz, K. B., McGuire, W. L., Pearson, O. H., and Segaloff, A. (1975): Predicting response

to endocrine therapy in human breast cancer: A hypothesis. *Science,* 189:726.

DISCUSSION

Anonymous: Is there any explanation for the significant change in receptor count between pre- and postmenopausal patients?

McGuire: Yes, we now know that postmenopausal patients have a higher estrogen receptor level than premenopausal patients. There may be many reasons for this, but at least one is the secretion of estrogen by the premenopausal patients and consequent occupation of receptor sites.

King: In relation to the analysis of estrogen receptors, we are getting approximately 80% positive results for the primaries and 60% for secondaries, which seems to be a fairly common experience. Using that as a predictive indicator for subsequent metastases gives a 20% difference, which is presumably positives going negative. Is this a real problem?

McGuire: In individual cases it could well be a problem. In the majority of cases, though, if the primary tumor is positive, the metastases will also be positive. Furthermore, if you can simultaneously measure several metastases, most will either be positive or negative. However, everyone has seen the positive primary tumor and negative metastases—and, in the same patient, two metastases that are different.

Juret: Why does the free interval in your studies correlate with estrogen receptor while many other studies disagree?

McGuire: My estrogen receptor data do correlate with free interval. What I was reporting was the combined experience of many institutions where that particular factor was examined, and the majority said that in their data it did not correlate. I have no explanation for this discrepancy.

Hayward: You indicated that one might be able to sharpen the prediction rate in positive cases by using dominant lesion-free interval and response to previous treatment. Have you in fact any evidence that this does sharpen prediction?

McGuire: Yes and no. With regard to the 381 patients reviewed by extramural reviewers, the data for dominant site, free interval, menopausal status, and estrogen receptor have now just been entered into a computer to sort out the role of each of those variables; we are then going to grade them according to response. The biostatisticians say the preliminary results are very interesting, and I think that within a month the people who contributed the data will receive some sort of an answer.

Carbone: If I remember rightly, the disease-free correlation was a measurement of many primary tumors in which the time to first recurrence did not correlate necessarily with the estrogen receptor. I am not sure that the receptor assay correlations would respond to the disease-free interval, since not all those patients were treated. There might be other answers.

Heuson: The free interval correlates very strongly with the presence or absence of invaded axillary nodes and there is no correlation whatsoever with the presence of estrogen receptor or receptor concentration in the primary, and presence or absence of invaded axillary nodes. It is therefore unlikely that estrogen receptors could be of any prognostic value in terms of free interval.

Powles: From a clinical point of view, is there any evidence that measuring estrogen binding improves the total time of remission or survival in patients with established metastatic disease? If not, is there a trial under way to test this?

McGuire Not that I know of, but the object here is not to look for a more effective endocrine therapy but for more effective timing perhaps, or selection—to use or not to use endocrine therapy. I hope my data are not misinterpreted as improving current therapies; they hopefully improve our decision when and if to use them. So the answer is no, we would not expect any survival data changes.

Powles: However, if you were using your treatment more optimally you would expect to get either longer or better remissions in patients with established disease, or longer survivors.

McGuire: That is the goal, of course. We know when to use cytotoxic agents, endocrine agents; and we do not expose patients to unnecessary risks and side effects, so in general I agree with you, but that specific information is not available.

Breast Cancer: Trends in Research and Treatment, edited by J. C. Heuson,
W. H. Mattheiem, and M. Rozencweig. Raven Press, New York © 1976.

Roundtable Discussion: Endocrine Aspects

Chairman: R. D. Bulbrook

Engelsman: I shall present a few data on the correlation between clinical response to treatment with estrogens or by castration in premenopausal women with advanced breast cancer, and the presence or absence of both estrogen and androgen receptors. First, the presence of estrogen receptor correlates very well to clinical response in patients treated with estrogens. The presence of androgen receptors in the same patients does not, or almost does not, predict response to estrogen treatment. With androgen treatment there is some correlation with estrogen receptor presence and with the presence of androgen receptors. What was surprising was that the response to castration in premenopausal women seems to correlate with the presence of androgen receptors. That is, in this series there were only four patients who responded to castration, and all four had androgen receptors in their tumors; of the patients who had no androgen receptors, no one responded. These numbers are small, but statistically the differences were very significant. If you look at the tumors which had both receptors present, there was an overall remission rate of 75%. With the tumors in which only estrogen receptors were present (and androgen receptors were absent), there was a remission rate of 56%. In the group without estrogen receptors but with androgen receptors, we still found a remission rate of 44%. Where no receptors at all could be found, there was a remission rate of only 8%.

This material I think suggests that to improve the correlation between receptor determinations and the chance of obtaining a remission by endocrine treatment you can do somewhat better if you also look at the presence or absence of androgen receptors.

Leclercq: Dr. Baulieu presented some data suggesting a correlation between progesterone receptors and estradiol receptors in the human uterus, which is true. We have now measured the amount of both estradiol and progesterone receptors in a series of human breast tumors to see if there was any correlation. Both receptors were measured by the well-known Scatchard plot technique using charcoal and dextran extraction. Estradiol receptor was evaluated using tritiated estradiol, and progesterone receptor using the Roussel compound R5020.

Most primary tumors were positive for estradiol receptor; there was no tumor containing progesterone receptors and lacking estradiol receptors. Finally, in the tumors positive for both receptors, there was no correlation between the levels of these receptors, unlike in the uterus. The same study in a group of metastatic breast cancer samples also showed no correlation. Apparently then, there is a difference between human breast cancer and human uterine cancer. We have also observed that there was a significant correlation between concentration of estradiol receptor in a given tumor and response to endocrine treatment in patients with advanced breast cancer. As there is no apparent correlation between the amounts of progesterone receptor and estradiol receptor, there should not be a relationship between the amount of progesterone receptor and the response to endocrine treatment, but it is too early yet to make any definite statement.

Anonymous: We have been told about three types of receptors in breast cancer cells, but would it not be more logical to speak about the amount of estrogen bound to these receptors?

McGuire: Most people do not find a correlation with the number of cytoplasmic binding sites and response. The question is really: Could all the sites in the cytoplasm be occupied in a premenopausal patient, and the test be negative, when in fact the tumor might contain receptor? Several people have developed and published assays now that could easily measure total cytoplasmic receptor, but if the receptor is occupied endogenously the receptor will migrate into the nucleus. What we need is a better assay of nuclear-bound receptor, and I have yet to see one that I think is satisfactory, although I know that many investigators including ourselves are working on this problem.

Breast Cancer: Trends in Research and Treatment, edited by J. C. Heuson,
W. H. Mattheiem, and M. Rozencweig. Raven Press, New York © 1976.

Role of Hormones in the Modern Treatment of Advanced Breast Cancer

Henri J. Tagnon

Service de Médecine Interne et Laboratoires d' Investigation Clinique,
Institut Jules Bordet, Brussels, Belgium

Hormonal treatment of breast cancer can no longer be used alone and should be considered in the general perspective of a resolute attempt to utilize all existing biological and pharmacological information available for the improvement of patient care. This is not a complete review of the subject but rather a chapter in the nomenclature and critical evaluation of methods of treatment now available to "task forces" with ambitious therapeutic aims. Recent progress in the treatment of Hodgkin's disease, leukemia, osteogenic sarcoma, etc. provided the encouragement for a renewed and concerted attack on breast cancer, a disease which affects 1 of every 20 women and has a mortality of probably over 75%, a rate that has remained practically unchanged during the last 50 years.

While primary breast cancer has traditionally been treated by surgical or roentgenological methods, the treatment of advanced breast cancer up to a few years ago was largely the responsibility of endocrinologists, especially the steroid endocrinologist. Administration of hormones 30 years ago represented one of the first really successful attempts at chemotherapy of a solid tumor. It is not surprising that much enthusiasm was generated by these early successful therapeutic trials, and that intensive research, continuing into the current period, took place on the endocrine control of breast tissue growth. However, in recent years the role of hormonal manipulation in the treatment of breast cancer has decreased comparatively in importance. The most recent clinical trials in our center as in others either discard hormones altogether or at best assign them limited participation in multidrug regimens comprising up to five or more chemotherapeutic agents. A current task for the clinical investigator is to find out whether such hormonal treatment, reduced as it is, is necessary and should be preserved. Although the more recently discovered and utilized antiestrogens appear to have definite advantages over other types of hormones, some think it unlikely that they will be maintained as therapeutic agents in view of the rapid progress of nonhormonal chemotherapy. (Cytotoxic chemotherapy is discussed in another chapter of this volume.) Nevertheless it is interesting to review briefly the evolution of the fundamental concepts which form the basis of the use of hormones in this disease.

Although the first regressions of breast cancer induced by administration of hormones were observed with the use of estrogens, the systematic search for active hormones was first carried out on androgenic compounds (1,2). No animal model was available for this search until rather recently, so it was based entirely on clinical observation. Around 1955-1956 the cooperative groups for breast cancer described and applied a very precise methodology for the objective evaluation of results of treatment, and we are still using practically the same criteria. A great number of androgenic compounds were tested in postmenopausal women, and few if any were found to be superior to the reference compound testosterone propionate, which gave 15–20% remissions with an average duration of 6–9 months (3,4). This modest achievement carried with it the heavy price of frightful virilization with most of these compounds, affecting nonresponders as well as responders. Nonvirilizing androgen derivatives like Δ-1-testololactone were also developed, but alone or in combination with testosterone they did not improve the response (4).

While oophorectomy produced a remission rate of approximately 30% (duration 9–15 months), the use of androgens in postmenopausal patients still produced a discouraging 20% regression rate with only a limited duration (6–9 months). Other hormonal treatments were of superior effectiveness in specific instances; for instance, high doses of estrogens for postmenopausal women were superior to androgens and were less objectionable (1). Estrogen effectiveness increased with the age of the patients and more specifically with postmenopausal age. The apparent paradox of this effect of estrogens compared with oophorectomy is probably explained by the dosage. Therapeutically used estrogens are administered in higher than physiological doses.

These unsatisfactory results stimulated investigators to explore more radical methods of hormonal treatment (5). The concept of hormone dependence is not discussed here, but it was the basis for introducing the major ablative procedures—bilateral adrenalectomy or hypophysectomy—which were the next step in the treatment of advanced breast cancer (6). The number of responders increased slightly with these procedures, but the rate still remained well under 50%. Against this definite but somewhat mediocre therapeutic gain, one had to weigh the operative risk and the inconvenience to the patient of a major endocrine imbalance during the postoperative period and the period of survival, although this could be corrected by the administration of cortisol. For all endocrine treatments, length of survival in responders is influenced by the anatomical site of the growth, the most favorable being the skin and the least favorable the visceral metastases, especially to the liver and brain.

The major inconvenience and the morbidity of these operations applied equally to nonresponders and responders. Since nonresponders comprised more than 60% of the treated patients, the use of the major ablative procedures represented imposition of a heavy burden without compensation in the form of improved health on a majority of patients in order to benefit only a relatively small number of responders. Justification for this therapeutic attitude was the lack of a better treatment and the low operative mortality when done by experienced surgeons (7).

However, there was a need for the development of predictive methods for selecting patients who respond to hormonal treatment, and this need became more pressing as improved chemotherapy with its higher percentage of responders made it more and more difficult to recommend a major operation without a guarantee of at least an even chance of improvement. Methods were proposed for such a prediction; they were based mainly on the measurement of urinary steroids or their metabolites and a mathematical treatment of the results (8). This is called the "discriminant" of Bulbrooks and Hayward. More recently, measurement of estrogen receptors directly in biopsy or surgical specimens of human breast cancer tissue has been introduced. The extensive literature on this subject is adequately reviewed in recent publications (9,10) and in other chapters in this volume. Estrogen receptors as well as other steroid receptors represent a notable advance in understanding the biochemistry and biology of breast cancer; ultimately this is bound to have an important influence on future therapeutic developments. As far as the current situation is concerned, the usefulness and clinical applications of receptor measurements in breast cancer are in the process of being evaluated; concepts are changing at a rapid rate because it now looks as if all patients, regardless of the presence or absence of receptors, should receive the same treatment. The present evolution in the treatment of cancer of the breast indicates a move away from a choice between hormonal or cytotoxic chemotherapy. This is so because while hormonal research was making progress, cytotoxic chemotherapy was also developing new concepts and possibilities. Multidrug clinical trials had shown the greatly increased effectiveness of the association of drugs. Furthermore the introduction of new and powerful drugs (e.g., CCNU, adriamycin, and others), as well as the progress of preclinical and clinical pharmacology, resulted in a dramatic increase in the effectiveness of cytotoxic chemotherapy (11). These developments are described in another chapter in this volume.

The net result is that hormonal therapy became relegated to a secondary role at the same time that methods were being developed to assure some degree of selectivity of patients. Furthermore, in at least one laboratory (Institut Jules Bordet), with improvement of the technique, receptors were found in an increasing percentage of breast cancers (albeit in variable amounts), some tumors containing many receptor sites and others only a few. During the final segment of the investigation, as many as 82% of all mammary cancers examined were found to be positive for estrogen receptors (10). This marked predominance of receptor-positive cancers appeared incompatible with a predictive usefulness of the measurement, since fewer than 40% of the patients are known to respond to hormonal manipulation. It is possible that rigorous quantitative assessment of receptor levels may result in the separation of a high-level group who always respond and a low-level group who never respond to hormonal treatment, with an intermediary group with unpredictable tumors. However, such a separation has not yet been demonstrated, and it should be noted that the concentrations of receptors in several hundred measurements represent a continuous spectrum and cannot be broken into two or even several classes. All one can say so far is that receptor-"negative" tumors do not respond to hormonal treatment. These tumors may be negative only in a relative way, and further refinement of detection methods may demonstrate that all breast tumors have some receptors. The same appears to be true for progesterone receptors, which are now also measured in breast cancer (12).

In view of the rapid development of cytotoxic chemotherapy in the treatment of breast cancer, estrogen receptor measurements—although probably representing the most accurate evaluation of the degree of hormone dependence of a tumor—may turn out to be of little practical value since treatment of advanced breast cancer no longer distinguishes between the hormonal and the cytotoxic approach. However, research on receptors remains very important because of the information provided on the essential hormonal factors at work in the genesis and maintenance of tumor growth.

Interpretation of tumor growth or regression under hormonal treatment could be expressed in the following concepts or hypotheses, based on the results of estrogen receptor measurements in humans: For the clinician, a tumor regresses when its volume decreases by a certain percentage (usually 50%), expressed in centimeters and millimeters; it is known that a 50% regression of a tumor mass may require a higher than 90% cell kill. Under these conditions it may well be that only the tumors containing an excess of receptors above a certain threshold will show a measurable decrease in size under hormonal therapy, corresponding to a number of killed cells sufficient to produce a visible decrease in size. These tumors are the "hormone-dependent" tumors of the clinician. In those lesions having a lower concentration of receptors, the number of killed cells under hormonal treatment could be insufficient to produce a measurable reduction in the size of the tumor. These tumors would be "hormone-independent." Actually, it is quite probable that all breast tumors are hormone-dependent for a fraction of their cells and hormone-independent for the rest. This concept explains the extreme rarity of complete (even if temporary) regression of all lesions with hormonal treatment. Another implication of this concept is that certain hormonal treatments may do some good despite the lack of measurable effects on the tumor.

It was well known that the steroid dependence of mammary cancer when clinically recognizable was always relative in the sense that regression under steroid treatment or after an ablative procedure was never complete and was of limited duration. The survey of estrogen receptors seems to reveal the biological basis for these clinical observations. Mammary cancer may tentatively be considered as essentially heterogeneous as far as receptors are concerned. It contains a variable number of receptor-negative cells, and these very likely are present in all cases and are not influenced by hormonal treatment. They probably constitute the starting point of the recurrence after hormonal treatment and the appearance of hormone-resistant tumor. This concept accounts for the narrow limitations of hormone therapy and the absolute necessity of adding cytotoxic agents to any hormonal treatment because it is certain to be incomplete if given alone. Conversely, there is every reason to add a hormonal agent of proved effectiveness to the cytotoxic regimen, since a proportion of cancer cells will be killed by this agent.

Therefore at the Institut Jules Bordet, we now tentatively accept the concepts based on the estrogen receptor survey and consider that the practical application resulting from the ubiquity or near ubiquity of receptors in all breast cancers justifies the use of hormone treatment of all cancers concomitantly with the chemotherapeutic regimen. Our present therapeutic protocol of advanced breast cancer comprises a cyclic type of cytotoxic chemotherapy associated with continuous administration of a hormonal agent.

This protocol is discussed elsewhere in the volume. The chemotherapy is analogous to that used in other institutions and consists of an association of the agents which given alone have proved to be the most effective in this particular form of cancer. The hormonal part of the treatment in our protocol is an antiestrogen, tamoxifen. Administered alone, tamoxifen gives a rate of objective remission approximating 35–40% with little or no toxicity, and it is preferred to nafoxidin, another antiestrogen with similar activity but exhibiting a notable degree of toxicity especially on the skin. These antiestrogens appear to be at least equivalent therapeutically to high-dosage estrogen administration while being better tolerated and more often free of the occasional growth-stimulating effect of stilbestrol and β-estradiol.

The first results of this method of treatment are analyzed elsewhere in this volume. Whether the addition of antiestrogen represents an improvement compared to cytotoxic chemotherapy alone should be the subject of a controlled clinical trial in the future. Other approaches to the treatment of advanced breast cancer by nonsteroid hormones, pituitary hormones, and neurendocrine active products remain at the experimental stage at present and have not yet proved useful (13).

CONCLUSION

Recent advances in chemotherapy with the introduction of new and potent drugs and the use of better associations of drugs are based on the progress of clinical pharmacology and the results of controlled clinical trials. These developments have led to a re-evaluation of the treatment of advanced breast cancer and have relegated hormonal treatment to the role of an adjuvant. Endocrine therapy by administering hormones as the only treatment may be indicated occasionally, as in elderly or very ill persons. The major ablative procedures seem to be gradually replaced by the new medical treatments, which give a larger percentage of remissions at a reduced cost in morbidity and mortality. Ultimately the control of breast cancer will probably depend on the acceptance by the medical profession of early, prolonged, and energetic administration of active drugs to all patients undergoing surgical excision of the mammary tumor.

Such treatment has already produced spectacular results in dramatically reducing the rate of recurrence after mastectomy (see Bonadonna et al., *this volume*). These forms of therapy should be generalized to all patients. The type and intensity of this adjuvant therapy should be adapted to the stage of the tumor. Early diagnosis by currently available methods, with its small yield of new cases and high expenditure of money, appears probably less important than support of research for the development of biochemical methods of diagnosis that permit detection before clinical manifestation. Perseverance in the development and utilization of adjuvant therapy seems to be the most promising approach to prevent the appearance of metastases, which when widespread and massive are very difficult to eradicate or treat. Endocrine research and exploration of the effect of hormones on breast cancer remain indispensable studies, even if at present they do not directly influence treatment.

REFERENCES

1. Council on Drugs (1960): Androgens and estrogens in the treatment of disseminated mammary carcinoma. *J.A.M.A.*, 172:1271–1283.
2. Cooperative Breast Cancer Group (1961): Progress report: Results of studies by the Cooperative Breast Cancer Group 1956–60. *Cancer Chemother. Rep.*, 11: 109–141.
3. Cooperative Breast Cancer Group (1964): Testosterone propionate therapy in breast cancer. *J.A.M.A.*, 188:1069–1072.
4. Groupe Européen du Cancer du Sein (1964): Le traitement hormonal du cancer du sein en phase avancée: Comparaison entre le propionate de testostérone et la combinaison propionate de testosterone-delta- 1-testololactone. *Rev. Fr. Etud. Clin. Biol.*, 9:88–90.
5. Fracchia, A. A., Farrow, J. H., Miller, T. R., Tollefsen, R. H., Greenberg, E. J., and Knapper, W. H. (1971): Hypophysectomy as compared with adrenalectomy in the treatment of advanced carcinoma of the breast. *Surg. Gynecol. Obstet.*, 133:241–246.
6. Cutler, S. J., Asire, A. J., and Taylor, S. G., III (1969): Classification of patients with disseminated cancer of the breast. *Cancer*, 24:861–869.
7. Plattner, P. A., editor (1964): *Chemotherapy of Cancer.* Elsevier, Amsterdam.
8. Bulbrook, R. D., Greenwood, F. C., and Hayward, J. L. (1960): Selection of breast cancer patients for adrenalectomy or hypophysectomy by determination of urinary 17-hydroxycorticosteroids and aetiocholanolone. *Lancet*, 1:1154–1157.
9. McGuire, W., Carbone, P. P., and Vollmer, E. P. (1975): *Estrogen Receptors in Human Breast Cancer.* Raven Press, New York.
10. Leclercq, G., Heuson, J. C., Deboel, M. C., and Mattheiem, W. H. (1975): Oestrogen receptors in breast cancer: A changing concept. *Br. Med. J.*, 1:185–189.
11. Staquet, M., Tagnon, H., Kenis, Y., Bonadonna, G., Carter, S. K., Sokal, G., Trouet, A., Ghione, M., Praga, C., Lenaz, L., and Karim, O. S., editors (1974): *EORTC International Symposium. Adriamycin Review.* European Press Medikon, Ghent.
12. Horwitz, K. B., McGuire, W. L., Pearson, O. H., and Segaloff, A. (1975): Predicting response to endocrine therapy in human breast cancer: A hypothesis. *Science*, 189:726–727.
13. Stoll, B. A., editor (1974): *Mammary Cancer and Neuroendocrine Therapy.* Butterworths, London.

Breast Cancer: Trends in Research and Treatment, edited by J. C. Heuson, W. H. Mattheiem, and M. Rozencweig. Raven Press, New York © 1976.

Chemotherapy of Breast Cancer: Current Status

Stephen K. Carter

Division of Cancer Treatment, National Cancer Institute, Bethesda, Maryland 20014

In terms of incidence and mortality, adenocarcinoma of the breast is the leading cancer among females in the United States (1). It is the leading cause of death among women in the 40- to 44-year age group and one of the leading causes in those 30–34 years of age and above (2). It is estimated that this tumor will be diagnosed in approximately 69,000 women in the United States during any given year. In 1968 in the United States 29,081 deaths were attributed to breast cancer, and the estimated number of deaths in 1971 was 31,000. The difference between 69,000 new cases and 31,000 deaths annually cannot be regarded as approximating the number of "cures" because many persons suffering with breast cancer die of other causes.

Breast cancer is a tumor that causes death by spreading throughout the body and not by virtue of local growth. A deadly dissemination can occur even when there is minimal local growth. After a breast cancer is initially diagnosed, it can follow a wide range of clinical courses. Some tumors kill quickly, regardless of the therapeutic intervention, whereas others progress slowly under almost any kind of therapy. This makes it difficult to evaluate the efficacy of any treatment modality in terms of survival.

Survival with breast cancer is usually correlated with such variables as size, histologic type, lymph node involvement, anatomic type, and grade of malignancy. One of the most extensively used variables is the extent of lymph node involvement. Fisher et al. (3) showed that after radical mastectomy women with four or more involved nodes have a 5-year survival rate of 31%. This increases to 45% when fewer than four nodes are involved and to 76% when there is no nodal involvement. The disease-free interval is similarly influenced. In the absence of axillary nodal metastasis, the 5-year recurrence rate is 21%; it rises to 66% in the presence of any nodal disease and to 81% with four or more involved nodes. The median time from first recurrence until death is 7 months (4). Fisher's data also indicate that when axillary nodes are uninvolved the location of the primary breast lesion does not influence the overall 5-year recurrence rate after a Halsted radical mastectomy.

For many tumors, survival for 5 years after treatment is a good indication that the disease has been controlled. Breast cancer, however, may recur as long as 20 or more years after therapy (5,6).

COMBINED MODALITY APPROACH TO THERAPY

Surgery with or without postoperative irradiation is the primary curative therapy for breast cancer in its early stages, but fully 60% or more of all breast cancer patients develop recurrent disease within 10 years after initial therapy (7). Only approximately 25% of all women treated for cancer of the breast are cured (8), while the remaining 75% later require treatment for incurable disease. These patients with systemic spread of disease fall into various categories.

More than half the women treated by mastectomy develop symptomatic metastatic disease without evidence of local recurrence. The current assumption is that small metastatic foci were present at the time of the attempted surgical cure. Since there is currently no means of measuring the number of these cells remaining after surgery, or of assessing their kinetic characteristics, any statement concerning their natural history must be hypothetical. It is hoped that systemic treatment with chemotherapeutic agents immediately after mastectomy will eradicate these remaining microfoci and increase the cure rates for the primary therapy. The assumptions and supporting data for this approach have been published previously (9,10) and are presented elsewhere in this volume.

A second category of advanced disease is recurrent local disease after mastectomy, either within the site of mastectomy or in the treated regional lymph nodes. Although extensive local recurrence may occur without evidence of metastatic disease elsewhere, it is assumed to be present; and if local recurrence is controlled by local therapy only, ultimately the metastases must be treated. Therefore the treatment of local recurrent disease should be undertaken with systemic adjunctive therapy after metastasis, which should control the microscopic clusters of remaining cells.

A third category is comprised of patients who have inoperable local disease when first seen, including those with large penetrating cancers and those with fixed axillary nodes. Mastectomy has no curative potential in this situation. The treatment is usually local radiotherapy, which can achieve total disappearance of all tumor for several years. Since local treatment does not produce a cure in this situation, systemic chemotherapy is being attempted (11).

Another interesting category of patients includes those with apparently early cancers (as assessed by the state of the primary tumors) but with evidence of silent asymptomatic distant metastases found by routine preoperative screening. This clearly represents a more advanced stage of the microscopic metastatic spread that leads to so many failures after mastectomy alone. Should these women be treated as having advanced and, by implication, incurable disease, or should they receive conventional local control therapy with adjunctive systemic therapy? This question was succinctly posed in 1972 by Welbourn and Burn (8), but there are no data to support a firm position in spite of recent successes of adjunctive treatment approaches that seem highly attractive.

The basis of the combined modality approach in breast carcinoma is the recognition that the capability of both surgery and radiotherapy to cure this tumor has plateaued. These local modalities kill or remove tumor cells only where applied, and it is not technically feasible to increase the scope of their application in patients in whom they are effective. They fail to cure many patients even when they remove all the tumor visible to the naked eye or diagnostic x-ray film. This failure is believed due to disseminated microscopic disease foci present at the time of surgical excision of the primary tumor, which many times includes the surrounding tissue and part of the regional lymph nodes. Used optimally, chemotherapy has the potential of eradicating these foci. It has been estimated that a 99% cell kill is required to produce a greater than 50% reduction of a large tumor mass. If this degree of cell kill could be directed against the relatively small tumor burden left after surgical excision, it would be theoretically possible to eradicate the last neoplastic cell.

The drug regimens that have shown the highest degree of activity and lowest morbidity in advanced disease are the prime candidates for use in a combined modality approach. The therapeutic strategy for increasing cure rates in solid tumors involves integration of drugs into combined modality therapy (9). In this approach, new drugs and drug combinations will be tested in advanced disease, and the effective regimens will be used in primary treatment of disseminated disease. The optimal regimen evolved in this situation would then be integrated into a combined modality approach for primary treatment of local and regional disease. Such an approach in the therapeutic attack against breast cancer is being made (through concerted efforts by the Division of Cancer Treatment, the Breast Cancer Task Force, and the Division of Cancer Resources and Centers) to integrate chemotherapy into the earlier stages of treatment (10).

STATUS OF CHEMOTHERAPY

In developing the building blocks for integrating chemotherapy into a combined modality strategy for breast cancer, one must consider the wide range of single agents that are active against this tumor (Table 1).

Single Agents

Almost all of the alkylating agents have similar patterns of effectiveness, but cyclophosphamide has been the most extensively studied drug of this class. Since both parenteral and oral formulations are available, cyclophosphamide can be used on a wide variety of dosage schedules. This is in contrast to other alkylating agents such as nitrogen mustard, thiotepa, and chlorambucil, which have been administered on schedules almost totally consistent for each given agent. The drug has been used clinically on both intermittent and chronic daily schedules with no difference observed based on schedule.

Phenylalanine mustard (L-PAM; melphalan, Alkeran) is the only other alkylating agent besides cyclophosphamide that has been used on a variety of schedules. Of the 177 patients treated, the majority have been on the daily for 5 days (× 5) schedule of ECOG (30) that gave a 20% response rate in 91 patients. Sears

TABLE 1. *Activity of single nonhormonal chemotherapeutic agents against breast cancer*

Drug	No. of literature series	No. of evaluable patients	Response	
			No.	%
Alkylating agents				
Cyclophosphamide (12–24)	13	529	182	34
Nitrogen mustard (25–27)	3	92	32	35
Phenylalanine mustard (28–30)	3	177	38	22
Chlorambucil (31,32)	2	54	11	20
Thiotepa (26,33–35)	4	162	48	30
Antimetabolites				
5-Fluorouracil (15,20,21,36–47)	15	1,263	324	26
Methotrexate (37,48–58)	14	356	120	34
6-Mercaptopurine (59)	1	44	6	14
Cytosine arabinoside (29)	4	64	6	9
Hydroxyurea (60)	1	16	2	12
Mitotic inhibitors				
Vincristine (35,61–64)	5	226	47	21
Vinblastine (61,65–69)	6	95	19	20
Antitumor antibiotics				
Adriamycin (70–73)	6	193	67	35
Mitomycin C (29)	2	60	23	38
Others (actinomycin D, Mithramycin, streptonigrin, Bleomycin, Daunomycin) (29,34,74)	9	99	13	13
Random synthetics				
BCNU (10)		76	16	21
CCNU (10)		155	18	12
Methyl CCNU (10)		33	2	6
Hexamethylmelamine (75)		39	11	28
Imidiazole carboxamide (29)		29	2	7
Dibromodulcitol (10)		22	6	27
Procarbazine (29)		21	1	5

et al. (28) reported a 30% response rate (12/40) for the oral loading course repeated at 3- to 6-week intervals. On the other hand, in a nonrandomized comparison she reported that chronic daily oral administration produced only an 11% response (1/9). In her hands the high-dose intravenous (i.v.) approach gave a 16% response rate with 4/25 achieving remission. Interest in this drug is now on an equal standing with that of cyclophosphamide because of its inclusion in adjuvant studies.

5-Fluorouracil (5-FU) has been the most extensively studied drug in the anti-metabolite group and is probably the most commonly used of the nonhormonal agents for standard breast cancer study. 5-FU exhibits no experimental schedule dependency, and the majority of testing has been on the 5-day loading course schedule originally devised by Ansfield and Curreri. On this schedule, the drug is administered intravenously at a dose of 15 mg/kg/day ×5, followed by one-half this dose given every other day until toxicity occurs. Severe toxicity has frequently been observed at this dose, and many clinicians now use a lower dose (12–13.5 mg/kg/day × 5).

Methotrexate is another antimetabolite that has been extensively studied in breast cancer. It has been used clinically on a wide range of dosage schedules, and it is of interest to evaluate the data in breast cancer on the basis of treatment schedule. When this is done, and recognizing all the dangers inherent in comparing pooled data from a variety of sources, it appears that an optimal schedule of methotrexate could be the single agent with the greatest potential for achieving tumor regression.

The vinca alkaloids (vincristine and vinblastine) comprise another group of compounds producing objective tumor regression in patients with breast cancer. Vincristine, the more intensively studied of the two compounds, has produced an overall response rate of 21%. When the two largest series (62,64) are examined in detail, a dose-response effect for regression is observed. At a dose level of 12.5 μg/kg no responses occurred in either series, but the response rate rises as the dose increases until a response rate of 33% is obtained at 75 μg/kg. In the study by Holland et al. (64), hormone treatments and endocrine ablation had no apparent effect on the frequency of partial remissions induced by vincristine.

When the antibiotics are reviewed, adriamycin immediately stands out as a new drug having activity comparable to any of the other standard agents. Adriamycin is a glycoside antibiotic originally isolated by aerobic fermentation of *Streptomyces peucetius* var. *caesius* followed by solvent extraction or chromatographic purification (76). Structurally it is an analogue of an earlier clinical compound (daunorubicin) and differs from it only by the hydroxylation of the 14th carbon. The proposed mechanism of the antineoplastic effect at the cellular level is drug-binding to DNA by intercalation between base pairs and inhibition of RNA synthesis by template disordering and steric obstruction. This mechanism is based predominantly on data obtained from investigations of daunorubicin (77). The evidence for binding of adriamycin to DNA is supported by the ultrastructural changes induced by it in mouse hepatic cell nucleoli (78).

The most commonly used dose schedule of adriamycin is an intermittent one of either 20–30 mg/m²/day × 3, 20–35 mg/m² once every 7 days, or 60–105 mg/m² once every 21 days (72,79–82). The currently recommended schedule evolved from clinical experience is 60–75 mg/m² given as a single rapid infusion and repeated at 21 days. This recommendation is based on the pharmacokinetics described above and the clinical observations of lower toxicities without apparent loss of therapeutic activity (70,72).

Reports are available showing 67 objective responses among 193 patients for a response rate of 35%, which is equivalent to results achieved with such standard agents as cyclophosphamide, methotrexate, and 5-FU (83). The efficacy of adriamycin is even more impressive in view of the fact that most of the treated patients had failed to respond to combination chemotherapy employing many of the standard agents.

Combination Chemotherapy

Many of the great advances in chemotherapy have been achieved using multiple drug combination regimens. The most notable progress has occurred in the hematologic malignancies, specifically acute lymphocytic leukemia of childhood and Hodgkin's disease. Some of the prerequisites for drugs to be used in a successful combination approach to a given tumor are: (a) the drugs should be active as single agents; (b) they should have independent mechanisms of action; and (c) they should not produce overlapping toxicity. Most of these conditions can be met in the chemotherapy of breast cancer. A number of drugs with differing mechanisms of action (e.g., cyclophosphamide, methotrexate, 5-FU, and vincristine) have significant activity as single agents. Although there is some degree of overlapping toxicity, the potential clearly exists for combination regimens employing doses of significant therapeutic potential.

Greenspan (84,85) was one of the first investigators to exploit successfully the potential of combination chemotherapy in breast cancer. He reported the results of two combination regimens dating back as far as 1963. With a five-drug combination involving three cytotoxic compounds and two hormonal compounds, he achieved an 81% response rate in 73 cases.

In 1969 Cooper (86) of the Buffalo Medical Group presented the results of a 5-drug combination (CMFVP) as follows:

C = cyclophosphamide	2.5 mg/kg/day orally (p.o.)
M = methotrexate	25–50 mg/week i.v.
F = 5-fluorouracil	12 mg/kg/day ×4, then 500 mg/week i.v.
V = vincristine	0.035 mg/kg/week i.v.
P = prednisone	0.75 mg/kg/day p.o.

Cooper reported a 90% complete remission rate in a group of 60 hormone-resistant patients with far-advanced breast cancer. This study deeply impressed the oncology community. During the past 5 years the major thrusts in the chemotherapy of advanced breast cancer can be grouped into the five categories shown in Table 2.

TABLE 2. *Major thrusts in chemotherapy of advanced breast cancer*

---

1. Follow-up of "CMFVP" regimen
    a. Dissection
    b. Substitution
    c. Addition
    d. Schedule manipulation
    e. Development of mutually noncross-resistant combinations
2. Integration of adriamycin in drug combinations
3. Integration of hormonal therapy with chemotherapy
4. Integration of immunotherapy with chemotherapy
5. Search for new drugs

The extensive follow-up of the CMFVP regimen includes 11 studies published after Cooper's original abstract (Table 3). Each study modified the original regimen to some extent, either the dose level or schedule of some or all of the drugs. Overall, 529 cases are reported with a cumulative response rate of 47%. The range of response rates is 20–70%, which is indicative of variations in factors such as patient selection, intensity of treatment, criteria of response, and data-reporting techniques. It is clear that no study has reproduced the original 90% response rate reported by Cooper, and in fact Cooper's abstract has never been followed by a full paper detailing his study. In view of the extensive data now accumulating for lesser combinations leading to similar response rates, it can be stated that all five of the drugs are not required to achieve objective remission in approximately 50% of women with advanced disease.

It is of interest that two of the studies in Table 3 (SWG 450 and SEG 339) examined continuous versus intermittent CMFVP. In both cases the results seem to favor the continuous regimen, although neither study has shown definitive differences. Dissection of CMFVP by removal of a single drug was investigated in five studies, i.e., deletion of prednisone in three studies, vincristine in one, and methotrexate in another (Table 4). The only studies controlled against the five-drug regimen are those of the Central Oncology Group (COG 7020B) and the Cooperative Breast Cancer Group (CBCG 7500), which are shown in Table 3. The COG study appears to indicate that prednisone adds nothing, and the CBCG study similarly indicates a lack of critical importance for vincristine. The latter study has not been fully analyzed, but the low overall response rate is disturbing.

Four different three-drug combinations based on the CMFVP regimen (i.e., CMF, CFP, FVP, and CFV) have been evaluated (Table 5). The CMF combination is a modification of the CMFP originally developed at the National Cancer Institute.

In a recently completed ECOG study (30), L-PAM alone was compared to CMF (Table 6). The study was conducted not only to examine the relative response rates with a single agent versus a combination, but also to establish a baseline of activity in advanced disease. Each of these programs form the basis of combined surgery and chemotherapy trials, one in the National Surgical Adjuvant Breast Program (96) and the other by the Istituto Nazionale Tumori in Milan, Italy (97). The response rates, median duration of remission, and survival in the L-PAM versus CMF trial indicate the superiority of the combination chemotherapy program.

In a controlled study (95) performed at the Istituto Nazionale Tumori, CMF was compared to a combination of adriamycin plus vincristine (AV). There was no statistical difference in the response rate (CR + PR) produced by CMF (55%) and AV (52%). Tumor regression, especially at the level of soft-tissue involvement, was more rapidly induced by AV than by CMF. In fact, after two cycles of treatment 58% of patients started on AV were already in PR compared to 38% of those given CMF.

The median duration of response after CMF was 7 months, compared to 9

TABLE 3. *CMFVP regimens in breast cancer*

Investigator[a]	Dose of drugs[b]					No. evaluable patients	Response	
	C	M	F	V	P		No.	%
Davis et al. (87)	100 mg/day	25 mg/wk	500 mg/wk	1 mg/wk	45 mg/day × 14, then taper	74	31	42
ALGB 6982 (88)	2 mg/kg/day	0.75 mg/kg/wk	12 mg/kg/wk	0.25 mg/kg/wk	0.75 mg/kg/day × 21, then taper	82	41	50
COG 7020B (89)	100 mg/day	25 mg/wk	500 mg/wk	1 mg/wk	45 mg/day × 14, then taper	46	27	59
SWG 450 (89)	60 mg/m²/day	15 mg/m²/wk	300 mg/m²/wk	0.625 mg/m²/wk	30 mg/m²/day, then taper	92[c]	53	58
	120 mg/m²/day i.v.	4 mg/m²/day × 5	180 mg/m²/day × 5	0.625 mg/m²/day × 5	40 mg/m²/day × 5	82[d]	42	51
CBCG 7500 (89)	100 mg/day	25 mg/wk	500 mg/wk	1 mg/wk	45 mg/day × 14, then taper	53	16	30
SEG 339 (89,90)	100 mg/m²/day	20 mg/m²/wk p.o.	400 mg/m²/wk	1 mg/m²/wk	45 mg/day, then taper	37[c]	14	38
	400 mg/m² i.v. day 1	30 mg/m² days 1 and 8	400 mg/m² days 1 and 8	1 mg/m² days 1 and 8	20 mg q.i.d. × 8	35[d]	7	20
Stutz et al. (91)	1.5 mg/kg/day	0.4 mg/kg/day	10 mg/kg/day	0.02 mg/kg/day	45 mg/day × 14, then taper	18	10	56
Lokich and Skarin (92)	3 mg/kg/day	0.3 mg/kg/day	10 mg/kg/wk	1 mg/wk	50 mg/day, then taper	10	7	70
Total						529	248	47

[a] Abbreviations: ALGB (Acute Leukemia Group B); COG (Central Oncology Group); SWG (Southwest Oncology Group); CBCG (Cooperative Breast Cancer Group); SEG (Southeastern Cancer Study Group).

[b] Route of administration, unless otherwise indicated: cyclophosphamide (C), p.o.; methotrexate (M), i.v.; 5-fluorouracil (F), i.v.; vincristine (V), i.v.; and prednisone (P), p.o.

[c] Continuous dose regimen.

[d] Intermittent dose regimen (every 28 days).

TABLE 4. *Four-drug regimens devised from CMFVP*

Investigator[a]	Dose of drug[b]					No. evaluable patients	Response	
	C	M	F	V	P		No.	%
Hanham et al. (93)	200–300 mg/kg i.v. days 1 and 5	0.25 mg/kg days 2 and 5	7.5 mg/kg/day × 5	0.015 mg/kg days 2 and 5	—	14	14	100
DeLena et al. (94)	5 mg/kg i.v. days 1 and 5	0.5 mg/kg days 1 and 4	10 mg/kg/day × 5	0.025 mg/kg days 2 and 5	—	55	25	45
COG 7020B (89)	100 mg/day	25 mg/wk	500 mg/wk	1 mg/wk	—	49	24	49
Total (CMFV)						118	63	53
CBCG 7500 (89)	100 mg/day	25 mg/wk	500 mg/wk	—	45 mg/day × 14, then taper	47	13	28
Mayo Clinic (89)	4 mg/kg/day × 5 i.v.	—	8 mg/kg/day × 5	1.4 mg/m² days 1 and 5	30 mg/day × 14, then taper	43	19	44

[a] Abbreviations: see footnote, Table 3.
[b] Routes of administration: see footnote, Table 3.

TABLE 5. Three-drug regimens devised from CMFVP

Investigator[a]	Dose of Drug[b]					No. of evaluable patients	Response	
	C	M	F	V	P		No.	%
Canellos et al. (30)	100 mg/m²/day ×14	40 mg/m² days 1 and 8	600 mg/m² days 1 and 8	—	—	93	—	53
DeLena et al. (95)	100 mg/m²/day ×14	40 mg/m² days 1 and 8	600 mg/m² days 1 and 8	—	—	53	26	49
Mayo Clinic (89)	4 mg/kg/day ×5 i.v.	—	8 mg/kg/day ×5	—	30 mg/day ×14, taper	49	21	43
Fisher et al. (96)	4 mg/kg/day ×5 i.v.	—	8 mg/kg/day ×5	—	30 mg/day ×14, taper	31	13	42
ALGB 6982 (88)	—	—	12 mg/kg/wk	0.25 mg/kg/wk	0.75 mg/kg/day ×21, taper	82	30	36
Michigan Univ. (89)	4 mg/kg/day ×5 i.v.	—	7.5 mg/kg/day ×5	0.015 mg/kg days 1 and 8	—	46	20	43

[a] Abbreviations: see footnote, Table 3.
[b] Route of administration: see footnote, Table 3.

TABLE 6. Comparative results in Eastern Cooperative Oncology Group Study No. 0971

Drugs	No. of patients[a]	Response rate (%)			Median duration CR (wk)	Median survival, all patients (wk)
		CR	PR	Overall		
L-PAM (6 mg/m²/day × 5 p.o., repeated q 42 days)	91[b]	5	15	20	21	38
versus						
"CMF" every 28 days Cyclophosphamide (100 mg/m²/day × 14 p.o.) Methotrexate (40 mg/m² i.v. days 1 and 8) 5-FU (600 mg/m² i.v. days 1 and 8)	93[c]	15	38	53	38	52

From ref. 30.
[a] Patients stratified by dominant disease site, performance status, and disease-free interval.
[b] Hematologic toxicity (platelets < 75,000/mm³; WBC < 3,000) was 32%. Gastrointestinal (GI) toxicity (vomiting, diarrhea, or mucositis) was 26%.
[c] Hematologic toxicity (as above) was 75%. GI toxicity (as above) was 59%.

months for AV followed after eight cycles by CMF to avoid cardiomyopathy. The analysis of survival revealed that the median was not yet reached in the CMF group compared to a median of 15.5 months for those started with AV. Secondary treatment after crossover for relapse or progression yielded a response rate of 28.5% for CMF and 26% for AV. The data indicate that CMF and AV lack cross resistance and are both effective against breast cancer. Furthermore, the data confirmed the ECOG results; i.e., CMF produces complete or partial response in at least 50% of patients. Therefore this finding represents a solid point of reference.

Two studies have evaluated the proposition that sequential use of the drugs in CMFVP might be as effective as concomitant administration (Table 7), but in both cases the sequential regimens proved inferior. The study of the Southeastern Group was controlled against CMFVP (Table 3), and the Western Group study is complicated by the fact that triiodothyronine was substituted for vincristine in both the combination and sequential regimens although the combination shows clear-cut superiority.

As pointed out earlier, the initial studies with adriamycin revealed it to be one of the most active single agents for the treatment of metastatic adenocarcinoma of the breast. A 36% response rate in 121 evaluable cases seen in the initial

TABLE 7. *Sequential regimens derived from CMFVP*

Investigator	Regimen	No. of evaluable patients	Response No.	%
Southeastern Cancer Study Group 339 (89, 90)	Sequential use at progressive disease: 5-FU (600 mg/m^2/wk × 8 i.v.) Methotrexate (20 mg/m^2 biwk × 8 wk p.o.) Cyclophosphamide (100 mg/m^2/day × 8 wk p.o.) Vincristine (1 mg/m^2/wk × 8 i.v.) Prednisone (45 mg/day, then taper)	34[a]	3	9
Western Cancer Study Group 115 (89)	Sequential use at progressive disease: 5-FU (15 mg/kg/wk i.v.)	47	13	28
	Cyclophosphamide (2 mg/kg/day p.o.)	25	7	28
	Prednisone (0.5 mg/kg/day p.o. + Triiodothyronine, 0.05 mg/day p.o.)	16	1	6
	Methotrexate (0.5 mg/kg/wk i.v.)	14	1	7

[a] Data reported only for initial response.

cumulative data review (98) has held in the larger analysis given earlier. This efficacy is particularly impressive because most of the patients had failed on prior chemotherapeutic approaches, most of which were intensive combinations.

Several studies examined adriamycin in comparison to combination regimens as initial chemotherapy for advanced breast cancer. The results of these studies are particularly impressive. The Southwest Oncology Group (SWOG) compared adriamycin (60 mg/m² every. 3 weeks) to the five-drug Cooper regimen given either continuously, as originally reported by Cooper, or intermittently (99). In 200 cases allocated to the three regimens, improvement was seen in 55% of cases treated with adriamycin, compared to 59% for the intermittent regimen and 65% for the continuous regimen. The median duration of remission was shorter for the adriamycin-treated group (5 months) compared to 9 and 13.5 months, respectively, for the combinations. Adriamycin was shown to have an inducing capacity equivalent to the aggressive five-drug combination and, despite the shorter duration of remission, is well established as perhaps the most active single agent.

In another study the Mayo Clinic group (100) compared adriamycin (60 mg/m² every 3 wks) to FCP (5-FU, cyclophosphamide, and prednisone), which has also been used by the Albany Medical College-Roswell Park group (101). Regressions were defined as a 50% reduction in the product of the perpendicular diameters of the measurable lesions. Nine of 20 patients responded to adriamycin (45%) compared to 12 of 28 (43%) on the combinations. The toxicity was comparable in both groups. Again the inducing ability of adriamycin was equivalent to the standard combination regimen in use in a particular group.

The Albany Medical College-Roswell Park group (102) recently updated their comparison of combination chemotherapy (FCP), adriamycin (ADM), and adrenalectomy (ADX). Patients were stratified and randomly assigned to one of three treatment sequences: (a) FCP → ADM → ADX; (b) ADM → ADX → FCP; and (c) ADX → FCP → ADM. The adriamycin was given at a dosage of 75 mg/m² i.v. every 3 weeks to a total dose of 550 mg/m². FCP consisted of cyclophosphamide (4 mg/kg/day ×5 i.v. every 4 weeks), 5-FU (8 mg/kg/day ×5 i.v. every 4 weeks), and prednisone (10 mg t.i.d. for 2 weeks and then tapered). The response rates to primary therapy were 42% (13/31) for FCP, 33% (11/33) for adriamycin, and 30% (9/30) for adrenalectomy. The median duration of response was 9 months for FCP, 7 months for adriamycin, and 5 months for the ablative hormonal procedure. These results suggest that adrenalectomy is inferior to chemotherapy as primary treatment in these patients.

Combination chemotherapy studies employing adriamycin have been undertaken on a large scale. There are 30 possible combinations of adriamycin with one or more of the five drugs in CMFVP, and clinical trials are progressing or completed with nine (30%) of these regimens (Table 8). Most of the studies involve combination with cyclophosphamide and 5-FU.

Salmon and Jones (103) developed a two-drug combination of adriamycin (40 mg/m² on day 1) and cyclophosphamide (200 mg/m² p.o. on days 3–6), with courses repeated every 21 days. In 26 consecutive patients having advanced breast

TABLE 8. *Possible combinations of adriamycin with CMFVP drugs*

Two-drug regimen	Four-drug regimen
AC (Southwest Oncology	ACMF (Eastern Cooperative Cancer
Group; Arizona)	Study Group; Southwest
AM (Mayo Clinic)	Oncology Group)
AF (Central Oncology Group)	ACMV
AV (NCI, Milan)	ACMP
AP	ACFV
Three-drug regimen	ACFP
ACM	ACVP
ACF (M.D. Anderson; Memorial-	AMFV
Sloan Kettering; NCI,	AMFP
Milan; others)	AFVP
ACV	Five-drug regimen
ACP	AMFVP
AMF	ACFVP (Acute Leukemia Group B)
AMV (Mayo Clinic)	ACMVP
AMP	ACMFV
AFV	ACMFP
AFP	Six-drug regimen
AVP (NCI, Milan)	ACMFVP

Clinical studies completed or in progress are shown in parentheses.

cancer, the treatment was well tolerated without serious myelosuppression. Of 23 evaluable cases 19 received an adequate trial of two courses, and 16 had excellent responses with greater than 50% tumor regression. Thus the ratio of responders to evaluable patients was 16/23 (70%); the ratio of responders to patients having adequate trial was 16/19 (84%). Only one responder with a remission duration of 3 months had relapsed at the time of the last report.

A regimen termed FAC, combining the three drugs, has also been developed at M. D. Anderson Hospital (104). The drugs are administered on a 21-day course as follows:

Adriamycin	50 mg/m^2 i.v. on day 1
Cyclophosphamide	500 mg/m^2 i.v. on day 1
5-FU	500 mg/m^2 i.v. on days 1 and 8

Twenty-five patients have been treated, with 3 complete and 15 partial remissions being observed for a 72% response rate. Of 13 patients completing three courses, 3 had CR and 8 had PR, for a response rate of 84%. This pilot study, which revealed significant but acceptable toxicity, shows major efficacy in metastatic breast cancer and will be further evaluated in a cooperative group study.

The Memorial Sloan-Kettering Cancer Center (105) has also examined the FAC combination on the following schedule repeated at 28-day intervals:

Cyclophosphamide	60 mg/m^2/day $\times$14 p.o.
Adriamycin	30 mg/m^2 i.v. on days 1 and 8
5-FU	400 mg/m^2 i.v. on days 1 and 8

Fifty-eight breast cancer patients were treated, but at the time of the report seven patients were in a category too early for evaluation and seven others had not completed one cycle of therapy. Among the 44 evaluable cases, 31 had never received nonhormonal drugs and 19 (61%) of them attained an objective response. Only 3 of 13 (23%) previously treated patients responded. The median duration of response was 3+ months. Alopecia occurred regularly, and there was moderate nausea and vomiting. The nadir of myelosuppression was at 15–18 days, with recovery in all instances.

The Southeastern Cancer Study Group has also evaluated FAC in metastatic breast cancer (106). Their dose schedule was administration of all three drugs as a single intravenous dose every 21 days, i.e., cyclophosphamide (500 mg/m^2), adriamycin (50 mg/m^2), and 5-FU (500 mg/m^2). The FAC produced marrow and gastrointestinal (GI) toxicity, with two septic deaths. Comparing the two regimens, results after two courses of each were as follows:

	Entered	Completed	Evaluable	CR+PR
FAC	37	21	17	8
CMFVP	35	21	18	2

The Albany Medical College-Roswell Park group (107) is currently comparing cyclophosphamide (500 mg/m^2) + adriamycin (40 mg/m^2) every 4 weeks (CA) versus cyclophosphamide (400 mg/m^2) + adriamycin (40 mg/m^2) + 5-FU (200 mg/m^2/day ×3) every 4 weeks (FAC) versus cyclophosphamide (150 mg/m^2/day ×5) + 5-FU (300 mg/m^2/day ×5) every 5 weeks + prednisone 30 mg tapering to 10 mg daily (CFP) versus CFP alternating with CA. The preliminary results are:

	Entered	Evaluable	PR>50%
CA	17	10	6
FAC	20	11	3
CFP	9	5	1
CFP/CA	7	4	4

Completion and full analysis of this controlled study will provide important comparative information.

Harvey et al. (108) at the Milton S. Hershey Medical Center used adriamycin sequentially with CMFVP in the following regimen:

5-FU	500 mg/week ×4
Methotrexate	25 mg/week ×4
Vincristine	1 mg/week ×4
Cyclophosphamide	100 mg/day ×28
Prednisone	20 mg daily
Adriamycin	60 mg/m^2 on day 29

The cycle was started again on days 60, 120, 180, etc. Among 23 evaluable patients, 5 had CR and 8 experienced greater than 50% tumor shrinkage, for an overall response rate of 56%, which is apparently not superior to the classic

CMFVP regimen. Mild to moderate hematologic, GI, and neural toxicity was noted, and there was no cardiotoxicity.

It is clear that combination chemotherapy can produce impressive response rates, although in every case these appear to be less than the additive effect of each component drug used optimally alone. Much work still remains to be done in elucidating the optimum drug combinations and sequences of drug administration. At this point no individual combination can be recommended as optimal, and the definitive value of combinations over sequential use of single agents for palliating advanced disease remains to be established. Despite this, the cell kill potential of combinations as evidenced by remission induction figures appears to be higher and makes this approach highly attractive for use in combined modality regimes.

COMBINED MODALITY STUDIES IN ADVANCED DISEASE

Since chemotherapy and hormonal therapy do not produce overlapping toxicity and probably work through different mechanisms of action, a combination of the two would seem an attractive concept and various studies are currently exploring this approach. In premenopausal females with recurrent tumor, remission rates ranging from 20% (109) to 40% (110) are reported for bilateral ovariectomy. Combination chemotherapy, which is generally used after ovariectomy or even after other therapies, gives response rates that appear to be superior or at least no worse.

It would be interesting to speculate on the results of a controlled trial comparing ovariectomy and chemotherapy, but this is not likely to be performed. However, several studies are comparing ovariectomy alone with this procedure plus chemotherapy (Table 9). The Acute Leukemia Group B and Mayo Clinic studies will test the possibility that chemotherapy given immediately after ovariectomy might increase the response rate, response duration, and survival over that achieved by ovariectomy alone. The National Cancer Institute (NCI) study will compare the effect of chemotherapy on the length of tumor response in patients who either respond to ovariectomy or show no change at 12 weeks. All patients in the NCI study will initially undergo ovariectomy. Patients showing evidence of progressive disease within 12 weeks will be removed from the study. Patients with either an objective response or no change postovariectomy will be randomized to either no therapy or a combination of cyclophosphamide, methotrexate, and 5-FU. When patients randomized to no further therapy relapse, they will receive the combination regimen. No data are currently available from any of these studies.

Immunotherapy is now of increasing importance in the therapeutic considerations for every tumor type. A wide range of materials are available for use as nonspecific immune stimulators (Table 10), and at least five chemoimmunotherapy trials are in progress (Table 11).

The importance of the immune response in controlling breast cancer has recently become increasingly evident. As early as 1922 MacCarty (111) showed that lymphoid infiltration of breast cancer tissue was a sign of good prognosis. Black et al. (112) and others demonstrated the importance of host immunological re-

TABLE 9. *Ovariectomy plus chemotherapy studies for treatment of metastatic or recurrent inoperable breast carcinoma currently supported by the National Cancer Institute*

Institution	Arm 1	Arm 2	Arm 3
Acute Leukemia Group B (Protocol No. 7382)	Ovariectomy alone	Ovariectomy + Cyclophosphamide (15 mg/kg i.v. 2 × weekly beginning within 14 days after ovariectomy)	Cooper regimen beginning within 14 days after ovariectomy
Mayo Clinic	Ovariectomy alone	Ovariectomy + 5-FU (8 mg/kg/day ×5) Cyclophosphamide (4 mg/kg/day × 5) Prednisone (30 mg/day × 7) Then taper, courses given q 5 wk	—
NCI, Bethesda	Ovariectomy alone	Ovariectomy + Cyclophosphamide (100 mg/m² /day × 14) 5-FU (600 mg/m² days 1–8) Methotrexate (40 mg/m² days 1–8) · Beginning 8–12 wk post-ovariectomy in patients with no response or no change status; repeated q 29 days	—

sponse in the prognosis of breast cancer, and tumor-associated immune responses have also been shown in this disease (113).

Following the observation that BCG could prolong chemotherapy-induced re-mission as well as overall survival in patients with acute myelogenous leuke-

TABLE 10. *Materials commonly used for nonspecific immunostimulation*

1. BCG
   a. Pasteur strain (lyophilized)
   b. Pasteur strain (fresh)
   c. Tice strain
   d. Connaught strain
2. *Corynebacterium parvum*
   a. Burroughs-Wellcome
   b. Merieux
3. MER-BCG
4. Transfer factor
5. Levamisole

TABLE 11. *Chemoimmunotherapy trials in breast cancer*

1. FAC + BCG (M.D. Anderson Hospital)
2. CMF + MER-BCG (Acute Leukemia Group B)
3. CMF +*C. parvum* (NCI)
4. CMF + BCG (UCLA)
5. CMF + BCG + tumor cell vaccine (UCLA)

mia (114) and disseminated melanoma (115), the M. D. Anderson group explored the question of whether BCG could increase remission rates, prolong remission duration, and prolong overall survival in metastatic breast cancer patients undergoing combination chemotherapy. Thus a program of chemoimmunotherapy was initiated by combining BCG and the FAC regimen (116).

Forty-seven consecutive patients received 5-FU (500 mg/m² i.v.) on days 1 and 8, adriamycin (50 mg/m² i.v.) and cyclophosphamide (500 mg/m² i.v.) on day 1 only, and BCG by scarification with 6×10^8 viable organisms on days 9, 13, and 17, with the entire regimen repeated every 3 weeks. After a total dose of 500 mg/m², adriamycin was replaced by methotrexate at 30 mg/m² i.v. or intramuscularly (i.m.) on days 1 and 8. The patients treated with chemoimmunotherapy were compared to an immediate historical control group of 44 consecutive patients who had received FAC alone. Overall response, response in nonvisceral areas, toxicity, and morbidity were similar in both programs, but patients achieving partial remission on FAC + BCG had a prolonged remission compared to those on FAC alone ($p=0.009$).

The group at M. D. Anderson (117) attempted sequential use of two mutually noncross-resistant drug combinations plus immunotherapy to improve the quality and duration of response and survival. Thirty-two consecutive patients were treated with three courses of VAC, consisting of vincristine (1.5 mg/m² on day 1 and weekly ×7), and adriamycin (50 mg/m²) and cyclophosphamide (750 mg/m² i.v.) given on day 2, with the courses repeated every 22 days. This was followed by three courses of FUM, consisting of 5-FU (500 mg/m²/day ×5 i.v.) and methotrexate (30 mg/m² i.v. or i.m. on days 1, 8, and 15), repeated every 28 days. BCG (6×10^8 organisms) was given by scarification on days 8 and 15 of VAC and on days 9, 16, and 23 of FUM. The recently reported findings show 3 complete and 19 partial remissions for an overall response rate of 69%, with 10 patients still on study with stable disease. The dose-limiting toxicity was predominantly granulocytopenia, which was more severe with VAC. Mild neurotoxicity occurred in 31% and moderate stomatitis in 9% of patients. It is too early in the study to determine if the duration of remission or survival will be longer than with older approaches.

CONCLUSION

The future of chemotherapy in treating breast cancer lies in its immediate use after surgical ablation of the primary lesion. A wide range of trials are in progress, and two already show positive results. The regimens active in advanced disease have been the ones chosen for the combined modality thrusts.

As more data are obtained from these combined studies, we will be able to evaluate how well advanced disease serves as a model for predicting dramatic effects in early disease. Chemotherapy can no longer be considered only a palliative modality. Its integration with surgery and radiotherapy, and perhaps immunotherapy, will be the curative approach of tomorrow.

REFERENCES

1. Silverberg, E., and Holleb, A. I. (1971): Cancer statistics—1971. *Cancer,* 21:13–31.
2. U.S. Public Health Service, National Vital Statistics Division (1934–1971): *Vital Statistics of the United States, Annual, 1930–1968.* Government Printing Office, Washington, D.C.
3. Fisher, B., Slack, N., Bross, I. D. J., and cooperating investigators (1969): Cancer of the breast: Size of neoplasm and prognosis. *Cancer,* 24:1071–1080.
4. Fisher, B., Ravdin, R. G., Ausman, R. K., Slack, N. H., Moore, G. E., and Noer, R. J. (1968): Surgical adjuvant chemotherapy in cancer of the breast: Results in a decade of cooperative investigation. *Ann. Surg.,* 168:337–356.
5. Ederer, R., Cutler, S. J., Goldenberg, I. S., and Eisenberg, H. (1963): Causes of death among long-term survivors from breast cancer in Connecticut. *J. Natl. Cancer Inst.,* 30:933–947.
6. Whitney, D. J., Smith, D. G., and Szilagyi, D. E. (1964): Meaning of five-year cure in cancer of the breast. *Arch. Surg.,* 88:637–644.
7. Seidman, H. (1969): Cancer of the breast: Statistical and epidemiological data. *Cancer,* 24:1355–1378.
8. Welbourn, M. A., and Burn, I. J. (1972): Current concepts—treatment of advanced mammary cancer. *N. Engl. J. Med.,* 287:398–400.
9. Carter, S. K., and Soper, W. T. (1974): Integration of chemotherapy into combined modality treatment of solid tumors. I. The overall strategy. *Cancer Treat. Rev.,* 1:1–13.
10. Carter, S. K. (1974): The chemical therapy of breast cancer. *Semin. Oncol.,* 1:131–144.
11. Bonadonna, G., Brusamolino, E., Valaqussa, P., and Veronesi, U. (1975): Adjuvant study with combination chemotherapy in operable breast cancer. *Proc. Am. Assoc. Cancer Res.,* 16:254 (abstract).
12. Wall, R., and Conrad, F. (1961): Cyclophosphamide therapy: Its use in leukemia, lymphoma and solid tumors. *Arch. Intern. Med.,* 108:456–482.
13. Anders, C., and Kemp, N. (1961): Cyclophosphamide in treatment of disseminated malignant disease. *Br. Med. J.,* 2:1516–1523.
14. Gordon, I., and McArthur, J. (1965): Thiotepa and cyclophosphamide in the treatment of advanced mammary cancer. *Scott. Med. J.,* 10:27–33.
15. Talley, R., Vaitkevicius, V., and Leighton, G. (1965): Comparison of cyclophosphamide and 5-fluorouracil in the treatment of patients with metastatic breast cancer. *Clin. Pharmacol. Ther.,* 6:740–748.
16. Firat, D., and Olshin, S. (1968): Treatment of metastatic carcinoma of the female breast with combination hormones and other chemotherapy. *Cancer Chemother. Rep.,* 52:743–750.
17. Rundles, R., Laszlo, J., Garrison, F. E., and Hobson, J. B. (1962): The antitumor spectrum of cyclophosphamide. *Cancer Chemother. Rep.,* 16:407–411.
18. Atkins, H., Gregg, H. G., and Hyman, G. A. (1962): Clinical appraisal of cyclophosphamide in malignant neoplasms. *Cancer,* 15:1076–1080.
19. Kunkler, P., Evans, I. H., June, L., et al. (1968): Cyclophosphamide in the management of advanced cancer. In: *Prognostic Factors in Breast Cancer,* pp. 221–227. Williams & Wilkins, Baltimore.
20. Nemoto, T., and Dao, T. (1971): 5-Fluorouracil and cyclophosphamide in disseminated breast cancer. *New York J. Med.,* 71:554–558.
21. Ravdin, R., and Eisman, S. (1967): Disseminated breast cancer: Relationship of response to endocrine manipulation; cytoxan and fluorouracil. In: *Current Concepts in Breast Cancer,* pp. 200–207. Williams & Wilkins, Baltimore.

22. Foley, J., and Kennedy, B. (1964): Effect of cyclophosphamide on far-advanced neoplasia. *Cancer Chemother. Rep.,* 34:55–58.

23. Gold, G., Salvin, L. G., and Schnider, B. (1962): Comparative study with three alkylating agents: Mechlorethamine, cyclophosphamide, and uracil mustard. *Cancer Chemother. Rep.,* 16:417–419.

24. Bersagel, D., Robertson, G. L., and Hasselback, R. (1968): Effect of cyclophosphamide on advanced lung cancer and the hematological toxicity of large, intermittent intravenous doses. *Can. Med. Assoc. J.,* 98:532–538.

25. Hurley, J., Ellison, E. H., Riesch, J., et al. (1960): Chemotherapy of solid carcinoma. *J.A.M.A.,* 174:1696–1701.

26. Zubrod, C., Schneiderman, M., Frei, E., et al. (1960): Appraisal of methods for the study of chemotherapy of cancer in man: Comparative therapeutic trial of nitrogen mustard and triethylene thiophosphoramide. *J. Chronic Dis.,* 11:7–33.

27. Rhoads, C. (1948): Report on a cooperative study of nitrogen mustard (HN_2) therapy of neoplastic disease. *Trans. Assoc. Am. Physicians,* 60:110–117.

28. Sears, M., Haut, A., and Eckles, N. (1966): Melphalan in advanced breast cancer. *Cancer Chemother. Rep.,* 50:271–279.

29. Livingston, R., and Carter, S. K. (1970): *Single Agents in Cancer Chemotherapy.* Plenum Press, New York.

30. Canellos, G. P., Taylor, S. G., Band, P., and Pocock, S. (1974): Combination chemotherapy for advanced breast cancer: Randomized comparison with single drug therapy. *Proc. XI Int. Cancer Congr.,* 3:596 (abstract).

31. Moore, G., Bross, I. D. J., Ausman, R., Nadler, S., et al. (1968): Effects of chlorambucil (NSC 3088) in 374 patients with advanced cancer. *Cancer Chemother. Rep.,* 52:661–666.

32. Gumport, S., Golomb, F., and Wright, J. (1958): Summary of results obtained with CB 1348. *Ann. N.Y. Acad. Sci.,* 68:1024–1034.

33. Moore, F. (1967): Thiotepa in breast cancer. *N. Engl. J. Med.,* 277:460–468.

34. Hurley, J. (1961): A method of selecting patients for cancer chemotherapy. *Arch. Surg.,* 83:611–619.

35. Silva, A., Smart, C. R., and Rochlin, D. B. (1965): Chemotherapy of breast cancer. *Surg. Gynecol. Obstet.,* 121:494–498.

36. Ansfield, F., Schroeder, J., and Curreri, A. (1962): Five years' clinical experience with 5-fluorouracil. *J.A.M.A.,* 181:295–299.

37. Hall, B., and Good, J. (1962): Treatment of far-advanced cancer with 5-fluorouracil, used alone and in combination with irradiation: Incidence and duration of remission and survival data in 223 patients. *Cancer Chemother. Rep.,* 16:369–386.

38. Moore, G., Bross, I., Ausman, R., et al. (1968): Effects of 5-fluorouracil (NSC 19893) in 389 patients with cancer. *Cancer Chemother. Rep.,* 52:641–653.

39. Eastern Cooperative Group in Solid Tumor Chemotherapy (1967): Comparison of antimetabolites in the treatment of breast and colon cancer. *J.A.M.A.,* 200:770–778.

40. Field, J. (1963): 5-Fluorouracil treatment of advanced cancer in ambulatory patients. *Cancer Chemother. Rep.,* 33:45–49.

41. Eyerly, R. (1962): The effects of 5-fluorouracil in patients with incurable cancer. *Cancer Chemother. Rep.,* 20:89–95.

42. Vaitkevicius, V., Brennan, M. J., Beckett, V. L., et al. (1961): Clinical evaluation of cancer chemotherapy with 5-fluorouracil. *Cancer,* 14:131–152.

43. Kennedy, B., and Theologides, A. (1961): The role of 5-fluorouracil in malignant disease. *Ann. Intern. Med.,* 55:719–730.

44. Jacobs, E., Luce, J., and Wood, D. (1968): Treatment of cancer with weekly intravenous 5-fluorouracil. *Cancer,* 22:1233–1238.

45. Horton, J. (1970): Comparison of 3 weekly dose schedules of 5-fluorouracil without a loading dose. In: *Proceedings of the Chemotherapy Conference on the Chemotherapy of Solid Tumors. An Appraisal of 5-Fluorouracil and BCNU,* pp. 112–127. National Cancer Institute, Bethesda.

46. Hall, T., Cavins, J. A., Khung, C. L., et al. (1966): Time and vehicle studies of a safe and effective method for administration of 5-fluorouracil. *Cancer,* 19:1008–1012.

47. Mackman, S., Ramirez, G., and Ansfield, F. (1967): Results of 5-fluorouracil given by the multiple daily dose method in disseminated breast cancer. *Cancer Chemother. Rep.,* 51:483–489.

48. Burchenal, J., Karnofsky, D., Kingsley-Pillers, E., et al. (1951): The effects of the folic acid

antagonists and 2, 6-diaminopurine on neoplastic disease. *Cancer,* 4:549–569.

49. Schoenbach, E., Colsky, J., and Greenspan, E. (1952): Observations on the effects of the folic acid antagonists, aminopterin and amethopterin, in patients with advanced neoplasms. *Cancer,* 5:1201–1220.

50. Wright, J., Cobb, J., Golomb, F., et al. (1959): Chemotherapy of disseminated carcinoma of the breast. *Ann. Surg.,* 150:221–240.

51. Greening, W. (1962): Methotrexate in the treatment of advanced cancer in the breast. In: *Methotrexate in the Treatment of Cancer,* edited by R. Porter and E. Wiltshaw, pp. 29–33, Williams & Wilkins, Baltimore.

52. Wilson, H., and Louis, J. (1965): The use of low dosage drug regimens in the treatments of neoplastic disease. *Ann. Intern. Med.,* 63:918 (abstract).

53. Sullivan, R., Miller, E., Zurek, W., et al. (1967): Re-evaluation of methotrexate as an anticancer drug. *Surg. Gynecol. Obstet.,* 125:819–824.

54. Vogler, W., Furtado, V., and Hugley, C. (1968): Methotrexate for advanced cancer of the breast. *Cancer,* 21:26–30.

55. Vogler, W., Huguley, C., and Kerr, W. (1965): Toxicity and antitumor effect of divided doses of methotrexate. *Arch. Intern. Med.,* 115:285–293.

56. Sears, M., Tucker, W., Coltman, C. A., and Bonnet, J. (1969): Effectiveness of various schedules of methotrexate in advanced breast carcinoma. *Cancer Chemother. Rep.,* 53:93 (abstract).

57. Andrews, N., and Wilson, W. (1967): Phase II study of methotrexate in solid tumors. *Cancer Chemother. Rep.,* 51:471–474.

58. Nevinny, H., Hall, T., Haines, C., et al. (1968): Comparison of methotrexate (NSC 740) and testosterone propionate (NSC 9166) in the treatment of breast cancer. *J. Clin. Pharmacol.,* 8:126–129.

59. Moore, G., Bross, I. D. J., Ausman, R., et al. (1968): Effects of 6-mercaptopurine in 290 patients with advanced cancer. *Cancer Chemother. Rep.,* 52:655–660.

60. Sears, M. (1964): Phase II studies of hydroxyurea (NSC 32065) in adults: Cancer of the breast. *Cancer Chemother. Rep.,* 40:43.

61. Gailani, S. (1963): Phase II studies of vincristine (VCR) in human cancer. *Proc. Am. Assoc. Cancer Res.,* 4:21 (abstract).

62. Grinberg, R., Nemoto, T., and Dao, T. L. (1965): Vincristine: Dosage and response in advanced breast cancer. *Cancer Chemother. Rep.,* 45:57–61.

63. Goldenberg, I. (1964): Vincristine therapy of women with advanced breast cancer. *Cancer Chemother. Rep.,* 41:7–9.

64. Holland, J., Sharlav, C., Galiani, S., et al. (1973): Vincristine treatment of advanced cancer: A comparative study of 392 cases. *Cancer Res.,* 33:1258–1264.

65. Johnston, B., and Novales, E. (1964): The use of vinblastine sulfate (Velban) in advanced malignancies of the female reproductive tract. *Proc. Am. Assoc. Cancer Res.,* 5:32 (abstract).

66. Bleehen, N., and Jelliffe, A. (1965): Vinblastine sulfate in the treatment of malignant disease. *Br. J. Cancer,* 19:268–273.

67. Goldenberg, I. (1963): Vinblastine sulfate therapy of women with advanced breast cancer. *Cancer Chemother. Rep.,* 29:111–113.

68. Wright, T., Hurley, J., Korst, D. R., et al. (Midwest Cooperative Chemotherapy Group) (1963): Vinblastine in neoplastic disease. *Cancer Res.,* 23:169–179.

69. Smart, C., Rochlin, D. B., Nahum, A. M., et al. (1964): Clinical experience with vinblastine sulfate in squamous cell carcinoma and other malignancies. *Cancer Chemother. Rep.,* 34:31–45.

70. Bonadonna, G., Monfardini, S., DeLena, M., et al. (1972): Clinical trials with adriamycin. Results of a three year study. In: *International Symposium on Adriamycin,* edited by S. K. Carter, A. DiMarco, M. Ghione, et al., pp. 139–152. Springer-Verlag, New York.

71. Tan, C., Etchubanas, E., Wollner, N., et al. (1973): Adriamycin, an antitumor antibiotic in the treatment of neoplastic disease. *Cancer,* 32:9–17.

72. Benjamin, R. S., Wiernick, P. H., and Bachur, N. R. (1973). Adriamycin—efficacy, safety, and pharmacologic basis of a single dose schedule. *Cancer Chemother. Rep.,* 57:98 (abstract).

73. Gottlieb, J. G., Bonnet, J. D., Hoogstraten, B., et al. (1973): Superiority of adriamycin over oral nitrosoureas in patients with breast cancer. *Cancer Chemother. Rep.,* 57:98 (abstract).

74. Blum, R. H., Carter, S. K., and Agre, K. (1973): A clinical review of bleomycin—a new antineoplastic agent. *Cancer,* 31:903–914.

75. Blum, R. H., Livingston, R. B., and Carter, S. K. (1973): Hexamethylmelamine—a new drug with activity in solid tumors. *Eur. J. Cancer*, 9:195–202.

76. Arcamone, F., Cassinelli, G., Franceschi, G., et al. (1972): Structure and physicochemical properties of adriamycin (Doxorubicin). In: *International Symposium on Adriamycin*, edited by S. K. Carter, A. DiMarco, M. Ghione, et al., pp. 9–22. Springer-Verlag, New York.

77. Calendi, E., DiMarco, A., Regiani, M., et al. (1965): On physico-chemical interactions between daunomycin and nucleic acids. *Biochim. Biophys. Acta*, 103:25–49.

78. Lambertenghi-Deliliers, G. (1972): Ultrastructural alterations induced in hepatic cell-nucleoli by adriamycin. In: *International Symposium on Adriamycin*, edited by S. K. Carter, A. DiMarco, M. Ghione, et al., pp. 26–34. Springer-Verlag, New York.

79. Middleman, E., Luce, J. K., and Frei, E. (1971): Clinical trials with adriamycin. *Cancer*, 28:844–850.

80. O'Bryan, R. M., Luce, J. K., Talley, R. W., et al. (1973): Phase II evaluation of adriamycin in human neoplasia. *Cancer*, 39:1–8.

81. Frei, E., Luce, J. K., and Middleman, E. (1972): Clinical trials of adriamycin. In: *International Symposium on Adriamycin*, edited by S. K. Carter, A. DiMarco, M. Ghione, et al., pp. 153–160. Springer-Verlag, New York.

82. Hahn, R. G., Ahmann, D. A., and Bisel, H. F. (1973): A phase II study of adriamycin as therapy for metastatic or inoperable sarcoma. *Cancer Chemother. Rep.*, 57:102 (abstract).

83. Carter, S. K. (1972): Single and combination nonhormonal chemotherapy in breast cancer. *Cancer*, 30:1543–1555.

84. Greenspan, E. (1966): Combination cytotoxic chemotherapy in advanced disseminated breast cancer. *J. Mt. Sinai Hosp. N.Y.*, 33:1–27.

85. Greenspan, E. (1963): Response of advanced breast cancer to the combination of the anti-metabolite, methotrexate, and the alkylating agent thiotepa. *J. Mt. Sinai Hosp. N.Y.*, 30:246–267.

86. Cooper, R. (1969): Combination chemotherapy in hormone resistant breast cancer. *Proc. Am. Assoc. Cancer Res.*, 10:15 (abstract).

87. Davis, H. L., Ramirez, G., Ellerby, R. A., and Ansfield, F. J. (1974): Five-drug therapy in advanced breast cancer: Factors influencing toxicity and response. *Cancer*, 34:239–245.

88. Leone, L. S., and Rege, V. (1973): Treatment of metastatic, recurrent or inoperable carcinoma of breast with VCR/PRED/5-FU/MTX/CYCLO (Reg. 1) vs VCR/PRED/5-FU (Reg II). *Proc. Am. Assoc. Cancer Res.*, 14:125 (abstract).

89. Broder, L. E., and Tormey, D. C. (1974): Combination chemotherapy of carcinoma of the breast. *Cancer Treat. Rev.*, 1:183–203.

90. Smalley, R. V., Murphy, S., Chan, Y. K., and Huguley, C. M. (1973): Comparison of two five-drug regimens vs sequential chemotherapy in metastatic breast carcinoma. *Cancer Chemother. Rep.*, 57:110 (abstract).

91. Stutz, F. H., Blom, J., and Tormey, D. C. (1974): Combination chemotherapy in disseminated carcinoma of the breast. *Oncology*, 29:139–146.

92. Lokich, J. J., and Skarin, A. T. (1972): Five-drug combination chemotherapy for disseminated adenocarcinoma. *Cancer Chemother. Rep.*, 56:761–767.

93. Hanham, I. W. F., Newton, K. A., and Westbury, G. (1971). Seventy-five cases of solid tumors treated by a modified quadruple chemotherapy regime. *Br. J. Cancer*, 25:462–478.

94. DeLena, M., DePalo, G. M., Bonadonna, G., Beretta, G., and Bajetta, E. (1973): Terapia del carcinoma mammario metastatizzato con ciclofosfamide, methotrexate, vincristina e fluoro-uracile. (Treatment of metastatic breast cancer with cyclophosphamide, methotrexate, vincristine, and fluorouracil.) *Tumori*, 59:11–24.

95. DeLena, M., Brambilla, C., Morabito, A., and Bonadonna, G. (1975): Adriamycin plus vincristine compared to and combined with cyclophosphamide, methotrexate and 5-fluorouracil for advanced breast cancer. *Cancer*, 35:1108–1115.

96. Fisher, B., Carbone, P. P., Economou, S. G., Frelick, R., Glass, A., Lerner, H., Redmond, C., Zelen, M., Katrych, D. L., Wolmark, N., Band, P., and Fisher, E. R. (1975): L-Phenylalanine mustard (L-PAM) in the management of primary breast cancer: A report of early findings. *N. Engl. J. Med.*, 292:117–122.

97. Brusamolino, E., Bonadonna, G., Morabito, A., and Veronesi, U. (1974): Controlled study for prolonged combination chemotherapy as an adjuvant in breast cancer. *Proc. XI Int. Cancer Congr.*, 3:532 (abstract).

98. Blum, R. H., and Carter, S. K. (1974). Review of adriamycin—a new anticancer drug with significant clinical activity. *Ann. Intern. Med.*, 80:249–259.

99. Hoogstraten, B., and George, S. (1974): Adriamycin and combination chemotherapy in breast cancer: A Southwest Oncology Group Study. *Proc. Am. Assoc. Cancer Res.,* 15:70 (abstract).

100. Ahmann, D., Bisel, H., and Hahn, R. G. (1974): Phase II evaluation of adriamycin (NSC 123127) as treatment for disseminated breast cancer. *Proc. Am. Assoc. Cancer Res.,* 15:100 (abstract).

101. Rosner, D., Dao, T., Horton, J., et al. (1974): Randomized study of adriamycin (ADM) vs. combined therapy (FCP) vs. adrenalectomy (ADX) in breast cancer. *Proc. Am. Assoc. Cancer Res.,* 15:63 (abstract).

102. Nemoto, T., Horton, J., Cunningham, T., Sponzo, R., Rosner, D., Diaz, R., and Dao, T. L. (1975): Update report: Comparison of combination chemotherapy (FCP) vs. adriamycin (ADM) vs. adrenalectomy (ADX) in breast cancer. *Proc. Am. Assoc. Cancer Res.,* 16:46 (abstract).

103. Salmon, S., and Jones, S. (1974): Chemotherapy of advanced breast cancer with a combination of adriamycin and cyclophosphamide. *Proc. Am. Assoc. Cancer Res.,* 15:90 (abstract).

104. Blumenschein, G., Cardenas, J., Freireich, E., and Gottlieb, J. (1974): FAC chemotherapy for breast cancer. *Proc. Am. Assoc. Cancer Res.,* 15:193 (abstract).

105. DeJager, R., Kaufman, R., Ochoa, M., and Krakoff, I. H. (1975): Chemotherapy of advanced breast cancer with a combination of cytoxan, adriamycin, and 5-FU (CAF). *Proc. Am. Assoc. Cancer Res.,* 16:273 (abstract).

106. Smalley, R., and Bornstein, R. (1975): C-A-F treatment of metastatic breast ca. *Proc. Am. Assoc. Cancer Res.,* 16:265 (abstract).

107. Horton, J., Dato, T., Cunningham, T., Nemoto, T., Sponzo, R., and Rosner, D. (1975): A comparison of 4 combination chemotherapies for metastatic breast cancer. *Proc. Am. Assoc. Cancer Res.,* 16:240 (abstract).

108. Harvey, H. A., White, D. S., and Lipton, A. (1975): Five drug regimen plus adriamycin in metastatic breast cancer. *Proc. Am. Assoc. Cancer Res.,* 16:255 (abstract).

109. Treves, N., and Finkbeiner, J. A. (1958): An evaluation of therapeutic surgical castration in the treatment of metastatic, recurrent, and primary inoperable mammary carcinoma in women: An analysis of 191 patients. *Cancer,* 11:421–438.

110. Kennedy, B. J. (1969): Hormone therapy in inoperable breast cancer. *Cancer,* 24:1345–1349.

111. MacCarty, W. C. (1922): Factors which influence longevity in cancer. *Ann. Surg.,* 76:9–12.

112. Black, M. M., Kerpe, S., and Speer, F. D. (1953): Lymph node structure in patients with cancer of the breast. *Am. J. Pathol.,* 29:505–521.

113. Hersh, E. M., Gutterman, J. U., and Mavligit, G. (1973): *Immunotherapy of Cancer in Man, Scientific Basis and Current Status.* Charles C Thomas, Springfield, Ill.

114. Mathe, G., Amiel, J. L., Schwarzenbert, L., et al. (1969): Active immunotherapy for acute lymphoblastic leukemia. *Lancet,* 1:697–699.

115. Gutterman, J. U., Mavligit, G., Gottlieb, J., et al. (1974): Chemoimmunotherapy of disseminated malignant melanoma with DTIC and BCG. *N. Engl. J. Med.,* 291:592–597.

116. Cardenas, J., Gutterman, J. U., Livingston, R. B., et al. (1975): 5-Fluorouracil, adriamycin, cyclophosphamide (FAC) with or without BCG maintenance chemotherapy for metastatic breast cancer. *J.A.M.A. (in press).*

117. Cardenas, J. O., Blumenschein, G. R., Gutterman, J. U., Freireich, E. J., and Gottlieb, J. A. (1975): Sequential combination chemotherapy for advanced metastatic breast carcinoma. *Proc. Am. Assoc. Cancer Res.,* 16:231 (abstract).

DISCUSSION

Levelle: What is the role of long-term Adriamycin treatment in regard to its toxicity?

Carter: It is important that Adriamycin has a total dose limitation of 550–600 mg/sq meter of body surface area (that is, 9 or 10 courses of treatment, depending on the dose level that is given. If you stay beneath that level you do not produce cardiomyopathy; if you go above it, there is a 20% incidence of a cardiomyopathy with congestive heart failure that is refractory to treatment in many cases and becomes quite dangerous.

Powles: Is there any information on the use of PAM with Adriamycin in breast cancer?

Carter: This has been tried in Italy, and while there was some experimental evidence to indicate that it might be valuable I have not seen any full analysis of the data to indicate whether it is going to be superior.

Breast Cancer: Trends in Research and Treatment, edited by J. C. Heuson,
W. H. Mattheiem, and M. Rozencweig. Raven Press, New York © 1976.

Current EORTC Trials

E. Engelsman

*Antoni van Leeuwenhoek Ziekenhuis, The Netherlands Cancer Institute,
Amsterdam, The Netherlands*

In 1974 two clinical trials by the EORTC Breast Cancer Cooperative Group
were concluded. In one the antiestrogen nafoxidine was shown to be at least as
effective as ethinyl estradiol in the treatment of advanced breast cancer; in the
other nafoxidine proved effective again, but L-DOPA failed to produce objective
remissions. The results of both trials were reported in 1975 (1,2) and are summarized in Table 1.

CHANGING VIEWS ON TREATMENT OF ADVANCED BREAST CANCER

By 1974 it was clear that remission rates in advanced breast cancer had begun
to move upward from the well-known 30% that could be expected from endocrine
treatment and from single-agent chemotherapy. In selected patients with estrogen
receptors present in their tumor tissue, a remission rate of approximately 60% can
be expected with endocrine treatment (3). In many advanced breast cancer patients, however, it is difficult or impossible to obtain tumor tissue specimens for
receptor assay, e.g., in patients presenting with lung, bone, or liver metastases.
Moreover, receptor assays are not available at all centers. More than 50%
remissions are achieved by combination chemotherapy, such as the CMF (cyclophosphamide, methotrexate, fluorouracil) combination or ADM (adriamycin) plus
VCR (vincristine) (4–6).

TABLE 1. *Trials concluded in 1974*

Comparative trial	Remitters/patients	% Remitters
Trial I		
Ethinyl estradiol	7/49	14
Nafoxidine	15/49	31
Trial II		
Nafoxidine	7/36	19
L-DOPA	0/40	0

DESIGN OF NEW TRIAL

The EORTC Breast Cancer Cooperative Group decided in 1974 that patients presenting with advanced breast cancer were entitled to treatment with at least a 50% chance of remission. A schedule was designed for combined treatment of advanced disease based on a number of considerations that should lead to a maximum effect:

1. Combination chemotherapy should be used.

2. The treatment should be intermittent to allow for sufficient recovery of the host tissues. In the time required for recovery of normal tissues, the tumor tissue is supposed to have not yet fully recovered from the effects of the preceding dose, with the result shown in Fig. 1.

3. Resistance against cytotoxic agents, if not present originally, develops sooner or later. In a number of tumors, resistance develops so early that clinically no objective remissions can be recorded, although the treatment may have been effective during a short phase.

The decision of the clinician that the result of a treatment must be regarded as a failure does not mean that there was no effect on the tumor. It seemed worthwhile to try to exploit these small "subclinical" effects by an alternating regimen (Fig. 2). Two treatments are shown in Fig. 2, each of which would fail to produce an objective remission if used on its own. Treatment A has some effect, but resistance develops soon and clinically the result would be recorded as "no change." When progression is evident again, treatment B is started. B is somewhat more effective than A and produces clinically recognizable tumor regression, but here also resistance develops and the result falls short of the criteria for objective remission: The measurable effects should have lasted for at least 3 months.

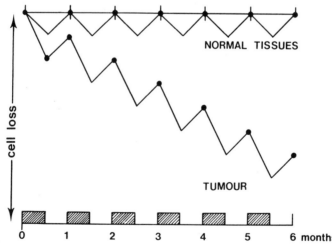

FIG. 1. Recovery in cyclical chemotherapy of EORTC breast cancer group.

If development of resistance could be prevented or at least postponed by giving alternating courses of A and B, the effect on tumor volume might be as indicated by the heavy lines in the figure. Since two almost equally effective combinations, probably without cross resistance, were available, the group decided to test this hypothesis by giving the CMF and the ADM-VCR combinations alternatingly.

4. Apart from the 30% of patients who achieve an objective remission on endocrine therapy, there are others in whom the treatment has some effect, although it is too small to meet the criteria of a remission. However, small, even "subclinical" effects of an endocrine treatment might add to the overall result in a combination hormone-cytotoxic therapy. We decided to include hormone therapy in the schedule and selected tamoxifen, an antiestrogen that is virtually nontoxic. Estrogen receptors should be assayed whenever possible for correlation with the results at the final evaluation.

5. Not all patients with advanced breast cancer can tolerate high doses of cytotoxic drugs. Age, extensive liver or bone metastases, and previous radiother-

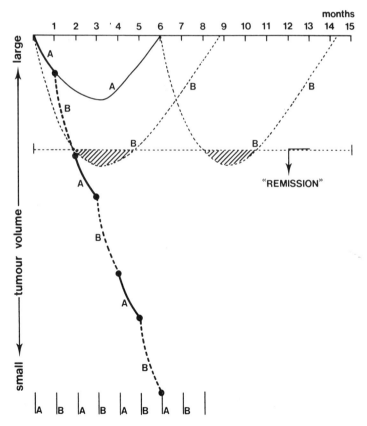

FIG. 2. Hypothetical effect of alternating cyclic chemotherapy (ABABABAB) of EORTC breast cancer group. A and B indicate different cytotoxic combinations.

TABLE 2. *Criteria of eligibility of patients for current trials*

Protocol 10741
Age: less than 68 years
No extensive bone involvement
No extensive bone irradiation
No extensive liver involvement
Protocol 10743
Age: 68–75 years
Extensive liver involvement
Previous endocrine treatment

apy to large areas of bone marrow are limiting factors. Therefore two separate protocols were designed: 10741 for patients who should be able to receive high doses of chemotherapy and 10743 for patients with expected impaired tolerance.

PROTOCOLS 10740, 10741, 10743

In 1974 the old general protocol of the EORTC Breast Cancer Cooperative Group was replaced by a new one (10740), describing the methodology of trials by the group. Protocols 10741 and 10743, for alternating intermittent hormonal-cytotoxic combination chemotherapy in postmenopausal patients, were started in July 1974. Selection criteria are listed in Table 2.

Table 3 shows the proposed dose schedule for protocol 10741. The main purpose of the trial is to establish the objective remission rate and the duration of remission; quality and duration of survival are also evaluated. Stratification is according to symptom-free interval and dominant site of metastatic lesions. A randomization takes place by which the alternating regimen starts with either combination A or B. If this should produce a difference for the induction of remission, it might come out at the final evaluation.

TABLE 3. *Dose schedule for protocol 10741*

Regimen	Dose
I (A): AV regimen	
Adriamycin	75 mg/m^2 on day 1
Vincristine	1.4 mg/m^2 on days 1 and 8
II (B): CMF regimen	
Cyclophosphamide	100 mg/m^2 on days 1–14
Methotrexate	60 mg/m^2 on days 1 and 8
5-Fluorouracil	600 mg/m^2 on days 1 and 8
Hormonal	
Tamoxifen	40 mg daily
	(Cyclus of 28 days)

The treatment is to be continued in all patients until clear progression is noted; the interval between two courses is lengthened to 6 weeks after 1 year. A problem will arise when the maximum safe dose for ADM has been reached (approximately 600 mg/m²), after eight courses of ADM-VCR, or after 20 months. At present we propose to continue, because this maximum dose has been found with ADM in a 3-week dose schedule, and it seems possible that the cardiac toxicity might be less if it is given at 2-month intervals, and later at 4-month intervals.

Very Preliminary Results

The trials were started in July 1974. By August 1975 there were 73 patients registered on protocol 10741 and 35 on protocol 10743. On more than 50% of the patients the intramural judgment of the treating clinicians is known, but the data have not yet been reviewed by two independent investigators, as is required for final evaluation by the general protocol.

The status of protocol 10741 by August 1975 is illustrated in Table 4. An acceptable remission rate of 67% has been reached in 40 evaluable patients. Table 5 shows the data for protocol 10743. The remission rate of 48% is not disappointing in these patients who were selected by expected impaired tolerance for chemotherapy.

I want to add my personal impression of this treatment, based on 18 patients registered on protocol 10741 in The Netherlands Cancer Institute so far (Table 6). Ten patients are evaluable now, and all 10 achieved a remission. The first three patients, entered 14 months ago, are still in remission (two complete, one partial). We saw two deaths by severe bone marrow toxicity, one in a patient who was not eligible.

For most patients the first two or three courses are not easily tolerable, but we find now that some of the long-term remitters help the beginners by explaining to

TABLE 4. *Protocol 10741: preliminary evaluation*
(August 1975)

Parameter	No. of patients
Patients registered	73
Not eligible	7
Not entered (toxicity)	2 (died)
Refused treatment	4
Insufficient data	6
Too early	14
Patients evaluable	40
Remission	27 (67%)
Partial	20
Complete	7
No change	4
Progression	9

TABLE 5. *Protocol 10743: preliminary evaluation*
(August 1975)

Parameter	No. of patients
Patients registered	35
Not eligible	2
Too early	3
Insufficient data	9
Patients evaluable	21
Remissions	10 (48%)
Partial	7
Complete	3
No change	6
Progression	5

them during their stay in the waiting room that it is worthwhile to persist. The loss of hair and wearing a wig is frightening at first but does not seem to be much of a problem once a remission has become evident.

My own impression is that the treatment schedule of protocol 10741 is surprisingly efficient, but that the toxicity is very severe in some patients. The use of this regimen for adjuvant chemotherapy of primary breast cancer is discussed by Mattheiem in another chapter.

PROTOCOL 10742

A separate protocol (10742) was started in 1974 to test the effectiveness of antiestrogens (tamoxifen) in premenopausal patients, instead of surgical or radiation castration. Twelve patients had been registered by June 1975, and at least two had shown a remission.

TABLE 6. *Protocol 10741: preliminary evaluation (Netherlands Cancer Institute, September 1975)*

Parameter	No. of patients
Patients registered	18
Not eligible	2
Toxicity	1 (died)
Too early	5
Patients evaluable	10
Remissions	10
Partial	8 (3–14 months; one death from toxicity)
Complete	2 (14 months)

REFERENCES

1. Heuson, J. C., Engelsman E., Blonk-van der Wijst, J., Maass, H., Drochmans, A., Michel, J., Nowakowski, H., and Gorins, A. (1975): *Br. Med. J.,* 2:711.
2. Engelsman, E., Heuson, J. C., Blonk-van der Wijst, J., Drochmans, A., Maass, H., Cheix, F., Sobrinho, L. G., and Nowakowski, H. (1975): *Br. Med. J.,* 2:714.
3. McGuire, W. L., Volmer, E. P., and Carbone, P. P., editors (1975): *Estrogen Receptors in Human Breast Cancer.* Raven Press, New York.
4. Carter, S. K. (1972): In: *The Design of Clinical Trials in Cancer Therapy,* edited by M. Staquet, p. 336. Editions Scientifiques Européennes, Brussels.
5. Carbone, P. A. (1974): In: *Report to the Profession: Breast Cancer,* p. 171. National Cancer Institute, N.I.H., Bethesda.
6. de Lena, M., Brambilla, C., Moralito, A., and Bonadonna, G. (1975): *Cancer,* 35:1108.

Breast Cancer: Trends in Research and Treatment, edited by J. C. Heuson, W. H. Mattheiem, and M. Rozencweig. Raven Press, New York © 1976.

Roundtable Discussion: Palliative Treatment

P. Alberto

Alberto: Dr. Bonadonna, will you give a short version of your results on your particular program of treatment?

Bonadonna: I would like to update some of the results on disseminated breast cancer that we published in *Cancer* this year. CMF and Adriamycin plus vincristine in combination were tested on a random basis to develop the concept of noncross resistant combinations. These data include both complete and partial remission and show rates of 52% with Adriamycin plus vincristine and approximately the same with CMF. On crossover, because of relapse or progression, about 30% of the patients did show some response, which was better in the soft tissues, but an appreciable number with bone involvement showed recalcification: 27% in the Adriamycin plus vincristine group and 21% in the CMF group.

Although the percentage of patients achieving complete plus partial remission is remarkable, as Dr. Carter mentioned before, the duration of complete response is still not what we would like to have. At least it is not yet comparable with what we see in a fraction of patients with malignant lymphomas. Again, though, as far as the two treatment groups are concerned, there is currently no difference and the same applies to median survival.

What we are doing at the moment is alternating cycles of therapy: (A) two cycles of Adriamycin plus vincristine followed by two of CMF, and in (B) just the opposite, two CMF cycles followed by two AV. The very preliminary data, which Dr. Christina Brambilla from this group has been putting together, shows that after four cycles with treatment A, complete plus partial remission is 38.5%, and with treatment B it is 40%. I would not take these data as definitive because the study has just been started, and we know that in a large number of patients it takes many cycles before achieving full remission. These new studies with alternating cycles were undertaken at our institute, as well as in other countries, not only to achieve a higher percent of complete response but also to try to prolong the duration of response. Increasing the response will be difficult unless we dramatically change the selection of patients.

Mouridsen: In our study in Copenhagen, patients with metastatic breast cancer were randomized to treatment either with continuous cyclophosphamide or the five-drug combination, according to Cooper. The patients were postmenopausal, ranging from less than 50 up to 75 years; they had a histologically proved diagnosis of metastatic disease, or measurable disease, and had been given no prior chemotherapy. There were 28 patients in one group and 27 in the other, the patients being matched for age, disease-free interval, previous radiotherapy, previous endocrine therapy, performance scale, and number of metastatic sites. The results showed 44% of partial remission on the Cooper regimen and only 21% with cyclophosphamide alone. Complete remission was seen in 19% on the Cooper regimen, and only 4% with cyclophosphamide. The duration of remission was 11 months with the Cooper regimen and only 7 months with cyclophosphamide. The conclusion of this trial is that the combined treatment is more than twice as effective as the single-drug treatment, and duration of remission is significantly longer.

Alberto: Dr. Band has a contribution showing a series of 40 cases treated with tamoxifen alone, in correlation with estrogen receptors.

Band: These are preliminary results of a phase 2 study carried out in conjunction with Dr. Harvey Lerner from Philadelphia and Prof. Lucien Israel. The patients had metastatic breast cancer, using the criteria for response defined by the Eastern Co-operative Oncology Group. Twenty patients were treated at a tamoxifen dose of 15 mg/sq meter twice daily, which is slightly higher than that which the EORTC group is currently using. Responses were seen for all the major sites of dominant disease, and 7 out of 20 patients had objective responses. Twenty-one patients were treated at a lower dose (10 mg twice daily) which represents the dose used by workers in the UK generally, and if anything there was a higher response at this lower regimen. The treatment was well tolerated with minimal toxicity. Of 10 patients in whom tissue was assayed for estrogen receptors, 6 out of 6 responded who had positive receptors, and none of 4 with negative receptors.

Alberto: First, is there a risk of stimulating the tumor with antihormonal compounds; and second, what is the risk of diminishing the remission rates when you combine chemotherapy and hormonal therapy?

Carter: I do not think that this is a great risk. There was a study, which the Eastern Co-operative Oncology Group published, in which Premarin (or conjugated estrogens) was compared in a controlled fashion to 5-Fu plus the conjugated estrogens. There was absolutely no difference in response rate or duration of response between the estrogens alone, and the estrogen plus chemotherapy. It was a negative study in that the chemotherapy did not do any better, but at least it answers the question that the chemotherapy did not make the situation worse in this particular controlled situation.

Anonymous: Following a relapse after remission with a hormonal treatment, are antihormonal treatments active?

Engelsman: For a number of years we have been giving all the endocrine treatments sequentially, and we have a number of patients who had relapsed after other endocrine therapies and who remitted again on antiestrogens, nafoxidine as well as tamoxifen.

Lucas: I am a renal transplant surgeon, and what we are hoping to achieve in immunotherapy or rather in immunosuppression is the opposite of what you are all trying to achieve with therapy of cancer. We want our foreign substance (the transplant) to survive, and you of course want your foreign substance (the cancer) to die. One of the problems that we have with kidney transplantation is that when we have induced prolonged immunosuppression after a year or more, we come up with an incidence of cancer in our patients of approximately 10–15%. In patients who are on chemotherapy for cancer, what is the incidence of second, totally new cancers? Is this going to be a significant problem that we must look forward to as chemotherapy for cancer becomes better and better?

Carter: Yes, it is a potential problem. I think, though, that it is very difficult to pin this down, because as patients live longer under treatment, we may expose a greater propensity to develop a second malignancy which is intrinsic in whatever factor induced the malignant process in the first place. For instance, if you keep acute multiple myeloma patients alive 2-3 years with PAM treatment and they develop acute myelocytic leukemia is it because of the alkylating agent? Or as a result of keeping such a patient alive long enough, is there a propensity to develop an acute myelocytic leukemia? It is an extremely difficult question to study in a controlled fashion. There is no doubt that we are dealing with carcinogenic, as well as immunosuppressive, agents. My feeling is that we will probably have a secondary tumor problem, although it will probably not be dramatic. The question then is: Is the tumor due to immunosuppression or to the intrinsic carcinogenicity of the compound? We are very concerned about that in the adjuvant studies where we are using long-term treatment. One of the things we are doing is giving intermittent courses of treatment, because it has been shown very clearly that you get immunosuppression and then a recovery, and occasionally even a rebound, depending on the sequence and schedule used. In all these studies we are not getting prolonged continuous immunosuppression without recovery. If we do come up with secondary tumors, we will have to judge the cross-benefit ratio of increasing survival and cures versus the problem of the second malignancy. We will certainly not be able to distinguish whether carcinogenicity or immunosuppression is the cause of it.

Alberto: Dr. Lucas, what in your opinion as a nonclinician oncologist is the place, if any, for immunotherapy in the treatment of breast cancer?

Lucas: We do not know enough about immunology to apply it to clinical trials. It depends on what your definition of immunotherapy is, and I am assuming that when you give BCG you are activating a nonspecific macrophage effect, which may have certain beneficial results. It is not the early macrophage-type work that I am critical of but the trials where various groups are now infusing lymphocytes into patients as a form of immunotherapy. One of the important facts is that there is no single kind of lymphocyte, there are many. You can classify them in many different ways: as T-cells, B-cells. You can classify them according to function, cytotoxic cells, suppressor cells; if you take a tumor and mix it with cytotoxic lymphocytes and inject the tumor subcutaneously into a susceptible animal, that tumor will not grow as fast as one that is injected alone. On the other hand, if you take a tumor and mix it with suppressor cells, that tumor will now grow faster, as much as two or three times as fast, measured by weights, as if you did not inject it with lymphocytes. At the present time we have no way of clearly separating suppressor cells, on the one hand, from cytotoxic cancer cells on the other.

Someone mentioned that one of the possibilities is to activate lymphocytes with PHA and then infuse activated lymphocytes in the patients. It is not generally known that during the first 36 hr following addition of PHA lymphocyte cultures, what one finds is an increase in cytotoxicity, which is all to the good; but if one waits 48 hr, the cytotoxic response fades away and a suppressor response comes on. This is now being investigated strongly, using cells which have been activated by using PHA or concanavalin A for 48 or 72 hr to shut down the immune response for antibody and cytotoxic cells. My conclusion is that we really need more basic work before we can apply it to the clinical patient.

Palshof: The preliminary results from protocol 10741 demonstrated a 5% mortality from treatment. Is that acceptable?

Engelsman: We realize that we are taking some risks with beginning heavy chemotherapy combinations, and that we must watch what we are doing constantly. We think that the toxic deaths have occurred at the beginning of treatment. It is very important to see why these patients died because there are many patients of approximately 70 years who may die of other causes. Of course, there are a number of patients who, despite having no extensive bone marrow involvement and not having undergone extensive irradiation, have a lower tolerance to chemotherapeutic drugs, and this is something I think you cannot completely predict. The two toxic deaths by chemotherapy in this trial were rather surprising to everybody, as we had no means of knowing beforehand that they would respond with such a heavy bone marrow depression. This is laying a heavy responsibility on the older patients, and maybe we should revise our schedule to start with a lower dose. Within the breast cancer group we have to talk through this problem, and one more toxic death at the beginning of treatment would probably be too much. No one knows if so many deaths are acceptable if they occur only at the beginning of the trial. If everybody had to get used to the treatment, it might be acceptable, but it certainly would not be if the death rate remained this high. We intend to continue this regimen until there is evidence of an increasing mortality rate. This means that if the patient is remitting, or even if there is no change we will continue the treatment. We decided to change the schedule after a year to one course of chemotherapy every 2 months, so that the time to reach potential accumulative toxicity of Adriamycin is postponed. By 20 months of treatment the patient will have reached a total Adriamycin dose of 600 mg/sq meter, and at the moment we are discussing whether to continue after that. It is possible that cumulative toxicity for Adriamycin will vary with different schedules.

Alberto: I noticed that you used methotrexate in a dose of 60 mg/sq meter, which would probably be considered very high. We have had long experience with the CMF regimen and in patients with good renal function tests and so on; with no extensive metastatic disease, we give 40 mg/sq meter. However, in patients with poor renal function or extensive metastatic lesions we start with 30 mg/sq meter.

Heuson: Dr. Bogden, would you comment on the feasibility of approaching the question of using alternating cycles of treatment more quickly in animal models? This would help the clinicians enormously.

Bogden: The animal model, especially a tumor model that is responsive to these agents, can be structured and utilized to match the required situation. We do not know if you can extrapolate to the clinical situation, but at least it can tell you something about what we do know—responses to a certain number of agents.

Alberto: Are there comments about the use of chemotherapy with surgery?

Carter: We have an ongoing series of controlled trials comparing oophorectomy to oophorectomy plus chemotherapy. In one trial the chemotherapy is given immediately after oophorectomy, and in another the chemotherapy is given only to those patients who are responding to oophorectomy—half of them getting chemotherapy, half not. These trials will give us the answers to the questions; we have no data yet, but we will have the answers pretty soon, empirically based on clinical results.

Breast Cancer: Trends in Research and Treatment, edited by J. C. Heuson, W. H. Mattheiem, and M. Rozencweig. Raven Press, New York © 1976.

Changing Strategy for Curative Treatment of Breast Cancer

Paul P. Carbone

Ecology Group, 850 Sligo Avenue, Suite 601, Silver Springs, Maryland 20910

Breast cancer presents clinically as a lump in the breast. In data collected from tumor registries by the National Cancer Institute (NCI) End Results Section, 45% of all patients present with disease limited to the breast, 43% have regional disease, and only 10% have metastatic disease (Table 1). Survival is related to disease extent, being best for localized breast cancer (84% at 5 years), 56% for regional, and 10% for metastatic disease (1) (Table 2).

Surgery alone or surgery and radiotherapy have been the traditional approaches to treatment in 80% or more of patients (Table 1). The radical mastectomy devised by Halsted over 80 years ago has been the classic operation (2). The results in many centers have been quite comparable, since the indications for this operation have been highly refined. However, two opposing approaches to treatment have been proposed. One school advocates expanding the operation and/or adding radiotherapy (3). Others have advocated less surgery, attempting to ascribe similar results with less mutilation (4,5). Radiotherapists likewise are suggesting

TABLE 1. *Female breast cancer: stage and treatment*

Parameter	1965–1969	1970–1971
No. of cases	14,493	5,600
Percent in stage classification		
Localized	47	45
Regional	41	43
Distant	10	10
Unknown	2	2
Percent treated by		
Surgery alone	53	53
Radiation alone	2	3
Surgery + radiation	27	31
Chemotherapy/hormonotherapy	3	2
Combined chemotherapy/surgery/radiation	12	8
None	3	3

From Axtell and Myers, ref. 1.

TABLE 2. *Breast cancer relative survival rates, 1965–1969*

Years of survival	% Survival in various stages			
	Total	Localized	Regional	Distant
1	80	97	92	45
3	74	91	70	17
5	64	84	56	10

From Axtell and Myers, ref. 1.

that postoperative radiotherapy combined with less surgery produces equivalent results (6).

The dilemma concerning the primary treatment of breast cancer can be examined as questions about surgical techniques, i.e., radical versus extended radical. Where adequate randomized clinical trials of these options have been done, the 5- and 10-year results are comparable (7). Does radiotherapy added to radical mastectomy increase the local or systemic control of breast cancer? Here the answer is clearly no (8). Does less extensive surgery give results comparable to a radical mastectomy? While the data are less clear, a simple mastectomy with or without radiotherapy has had failure rates similar to those associated with radical mastectomy. For patients with a clinically negative axilla, less extensive surgery combined with removal of the tumor and a small portion of the breast combined with X-ray therapy is equivalent to a radical mastectomy. In patients with clinically involved axillae (stage II), the lesser surgical procedure is not as effective as a radical mastectomy and postoperative X-ray therapy (6).

If we examine the same problem as a biological question (i.e., why patients fail to be cured), we find that failure of cure is related not to the type of primary treatment but rather to the inability of all these procedures to affect occult metastases that become manifest in the bones, liver, or lungs. While removal of the axillary contents and the chest wall muscles are not clearly superior to leaving them in, we know that prognosis and disease failure is related to the presence or absence of histological involvement of the axilla (9). For patients with histologically negative nodes, 75% are disease-free at 10 years. For positive-node patients, only 25% are without recurrence at 10 years. Most impressive are the dire results in women with four or more axillary nodes; recurrence is found in 90% at 10 years, and survival is approximately 10%. Thus patients fail to be cured despite an aggressive attack on their local disease and lymph nodes because metastases are already present at the time of diagnosis. One of the best indications of a dire prognosis is the presence of tumor in the axillary nodes *(vide supra)*. The mortality due to breast cancer continues to be greater than expected until 20 years or more after primary treatment (10).

Experimental studies have shown that even small tumors shed cancer cells into the circulation. Many of these cells do not give rise to metastases. The local lymph nodes are not efficient mechanical traps of cancer cells (11). Yet the basis for radical mastectomy was that cancer cells develop as a localized tumor deposit that first spreads locally. With time, these cells invade local tissues by contiguous extension. With more time, the cancer cells enter the lymphatics and spread to the lymph nodes, and eventually *late* in the course they invade the bloodstream to disseminate and develop metastases. While the radical mastectomy and/or local radiotherapy can control the primary tumor growth, they clearly have no effect on systemic micrometastases. Therefore one can logically deduce that any one of several surgical or surgery/radiotherapy maneuvers can control local disease. Moreover, since the reason patients fail to be cured is that they have occult metastases, then some effective systemic therapy combined with local therapy offers the best chance of cure. The number and size of these tumor deposits, along with the effectiveness of systemic treatment, determine the curability.

The principles for systemic treatment of micrometastases by drug treatment have been worked out in experimental systems by Schabel (12), Stolfi et al. (13), and Bogden et al. (14). Cancer chemotherapeutic drugs kill by first-order kinetics (15). Wilcox (15) ably described the analogy of first-order cell kill by drugs as being like a small boy standing outside a hen house with an unlimited supply of nails. Without aiming he throws the nails through the chicken wire. Only those nails which go through without touching the wire and strike the egg point first will break an egg. He states, "Most of the nails will strike the wire and be going too slow to 'react.' Of the few that go directly through, most will not be traveling point first. Each egg is likely to be struck many times before it is broken, but sooner or later it [the egg] will receive a fatal blow. Let us suppose that by the time the boy has thrown a bushel of nails, 900 of the 1,000 eggs have been broken. The nails continue...but each nail has a smaller chance of breaking an egg because there are only a 10th as many eggs...so we may expect the second bushel of nails to break only 90 of the remaining eggs. The third bushel will probably break about 9 of the last 10 eggs. There are then 9 chances in 10 that the last egg will not survive the next bushel of nails and the chance that it will survive two or more bushels is no better than 1 in 100." Thus in the treatment of these small tumors, treatment must be sufficiently long that the probability of killing all cells is 100%. It obviously depends on getting enough drug to the tumor to kill each cell.

The sensitivity of tumor cells to killing by drugs is also related to their growth kinetics. Reduction of the body burden by removing gross tumor has been shown to increase the growth fraction and shorten the average cell cycle time (12). The response of the clinically apparent tumor does not predict for the sensitivity of the micrometastases; these are more vulnerable to chemotherapy. Experimental data are available to demonstrate this principle in a variety of systems, including a spontaneously metastasizing mammary cancer.

Systemic therapeutic approaches to human breast cancer include the use of chemotherapy, hormonotherapy, and immunotherapy. Chemotherapy and hormonotherapy have had the widest application. A variety of antineoplastic drugs alone (16) and in combination (17) have a wide range of effectiveness in patients with advanced disease. Combinations have been shown to produce higher response rates than single agents. In this chapter several aspects of systemic treatment are relevant to the problem of developing a meaningful new biology in the curative treatment of breast cancer.

One of the first questions relates to which drugs to use. Secondly, how much effectiveness and/or toxicity is required to produce an effect in the adjuvant situation as compared to late disease? Thirdly, how does one combine chemotherapy and hormonotherapy?

Regarding the problem of which drug(s) to use, one must consider efficacy, safety, and tolerability, as well as more practical aspects of acceptability to the doctor and the patient. Breast cancer responds to a variety of single agents and combinations (16,17). The response rates to the single agents adriamycin (ADR), methotrexate (MTX), cyclophosphamide (CTX), L-phenylalanine mustard (L-PAM), vincristine (VCR), and 5-fluorouracil (FU) varies from 18% to 37% when used as treatment in advanced disease patients. Combinations of the more active agents with or without prednisone ranges from 50% to 80%. Yet few patients with advanced disease achieve complete disappearance of all tumor, and response, when it occurs, lasts only a few months. Survival gain is measured likewise in terms of 1 year or less. Prednisone and VCR are frequently used in combination chemotherapy programs in patients with advanced disease and have adverse long-term effects on normal tissues. Ahmann (18) and Ramirez (19) and their associates reported that prednisone and VCR may not add significantly to the response rates of multiple drug combinations in advanced disease, thereby decreasing the necessity of using these drugs in an adjuvant or combined modality mode. ADR, a relative newcomer, has many adverse side effects including cardiotoxicity, although additions of ADR to FU, CTX, and MTX in various combinations have proved to be very active in patients with advanced breast cancer (20–22).

One of the major factors in the choice of drugs for use with surgery rests on the acceptability of the drug(s) to surgeons, particularly their attitudes on its safety. As mentioned previously, primary breast cancer is a localized disease most often treated and seen by surgeons. Therefore any regimen suggested for an adjuvant situation must be acceptable to them. Avoidance of severe side effects in the testing of the initial combined modality therapy is an absolute necessity. Once efficacy has been shown, willingness by the surgeons to accept more toxicity to increase effectiveness is a natural consequence. The tolerance and oral administration of L-PAM were major deciding factors in the choice of L-PAM for the NSABP-ECOG trial (23).

Another important element of combined modality trials relates to the degree of activity in advanced disease patients (a logical test system) needed to be translated into an effective regimen in early disease (adjuvant situation). From the experimental systems we see that there may be little relationship between activity against advanced tumors and effectiveness of the same regimen in the adjuvant or combined modality mode (12). After surgery there is a wide variation in the tumor load, but by definition all the bulky tumor sites have been cleared. Thus highly curative regimens are not needed in advanced disease to be effective against the micrometastases.

The correlative data of advanced disease activity and adjuvant activity become extremely important, not only for the treatment of breast cancer but also for the design of adjuvant trials with other solid tumors. The Eastern Group recently reported that the results of their study utilizing L-PAM produced responses in 19% of patients and CMF in 53% (24). Both of these regimens have been used in the adjuvant situation and have been shown to delay recurrence significantly (23,25). While these studies are still early, the data collected will prove to be very important in determining the goals for developing adjuvant trials for other solid tumors. A preliminary comparison of these two trials is shown in Table 3. Response rates of 19–50% are achievable in other solid tumors, thus setting the stage for further adjuvant trials.

Endocrine therapy has been a major therapeutic tool in the management of human breast cancer. Estrogen therapy in postmenopausal women results in responses in 16–37% of patients (26). Ablative hormonal therapy (i.e., castration, hypophysectomy, and/or adrenalectomy) likewise can induce significant regression in 20–40% of patients. As reported recently, estrogen receptors (ER) have been found in human breast cancers (27). Response to hormone treatment is highly unlikely if the receptor is absent. A positive ER test does not guarantee a response but does confer a better probability of response. Hormone treatment, particularly in ER-positive women, therefore would be desirable to enhance response when combined with chemotherapy. Combinations of hormone and chemotherapy may employ two possible strategies.

First, since breast cancer growth can be stimulated by estrogens, hormones can be used to induce cells into initiating DNA synthesis. This should increase the growth fraction and increase the cell kill by cycle-specific agents. A trial done by the Eastern Cooperative Oncology Group (ECOG) proved to be unsuccessful (28). Estrogen stimulation is dose-dependent and may be short-lived.

A second approach is to combine cytotoxic agents and hormonal treatment as if they were two independent agents. Some trials have already indicated that this can be done successfully (29). Other trials are currently underway to test this approach (Table 4). However, as tumors may be stimulated by estrogens, removal of estrogens or large pharmacological doses may shut off DNA synthesis and compete with cytotoxic killing by drugs (30). Moreover, if there are two populations of cells (ER+ and ER−, as contrasted to ER+ monoclonal populations that lose their ER activity), the strategy employed may need to be different. In the listed trials attempts are being made to look at the question of sequencing versus simultaneous combinations to examine the possible interference or synergism.

In trials now underway in combined modality treatment of primary breast cancer, a variety of regimens, using combinations of chemotherapy and immunotherapy, and chemotherapy and hormonotherapy, are being tried (Table 5). They are all based on the assumption that breast cancer is a systemic disease. They will determine whether the principle of combined modality treatment is valid for breast

TABLE 3. Recurrence rates for *L-PAM and CMF adjuvant trials*

	One to three positive nodes		Four or more positive nodes		Premenopausal		Postmenopausal	
	No. of pts.	%	No. of pts.	%	No. of pts.	%	No. of pts.	%
Surgery alone								
Fisher (23)	74	8	74	31	54	24	85	18
Bonadonna (25)	92	10	36	33	42	17	86	16
Surgery and chemotherapy								
Fisher	75	3	73	16	50	10	86	10
Bonadonna	70	1.4	33	3	48	0	55	4

Data as of February 1975.

TABLE 4. *Hormone and chemotherapy trials*

Regimens	Investigators	Group
Oophorectomy ± cyclophosphamide, fluorouracil, prednisone	Ahmann	Mayo Clinic
Oophorectomy ± cyclophosphamide, methotrexate, fluorouracil	Perlia-Carbone	Eastern Cooperative Oncology Group
Oophorectomy with and without cyclophosphamide or cyclophosphamide, methotrexate, fluorouracil, vincristine, prednisone, methotrexate	Tormey-Holland	Acute Leukemia Group B
Estrogen ± cyclophosphamide, methotrexate, fluorouracil	Tormey	National Cancer Institute, Bethesda
Estrogens ± cyclophosphamide, adriamycin, fluorouracil	Vogel	Emory University

TABLE 5. *Controlled combined modality trials in primary breast cancer*

Group	Treatment	Investigators
NSABP (USA)		
Protocol 5	RM vs. RM + L-PAM	Fisher
Protocol 7	RM + L-PAM vs. L-PAM + FU	Fisher
NCI-Milan (Italy)	RM vs. RM + CMF	Bonadonna, Veronese
Mayo Clinic (USA)	RM + L-PAM RM + CFP RM + CFP + XRT	Ahmann, Paine
Northwestern U. (USA)	RM + L-PAM RM + CFP RM + CFP + BCG	Scanlon
UCLA (USA)	RM + CMF + BCG RM + CMF + BCG + TC	Sparks, Morton
Case Western Reserve (USA)	RM RM + CMF + AE RM + CMF + AE + BCG	
ALGB (USA)	RM + CMFVP RM + CMF RM + CMF + MER	Tormey, Holland
Guy's Hospital (England)	RM vs. RM + L-PAM	Hayward
British Breast Group	RM vs. RM + FU	Forrest

Abbreviations: RM=radical mastectomy. L-PAM =L-phenylalanine mustard. FU=fluorouracil. CMF=cyclophosphamide, methotrexate, fluorouracil. XRT=irradiation. CFP= cyclophosphamide, fluorouracil, prednisone. BCG=Bacillus Calmette-Guérin. TC=allogeneic tumor cells. AE=antiestrogens. CMFVP=cyclophosphamide, methotrexate, fluorouracil, vincristine, prednisone. MER=methanol-extractable residue of BCG.

cancer. Moreover, the success of any of these advanced disease regimens used in the early clinical stage then sets the bench mark against which we will measure our achievements in treating other solid tumors. So far it appears that the experimental principle—that activity is accentuated when used against early disease—is a valid one. The results indicate that we have the tools in hand to decrease significantly the morbidity and mortality of breast cancer. The challenge is to perform well-designed clinical trials to obtain the best data. The most obvious questions are:

1. What is the best treatment producing the best results with the least toxicity when combined with surgery?

2. Can immunotherapy or endocrine therapy add significantly to chemotherapy regimens?

3. How can these other modalities most effectively be combined with chemotherapy?

4. What is the optimal duration of treatment?

5. Can we identify those patients with no positive histological nodes who are bound to fail so that they can be treated? Likewise, can we avoid treatment in the positive-node patients who are not going to experience recurrence?

The answer to some of these questions may be aided by the identification of a specific breast tumor cell marker. Several studies have indicated that CEA and other products of tumor cells may be useful as markers of active disease (31,32). If we had a good tumor cell product like paraproteins in myeloma and HCG in choriocarcinoma, questions like identifying high-risk patients and duration and intensity of treatment would be answered more expeditiously. The ER assay modified to be more selective will help to identify the best treatment. The recent developments indicating that breast cancer cells grow readily in tissue culture and thymus-deficient mice will help in developing laboratory models to select specific chemotherapy for individual patients (33).

REFERENCES

1. Axtell, L. M., and Myers, M. H. (1975): Recent trends in survival of cancer patients 1960–1971. In: *End Results in Cancer Report #4.* D.H.E.W. Publication No. (N.I.H.) 767.
2. Halsted, W. S. (1894–1895): The results of operations for the cure of cancer of the breast performed at The Johns Hopkins Hospital from June 1889 to January 1894. *Johns Hopkins Hosp. Rep.,* 4:297–350.
3. Urban, J. A., and Castro, E. B. (1971): Selecting variations in extent of surgical procedure for breast cancer. *Cancer,* 28:1615–1623.
4. Crile, G. (1975): Results of conservative treatment of breast cancer at ten and fifteen years. *Ann. Surg.,* 181:26–30.
5. Hayward, J. (1974): The conservative treatment of early breast cancer. *Cancer,* 33:593–599.
6. Atkins, H., Hayward, J. L., Klugman, D. J., and Wayte, A. B. (1972): Treatment of early breast cancer; a report after 10 years of a clinical trial. *Br. Med. J.,* 2:423–429.
7. Caceres, E. (1967): An evaluation of radical mastectomy and extended radical mastectomy for cancer of the breast. *Surg. Gynecol. Obstet.,* 125:337–341.
8. Fisher, B., Slack, N. H., Cavanaugh, P. J., Gardner, B., Ravdin, R. G., et al. (1970): Postoperative radiotherapy in the treatment of breast cancer: Results of the NSABP clinical trial. *Ann. Surg.,* 172:711–732.

9. Fisher, B., Slack, N., Katrych, D., and Wolmark, N. (1975): Ten year followup results of patients with carcinoma of the breast in a cooperative clinical trial evaluating surgical adjuvant therapy. *Surg. Gynecol. Obstet.*, 140:528–534.
10. Forrest, P. (1974): Primary cancer of the breast—indications for therapy. In: *The Treatment of Breast Cancer*, edited by H. Atkins, pp. 9–48. University Park Press, Baltimore.
11. Fisher, B. (1970): The surgical dilemma in the primary therapy of invasive breast cancer: A critical appraisal. *Curr. Probl. Surg.*, October.
12. Schabel, F. M. (1975): Concepts for systemic treatment of micrometastases. *Cancer*, 35:15–24.
13. Stolfi, R. L., Martin, D. S., and Fugmann, R. A. (1971): Spontaneous murine mammary adenocarcinoma: Model system for evaluation of combined methods of therapy. *Cancer Chemother. Rep.*, 55:239–249.
14. Bogden, A. E., Ebber, H. J., Taylor, D. J., and Gray, J. H. (1974): Comparative study of surgery, chemotherapy and immunotherapy alone and in combination on metastases of 13762 mammary adenocarcinoma. *Cancer Res.*, 34:1627–1631.
15. Wilcox, W. S. (1966): The last surviving cancer cell: The chances of killing it. *Cancer Chemother. Rep.*, 50:541–542.
16. Carter, S. K. (1974): The chemical therapy of breast cancer. *Semin. Oncol.*, 1:131–144.
17. Broder, L. E., and Tormey, D. C. (1974): Combination chemotherapy of carcinoma of the breast. *Cancer Treat. Rev.*, 1:183–203.
18. Ahmann, D. L., Bisel, H. S., and Hahn, R. G. (1974): A phase II evaluation of adriamycin as treatment for disseminated breast cancer. *Proc. Am. Assoc. Cancer Res.*, 15:100.
19. Rameriz, G., Strawitz, J. G., Wilson, W. L., Cornell, G. N., Madden, R. E., and The Central Oncology Group (1975): Multiple drug therapy in disseminated breast carcinoma—a randomized study. *Proc. Am. Assoc. Cancer Res.*, 16:33.
20. Blumenschein, G. R., Cardenos, J. O., Livingston, R. B., Einhorn, L. H., Freireich, E. J., and Gottlieb, J. A. (1975): 5-Fluorouracil, adriamycin and cyclophosphamide combination chemotherapy for metastatic breast cancer. *Clin. Res.*, 23:336.
21. Bull, J., Tormey, D., Falkson, G., Blom, J., Perlin, E., and Carbone, P. (1975): A comparison of cyclophosphamide, adriamycin and 5-fluorouracil versus cyclophosphamide, methotrexate and 5-fluorouracil in metastatic breast cancer. *Proc. Am. Assoc. Cancer Res.*, 15:246.
22. DeJagar, R. L., Kaufman, R., Ochoa, M., and Krakoff, I. H. (1975): Chemotherapy of advanced breast cancer with a combination of Cytoxan, adriamycin and 5-fluorouracil. *Proc. Am. Assoc. Cancer Res.*, 16:273.
23. Fisher, B., Carbone, P. P., Economou, S. G., Frelick, R., Glass, A., Lerner, H., Redmond, C., Zelen, M., Katrych, D. L., Wolmark, N., Band, P., and Fisher, E. R. (1975): L-Phenylalanine mustard (L-PAM) in the management of primary breast cancer: A report of early findings. *N. Engl. J. Med.*, 292:117–122.
24. Canellos, G. P., Pocock, S. J., Taylor, S. G., III, Sears, M. E., Klaassen, D. J., and Band, P. R. (1975): Combination chemotherapy for metastatic breast carcinoma: Prospective comparison of multiple drug therapy with L-phenylalanine mustard. *(In preparation.)*
25. Bonadonna, G., Brusamolino, E., Valagussa, P., and Veronesi, U. (1975): Adjuvant therapy with combination chemotherapy in operable breast ca. *Proc. Am. Assoc. Cancer Res.*, 16:254.
26. Heuson, J. C. (1974): Hormones by administration. In: *Treatment of Breast Cancer*, edited by H. Atkins, pp. 113–164. University Park Press, Baltimore.
27. McGuire, W. L., Carbone, P. P., and Vollmer, E. P. (1975): *Estrogen Receptors in Breast Cancer*. Raven Press, New York.
28. Taylor, S. G., III, Pocock, S. J., Shnider, B. I., Colsky, J., and Hall, T. C. (1975): Clinical studies of 5-fluorouracil + premarin in the treatment of breast cancer. *Med. Pediatr. Oncol. (in press)*.
29. van Dyk, J. J., and Falkson, G. (1971): Extended survival and remission rates in metastatic breast cancer. *Cancer*, 27:300–303.
30. Simpson-Herren, L., and Griswold, D. P. (1970): Studies on the kinetics of growth and regression of 7,12 dimethylbenz (α) anthrocene induced mammary adenocarcinoma in Sprague-Dawley rats. *Cancer Res.*, 30:813–818.
31. Tormey, D. C., Waalkes, T. P., Ahmann, D., Gehrke, C. W., Zumwatt, R. W., Snyder, J., and Hansen, H. (1975): Biological markers in breast cancer. I. Incidence of abnormalities of CEA, HCG, three polyamines and three minor nucleosides. *Cancer*, 35:1095–1100.
32. Steward, A. M., Nixon, D., Zamchek, N., and Aisenberg, A. (1974): Carcinoembryonic antigen in breast cancer patients: Serum levels in disease progress. *Cancer*, 33:1246–1252.

33. Giovanella, B. C., Stëhlin, J. S., and Williams, L. J., Jr. (1974): Heterotransplantation of human malignant tumor in nude thymusless mice. II. Malignant tumors induced by injection of cell cultures derived from human solid tumors. *J. Natl. Cancer Inst.*, 52:921–930.

Breast Cancer: Trends in Research and Treatment, edited by J. C. Heuson, W. H. Mattheiem, and M. Rozencweig. Raven Press, New York © 1976.

Results of Ongoing Clinical Trials with Adjuvant Chemotherapy in Operable Breast Cancer

Gianni Bonadonna, Pinuccia Valagussa, and Umberto Veronesi

Istituto Nazionale Tumori, Milan 20133, Italy

During the past three decades a lack of significant change was documented in the overall cure rate of breast cancer (1). In patients with disease apparently localized to breast and homolateral axillary lymph nodes, different surgical techniques and combined surgical-radiotherapeutic approaches have substantially failed to improve the long-term tumor-free survival. In particular, controlled studies have demonstrated that preoperative (2) and postoperative radiotherapy (3–5) did not alter the incidence of distant metastases. On the contrary, in one retrospective analysis a statistically significant increased mortality in early operable breast cancer was correlated to the routine use of local postoperative irradiation (6).

The plateau reached by radical surgery and radiotherapy in their ability to cure breast cancer, as well as the observation that relapsed patients almost invariably died of subsequent progressive metastatic disease, stimulated several investigators during the past 20 years to attempt new approaches with a variety of systemic treatments. The first modalities included postoperative endocrine therapy (oophorectomy, radiotherapeutic castration, androgens). The results were conflicting. Few prospective controlled studies showed that adjuvant endocrine therapy may delay the clinical appearance of metastases although it failed to improve the disease-free survival (7,8). More recently Dao et al. (9) performed bilateral adrenalectomy with radical mastectomy in a series of 17 postmenopausal women with breast cancer having metastases in four or more axillary nodes. Results to date showed that both recurrence and mortality rate were significantly lowered by the combined treatment. This pilot study lacks a control group, however, and the authors believe that their findings should be considered as a guide to future clinical trials rather than an immediate recommendation for general therapy.

The initial promising results obtained with the administration of growth-inhibiting drugs in disseminated tumor cells of experimental animals and in some forms of human neoplasia moved a new generation of investigators to turn their attention to chemotherapy as a potentially useful adjuvant treatment.

EARLY STUDIES WITH ADJUVANT CHEMOTHERAPY

The main rationale for administering a chemotherapeutic agent systemically in conjunction with radical mastectomy was derived from the opinion that surgical-radiotherapeutic treatment failures were in part due to neoplastic cells dislodged into the circulation during operative manipulation of the lesion. In addition, it was believed at that time that the tumor cell killed by anticancer drugs occurred as zero-order reaction kinetics. These were the reasons chemotherapy was administered for a short period of time (usually up to 2 months) after mastectomy (perioperative chemotherapy).

The results of published controlled studies were inconsistent. They were recently reviewed in detail by Tormey (10). As summarized in Table 1, in five of eight trials the authors reported a decreased relapse rate in the chemotherapy arm, at least for some patient subsets. This was associated with improved survival in only two studies and for a limited subgroup of patients. The case series are difficult to compare, mainly because of the different criteria of patient selection (extent of primary tumor and regional nodes) and the different approach utilized to treat the local disease (type of mastectomy, postoperative radiotherapy). Furthermore, the various series comprise different numbers of patients, the data were not always reported in detail, and an accurate statistical evaluation was carried out in the minority of studies. In general, the short-term chemotherapy course was believed to represent the major cause for treatment failure.

The results of a few more studies in which adjuvant chemotherapy was administered over 2 months postoperatively are summarized in Table 2. Again results are difficult to analyze for most of the reasons reported above as well as for lack of controls in three studies. All authors but Donegan (17) report a decreased relapse rate, which was associated with improved survival in three of five studies.

ONGOING STUDIES WITH ADJUVANT CHEMOTHERAPY

During the past 3 years the interest for adjuvant postoperative chemotherapy has been revitalized on the basis of new concepts. The clinical and biological considerations that stimulated the ongoing trials are summarized in Table 3.

Strategic Approach

Current knowledge on the natural history of breast cancer has well established that not only the presence of homolateral axillary nodes but the number of histologically positive nodes at the time of radical mastectomy represents the most useful indicator for prognosticating the course of the disease (Table 4). This finding, coupled with the observation that super-radical operations and postoperative irradiation do not significantly alter the occurrence of distant metastases (22), led to the conclusion that at the time of radical mastectomy most patients with involved nodes have subclinical disseminated foci of disease requiring a systemic approach. Furthermore, in metabolically homogeneous cell populations, the ef-

TABLE 1. Summary of results obtained with perioperative short-term single-agent chemotherapy

Country	Principal author	Stage	No. of patients		Treatment[a]	Relapse rate[b]	Survival
			Control	Treated			
USA	Fisher (11)	T_{1-4}, N_{0-1}	207	450	RM + FU	Decreased at 3 yr. in ≥ 4 N+	Not reported
			603	1,078	RM + TSPA	Delayed in ≥ 4 N+ premenop.	Increased in ≥ 4 N+ premenop.
USSR	Garin (12)	I-II-IIb	Total 698		RM + TSPA	Decreased	Not available
					RM + CTX	Increased	Not available
Denmark	Nissen-Meyer (13)	I-II	554	534	M + CTX	Decreased	No difference
England	Finney (14)	I-II	40	43	M + CTX	Increased	Decreased in stage II
Germany	Rieche (15)	I-III	144	143	RM + CTX	Decreased in N+	Increased in N+
Japan	Yoshida (16)	Data not available	Total 167		RM + MITO	Data not available	No difference

[a]M, single, modified radical, conventional radical. RM, radical mastectomy. FU, 5-fluorouracil. TSPA, triethylenthiophosphoramide. CTX, cyclophosphamide. MITO, mitomycin C.
[b]N+, positive nodes.

TABLE 2. *Summary of results obtained with postoperative chemotherapy*

Country	Principal author	Axillary Nodes	No. of patients		Treatment[a]	Relapse Rate	Survival
			Control	Treated			
USA	Donegan (17)	N−, N+	90	76	RM + TSPA	No difference	No difference
USA	Mrazek (18)	N−, N+	78	78	RM + HN2	Decreased	Increased
USSR	Kholdin (19)	N−, N+	Historical	392	RM + TSPA + CTX (± endocrine therapy)	Decreased	Increased
USA	Ansfield (20)	N+	None	60	RM + FU	Decreased	Increased
USA	Ramirez (21)	N+	None	35	RM + FU	Decreased	Too early to evaluate

[a]See Table 1 for explanation of abbreviations.

TABLE 3. *Critical clinical and biological findings stimulating recent adjuvant trials in primary breast cancer*

1. Postoperative radiotherapy does not improve the prognosis.
2. The presence of histologically positive axillary nodes (especially ≥ 4) is associated to an increased incidence of relapse.
3. Prolonged adjuvant chemotherapy has produced favorable results in other human neoplasms.
4. Tumor cell population growth kinetics indicates that the fraction of viable cells undergoing active replication is inversely related to population size.
5. First-order cell-kill kinetics characterizes effective drug cell kill of tumor cells.
6. Cell cure by effective drugs is dependent on the size of a kinetically homogeneous cell population at the start of treatment.

fective drug kill of tumor cells is better described by first-order reaction kinetics (23). The study of population growth kinetics has revealed that the relative proportion of tumor cells in the compartment of dividing cells is highest when the tumor is small. Furthermore, in experimental animals cell cure by effective drugs is dependent on the size of the kinetically homogeneous cell population at the start of treatment (23). These optimal conditions theoretically exist in breast cancer when microscopic foci of disease are present after curative surgery. The suggestions derived from the above-mentioned studies were the following: (a) systemic treatment is indicated in the subgroup of patients at high risk of relapse in the hope of suppressing or eradicating the minimal residual disease; (b) chemotherapy should be started as soon as possible after mastectomy; (c) the administration of adjuvant chemotherapy must be prolonged, since the long doubling time of breast cancer cells is due to a fraction of cells temporarily entering a nonproliferative state.

Experimental Design

The new generation of prospective randomized adjuvant treatments began with the studies started in the United States in September 1972 (24) and in Milan in June 1973 (25), respectively. The activity of both chemotherapeutic regimens

TABLE 4. *Effect of lymph node involvement on recurrence rate and survival*

Ipsilateral axillary nodes	Relapse rate (%)			Survival (%)	
	18 mo	5 yr	10 yr	5 hr	10 yr
N−	5	21	24	76	65
N+	33	67	76	46	25
N+ (1–3)	13	53	65	62	38
N+ (≥ 4)	52	80	86	31	13
All patients	17	45	50	61	46

Modified from Fisher, ref. 11.

employed as adjuvant therapy were tested in clinically advanced breast cancer by members of the Eastern Cooperative Oncology Group (ECOG). In advanced disease L-phenylalanine mustard (L-PAM) demonstrated a complete plus partial remission in 19% of patients, while CMF treatment resulted in a 53% response rate. L-PAM was selected by the American group because it could be administered orally by a simple intermittent schedule with only moderate toxicity. The combination of cyclophosphamide, methotrexate, and fluorouracil (CMF) originally designed by the NCI–Medicine Branch for breast cancer included prednisone (CMFP). CMFP was reported to be effective in 68% of patients with advanced disease (26). Subsequently the ECOG study dropped prednisone from the combination, which then became known as CMF. Prednisone administration was not felt to be important in a regimen used in an adjuvant situation. On the base of initial results showing the efficacy of CMF (27,28) and its superiority over L-PAM (27), Carbone suggested that this triple combination be tested as adjuvant therapy in patients with operable breast carcinoma and histologically positive axillary nodes.

The trials with L-PAM and CMF were identical in terms of criteria for patient selection (Table 5). They differed as far as chemotherapy was concerned (Fig. 1). Within 4 weeks of the time of radical or modified radical mastectomy, the study (performed by members of NSABP, ECOG, and COG under the chairmanship of Fisher) randomized patients between placebo and cyclic single-agent chemotherapy. L-PAM was administered orally at the dose of 0.15 mg/kg/day for 5

TABLE 5. *Main conditions for patient eligibility and ineligibility in study protocols adopted by NSABP, ECOG, COG, and Milan Cancer Institute*

	Eligibility		Ineligibility
1.	Primary breast carcinoma with no fixation to underlying pectoral fascia and/or muscle ($T_{1a}-T_{2a}-T_{3a}$)	1.	Primary breast carcinoma with fixation to pectoral fascia, muscle, chest wall, or skin ($T_{3b}-T_4$)
2.	No palpable homolateral axillary nodes or palpable and movable ($N_0-N_{1a}-N_{1b}$)	2.	Homolateral axillary nodes fixed to one another or to other structures; or supraclavicular nodes; or arm edema (N_2-N_3)
3.	Histologically positive homolateral axillary nodes (N+)	3.	Previously treated tumor; or malignant breast tumor other than carcinoma
4.	Negative radiological studies	4.	Bilateral malignancy
5.	Age less than 75 years	5.	Previous or concomitant malignancy
6.	Adequate marrow reserve and blood urea nitrogen ≤ 25 mg	6.	Concomitant systemic disease (cardiovascular, renal, etc.)
7.	Geographic accessibility	7.	Pregnancy or lactation

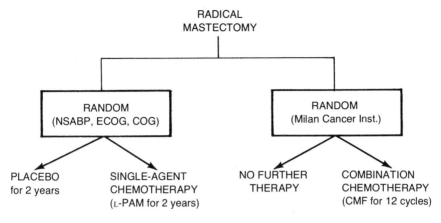

STRATIFICATION

Age: ≤ 49 or 50–75 years Axillary nodes: 1–3 or ≥ 4	≤ 49 or 50–75 years 1–3 or ≥ 4

Mastectomy: conventional radical or extended radical

ENDPOINT

Treatment failure is defined as the presence of tumor in local, regional, or distant sites—confirmed by biopsy when possible or by acceptable clinical, pathological, radiological, or radioisotopic evidence.

FIG. 1. Outline of protocol studies for adjuvant chemotherapy of NSABP, ECOG, COG, and Milan Cancer Institute.

consecutive days every 6 weeks. In the absence of documented evidence of treatment failure, chemotherapy and placebo were given for 2 consecutive years.

In the study performed at the Istituto Nazionale Tumori of Milan, patients were randomly allocated to no further therapy after mastectomy or to CMF (Table 6). The dosage of CMF was temporarily reduced in the presence of toxicity, espe-

TABLE 6. *Outline of CMF regimen*

Drugs	1	2	3	4	5	6	7	8	9	10	11	12	13	14	15 → 28
Cyclophosphamide, 100 mg/m² p.o.	———————————————————————————————————→														No therapy
Methotrexate, 40 mg/m² i.v.[a]	↑							↑							
Fluorouracil, 600 mg/m² i.v.[b]	↑							↑							

[a],[b] Doses of [a]30 mg/m² and [b]400 mg/m² are recommended in patients older than 65 years. Subsequent doses should be temporarily lowered in the presence of hematosuppression.

cially myelosuppression. In particular, as also employed in the L-PAM study, if no toxicity was evident (grade 0: WBC>4,000/mm³ and platelet count>130,000/mm³), 100% of each drug was administered. For grade 1 toxicity (WBC 2,500–3,999/mm³ and/or platelet count 75,000–129,000/mm³), 50% of the calculated dose was given. In the presence of grade 2 toxicity (WBC<2,500/mm³ and/or platelet count < 75,000/mm³), no drug was administered until at least grade 1 toxicity was reached. In the presence of cystitis secondary to cyclophosphamide, the drug was temporarily discontinued and resumed as soon as the side effect had disappeared. In the absence of relapse, CMF was continued for 12 cycles, i.e., for approximately 12 months.

In both trials patients received a follow-up examination, including evaluation of hemograms, blood chemistries, and X-ray studies. The endpoint was represented by documented evidence of treatment failure.

Significant Results

In the L-PAM study the results published in January 1975 (24) can be summarized as follows. Failure occurred after approximately 18 months from the beginning of therapy in 22% of 108 patients receiving placebo and in 9.7% of 103 women receiving L-PAM. A statistically significant difference existed in favor of L-PAM relative to disease-free survival. In premenopausal women the difference with respect to disease-free interval of treated and placebo group was significant ($p = 0.008$). Treatment failed in 30% of premenopausal patients receiving placebo and in 3% of those treated with L-PAM. Where a similar trend was observed in postmenopausal women, the difference at the time of analysis was not statistically significant.

Table 7 presents the characteristics of patients with treatment failure in the CMF study after approximately 2 years from the beginning of the trial. It appears evident that all subgroups present a significant difference in favor of adjuvant chemotherapy. In particular, the difference in the relapse rate between CMF and controls was highly significant in the group of patients with four or more axillary nodes. As detailed in Table 8, the observed failure proportions are almost directly proportional to the number of involved lymph nodes. However, it is worthwhile noting the failure rate of control patients with only one positive node. Contrary to what was reported in the L-PAM study, combination chemotherapy was active irrespective of menopausal status. The only statistical difference between pre- and postmenopausal control patients was related to the number of positive nodes (premenopause: one to three versus four or more nodes: $p<0.001$; postmenopause one to three versus four or more nodes: $p<0.05$).

In the present series the proportion of failures and control patients occurred more often in those subjected to extended radical mastectomy compared to those who underwent conventional (Halsted) radical mastectomy.

The most important results obtained so far with L-PAM and CMF are compared in Table 9. With the limits of a retrospective comparison, available data

TABLE 7. *Characteristics of patients with treatment failure in the CMF study*

Parameter	Evaluable controls		Evaluable CMF patients		Level of significance (*p*)
	No.	%	No.	%	
Total with relapse	38/165	23	5/185	2.7	10^{-8}
Axillary nodes					
1–3	17/115	15[a]	2/124	1.6	$< 10^{-3}$
≥ 4	21/50	42[a]	3/61	5	$< 10^{-5}$
Age (years)					
≤ 49	15/63	24	3/86	3.4	$< 10^{-3}$
≥ 50	23/102	22.5	2/99	2	10^{-5}
Menopause					
Pre	17/71	24	3/85	3.5	$< 10^{-3}$
Post	21/94	22	2/100	2	$< 10^{-4}$
Mastectomy					
Radical	21/120	17.5[b]	4/128	3.1	$< 10^{-3}$
Enlarged	17/45	38[b]	1/57	1.7	$< 10^{-5}$

[a]One to three versus four or more: $p < 10^{-3}$.
[b]Radical versus enlarged: $p < 10^{-2}$.

TABLE 8. *Observed failure proportions related to the number of histologically involved axillary lymph nodes*

Patient group	Failure proportions		Failure rate[a]	Ratio
	No.	%		
One positive node				
Controls	11/69	16	130	
CMF	1/59	1.6	15	8.7
Two positive nodes				
Controls	2/28	7.1	58	
CMF	0/43	—	—	—
Three positive nodes				
Controls	4/18	22	197	
CMF	1/22	4.5	42	4.7
Four positive nodes				
Controls	3/16	18	171	
CMF	1/17	5.8	54	3.2
Five or six positive nodes				
Controls	9/16	56	675	
CMF	1/11	9	104	6.5
Seven or more positive nodes				
Controls	6/18	33	481	
CMF	1/33	3	35	13.7

[a]Per year per thousand patients.

TABLE 9. *Observed failure proportions after single-agent chemotherapy (L-PAM) and combination chemotherapy (CMF)*

Treatment	No. of evaluable patients	Proportion of recurrence observed[a] (Controls vs. chemotherapy group)				
		Total	1–3 positive nodes	≥ 4 positive nodes	Premenopause	Postmenopause
RM ± L-PAM[b]	211	22 vs. 9.7	6.1 vs. 1.9	34 vs. 18	30 vs. 3	21 vs. 11
RM ± CMF	350	23 vs. 2.7	15 vs. 1.6	42 vs. 5	24 vs. 3.5	22 vs. 2

[a] Average follow-up times for L-PAM and CMF studies are 8.4 months as of September 1, 1974 and 13.5 months as of August 31, 1975, respectively.

[b] From Fisher et al., ref. 24. RM, radical mastectomy.

indicate that at this point of analysis multiple drug treatment is superior to single-agent chemotherapy in decreasing the total failure rate after radical mastectomy. The advantage in favor of CMF appears evident in all subgroups of patients, while no appreciable difference is detectable between L-PAM and CMF in premenopausal women.

Figure 2 presents the treatment failure time distribution for all patients in the CMF program. The progressive relapse rate with time in the control group is evident, as is the advantage in favor of the CMF-treated patients. This finding is particularly prominent in the subgroup of patients with four or more axillary nodes (Fig. 3). In fact at 25 months from mastectomy, only 24% of controls remain clinically free of disease compared to 93% of those treated with combination chemotherapy. The comparative findings for those with one to three involved nodes are 72% and 97%, respectively (Fig. 4).

Figure 5 reports the sites of relapse. Treatment failure was documented at distant sites in 33 of 43 patients with recurrence. Furthermore, multiple relapses were observed in 28% of patients. In only 23% of all the patients with treatment failure did the initial recurrence appear in local and regional areas (i.e., those usually encompassed by postoperative irradiation). However, in 4 of 10 patients, disseminated disease was detected within 2 months of the initial recurrence. The site of distribution of local and distant recurrences was not reported in the L-PAM study.

Although at the time of this writing the analysis of survival is premature, it should be mentioned that 8 of 38 (21%) relapsing patients in the control group have already died of progressive cancer after a median of 14.5 months from mastectomy. To date one of five patients relapsing during CMF therapy expired.

Drug Tolerance

Among the L-PAM-treated group, the white cell count decreased at some time during therapy in 60% of patients. A grade 2 toxicity was observed in 12.6%. The level of platelets during L-PAM therapy was not reported. Thirty percent of patients complained of nausea and vomiting during chemotherapy, and in some instances the discomfort occurred more than once.

In the CMF study side effects were more numerous. Most patients complained of nausea and vomiting within a few hours of drug injection. Furthermore, in more than half of the patients the daily administration of cyclophosphamide caused prolonged nausea and loss of appetite. Unless encouraged to take the drug regularly, about one-third of the patients showed a repeated tendency to discontinue treatment or to diminish the dose in an attempt to alleviate the abdominal discomfort. The episodes of stomatitis were few (18%), and mild. Loss of hair occurred in 57% of patients and in about one-third this esthetically undesirable side effect was minimal and pronounced alopecia was rare. Mild chemical cystitis secondary to cyclophosphamide was observed in 30%, and in some patients this occurred more than once. Treatment produced amenorrhea in 54% of pre-

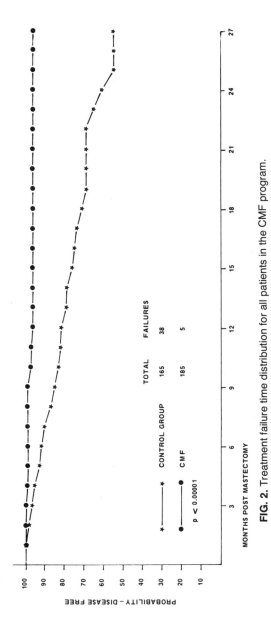

FIG. 2. Treatment failure time distribution for all patients in the CMF program.

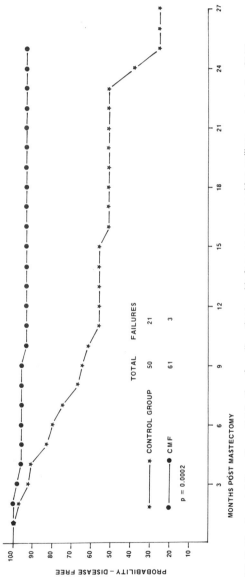

FIG. 3. Treatment failure time distribution for all patients with four or more positive axillary nodes in the CMF program.

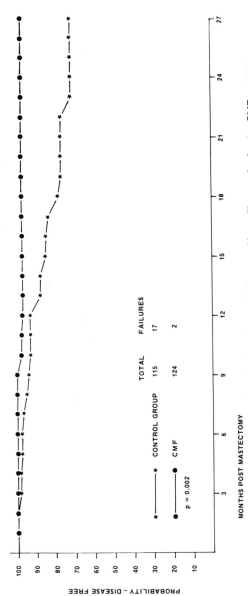

FIG. 4. Treatment failure time distribution for patients with one to three positive axillary nodes in the CMF program.

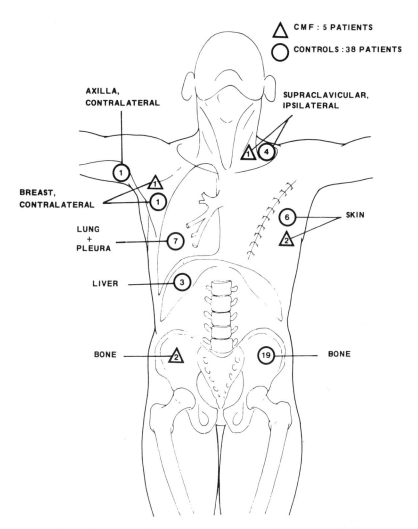

FIG. 5. Distribution of sites of relapse, reporting the number of findings.

menopausal patients, and in 30% the suppression of menses was reversible. In the remaining patients, the duration of amenorrhea cannot be estimated at present. However, it is conceivable that cyclophosphamide, which is most probably responsible for this side effect, induced a permanent ovarian failure in some patients (29). Myelosuppression represented the dose-limiting factor. At some time during therapy leukopenia occurred in a total of 68% of patients (grade 1, 64%; grade 2, 4%) and thrombocytopenia in 66% (grade 1, 54%; grade 2, 12%). No episodes of infections or bleeding secondary to drug-induced hematosuppression were documented.

Despite a variety of toxic manifestations, treatment was in general fairly well tolerated. This statement is supported by the fact that the optimal dose administered for each drug was high (cyclophosphamide 76%, methotrexate 81%, fluorouracil 81%). Approximately half of the patients who have completed 12 cycles of CMF have received a total dose of each drug ranging from 81% to 100% (Table 10). Only 10 patients refused to complete the chemical treatment—and this mainly for psychological reasons rather than because of severe side effects.

CONCLUSIONS

The preliminary results of new controlled adjuvant studies based on the contemporary strategic approach for local-regional disease at high risk of relapse suggest that chemotherapy can significantly decrease the recurrence rate during the first 18–24 months after radical mastectomy. Available results indicate that, as already documented for clinically disseminated disease (27), CMF is more effective than L-PAM. However, as previously observed in animal studies (23), a single agent such as L-PAM, which is only moderately effective in clinically disseminated disease, can exert significant anticancer activity in a kinetically optimal situation as represented by its use as adjuvant treatment. Although the effects of adjuvant therapy appear to be more significant in patients with four or more axillary nodes, there is significant evidence that CMF is also effective in the patient subset with one to three involved nodes. At the time of this analysis, in premenopausal women L-PAM and CMF appear to be equally effective, whereas in postmenopausal patients CMF is more effective than L-PAM. The reason for this difference is unknown. The fact that a significant trend in favor of CMF was observed also in postmenopausal patients indicates that the positive effect of chemotherapy was independent of ovarian activity suppression ("chemotherapeutic oophorectomy"). In an attempt to provide general directions about when to use single-agent or combination chemotherapy in clinical practice, a statistical

TABLE 10. *Patients who completed 12 cycles of CMF (72 cases) with different amounts of dose administered*

Percent of dose administered	Cyclophosphamide		Methotrexate		Fluorouracil	
	No.	%	No.	%	No.	%
91–100	8	11	16	22	17	24
81–90	25	35	23	32	28	39
71–80	22	31	20	28	18	25
61–70	8	11	10	14	6	8
51–60	8	11	2	3	3	4
< 50	1[a]	1	1[b]	1		

[a] Twenty-five percent.
[b] Thirty-one percent.

updated comparative analysis of L-PAM and CMF series is highly desirable since the criteria for patient selection were identical in both protocols.

Prolonged treatment was administered at the expense of minimal (L-PAM) or moderate (CMF) toxicity. Side effects were reversible, with the possible exception of some patients having amenorrhea after CMF therapy. Their occurrence did not prevent the administration of a high drug dosage over a long period of time.

At present many institutions all over the world are engaged in controlled adjuvant treatments for patients having histologically positive axillary nodes after radical mastectomy. A few representative examples are shown in Table 11. As can be seen, different treatments have been designed to include immunotherapy in three studies. It will take a few years to document the effect of new therapies and to compare the results with those achieved after L-PAM or CMF.

Despite favorable preliminary results, many questions remain to be answered. First of all, the natural history of breast cancer does not allow us to state, with the

TABLE 11. *Examples of ongoing controlled trials with prolonged adjuvant therapy in primary breast cancer with positive axillary nodes*

Group	Type of treatment [a]	Duration
NSABP, ECOG, COG (USA)	R → Placebo / L-PAM	2 years
Guy's Hospital (England)	R → Placebo / L-PAM	12 cycles
Milan Cancer Institute (Italy)	R → Control / CMF	12 cycles
NSABP, ECOG, COG (USA)	R → L-PAM / L-PAM + FU	2 years
Mayo Clinic (USA)	R → RT / CFP / RT + CFP	1 year
University of California UCLA (USA)	R → BCG + CMF / BCG + CMF plus TC	1 year
Memorial Hospital (USA)	R → RT / CbMF / Levamisole	2 years
Case Western Reserve (USA)	R → Control / CMF + tamoxifen / CMF + tamoxifen + BCG	2 years

[a]RT, radiotherapy. L-PAM, melphalan. C, cyclophosphamide. M, methotrexate. F, fluorouracil. P, prednisone. Cb, chlorambucil. TC, allogeneic tumor cell.
Modified from Carbone, ref. 33.

available data, whether subclinical disease was eradicated or merely suppressed in the chemotherapy group. In fact, in many patients, breast cancer shows a pattern of continuous relapse over time. For this reason the definition of cure for breast cancer becomes very difficult compared to other neoplasms such as childhood tumors, Hodgkin's disease, and histiocytic lymphoma. The ultimate goal of adjuvant therapy is to improve the disease-free survival, and only prolonged follow-up will tell us if we have achieved our aim. Furthermore, the long-term side effects are still unknown. On the basis of findings observed in malignant lymphomas (30,31), it is conceivable that some patients might develop a secondary neoplasm as a result of prolonged chemotherapy. However, it should be recalled that in a recent retrospective study (32) the risk of second primary malignancies after prolonged thiotepa in breast cancer patients was no greater than the inherent susceptibility of developing second primaries in these patients.

The above-mentioned considerations suggest that we maintain a cautious attitude toward our present results until more solid data become available through long-term analysis. Nevertheless, the evidence that new lines are constantly emerging from new, controlled studies should not be minimized. Adjuvant treatment is gradually becoming a widespread therapeutic approach for breast cancer. Its clinical usefulness depends on a few important areas in the design of study protocols (Table 12). Current knowledge of tumor cell population growth kinetics, tumor cell kill as related to classes of anticancer drugs, and the known relationship between chemotherapeutic toxicity and immune competence provide ample possibilities for testing different types of adjuvant therapies.

The strategy for curative treatment of breast cancer is changing (33), and the field is now open to new enterprises. A few milestones, however, should remain unchanged. The first deals with the role of radical surgery. For the time being, radical or modified radical mastectomy offers the best chance of eradicating the local-regional disease. To limit the extent of surgery to a segmental mastectomy without removal of homolateral axillary nodes should be regarded as unwise. The second point deals with adjuvant therapy. The regimen to be employed should not only be effective but safe, tolerable, and feasible on an outpatient basis. The type

TABLE 12. *Attributes for useful adjuvant chemotherapy in primary breast cancer with axillary nodes*

---

1. The primary neoplasm and regional nodes must be surgically removed because of the known biological interrelationship between tumor size, host defense, and chemotherapeutic response.
2. Chemotherapy should be started as soon as possible after surgery and must be prolonged to encompass the expected doubling time of neoplastic cells.
3. Chemotherapy should include cell cycle-specific drugs to which growing micrometastases should be very sensitive.
4. Chemotherapy should be administered via an intermittent high-dose schedule to maximize tumor damage and minimize host immune competence.
5. The regimen should be safe (no long-term side effects), tolerable (reversible toxicity), and simple (feasible on an outpatient basis).

---

of adjuvant chemotherapy and/or immunotherapy to be tested should be based on results obtained in patients with advanced disease, and theoretically systemic adjuvant treatment should provide the maximum tumor cell kill with tolerable toxicity.

In the future better knowledge of the natural history of breast cancer, particularly identifying specifically which patients are going to relapse irrespective of their node status and the clinical use of biological markers such as CEA, HCG, methylated transfer RNA (34), and hydroxyproline (35), may allow delineation of more specific surgical and adjuvant systemic treatments for specific subsets of patients (33).

ACKNOWLEDGMENTS

The work reported herein was partially supported by Contract N01-CM-33714 with DCT, NCI, NIH.

REFERENCES

1. Cutler, S. J., Myers, M. H., Green, S. B. (1975): Trends in survival rates of patients with cancer. *N. Engl. J. Med.*, 293:122–124.
2. De Schryver, A. (1975): La radiothérapie préopératoire dans le cancer du sein: Description d'un protocole d'essai clinique et premiers résultats. *Bull. Cancer (Paris)*, 62:175–182.
3. Easson, E. C. (1968): Post-operative radiotherapy in breast cancer. In: *Tenovous Symposium, 1st, Cardiff, 1967. Prognostic Factors in Breast Cancer, Proceedings of the Symposium*, edited by A. P. M. Forrest and P. B. Kunkler, pp. 118–127. Livingstone, Edinburgh.
4. Fisher, B., Slack, N. H., Cavanaugh, P. J., et al. (1970): Postoperative radiotherapy in the treatment of breast cancer: Results of the NSABP clinical trial. *Ann. Surg.*, 172:711–732.
5. Host, H., and Brennhovd, I. (1971): Combined surgery and radiotherapy vs. surgery alone in primary breast cancer. In: *International Cancer Congress, 10th, Houston, 1970*, pp. 603–604 (abstract). Year Book, Chicago.
6. Stjernswärd, J. (1974): Decreased survival related to irradiation postoperatively in early operable breast cancer. *Lancet*, 2:1285–1286.
7. Kennedy, B. J., Mielke, P. W., and Fortuny, I. E. (1964): Therapeutic castration versus prophylactic castration in breast cancer. *Surg. Gynecol. Obstet.*, 118:524–540.
8. Ravdin, R. G., Lewison, E. F., Slack, N. H., et al. (1970): Results of a clinical trial concerning the worth of prophylactic oophorectomy for breast carcinoma. *Surg. Gynecol. Obstet.*, 131:1055–1064.
9. Dao, T. L., Nemoto, T., Chamberlain, A., et al. (1975): Adrenalectomy with radical mastectomy in the treatment of high-risk breast cancer. *Cancer*, 35:478–482.
10. Tormey, D. C. (1975): Combined chemotherapy and surgery in breast cancer: A review. *Cancer* 36:881–892.
11. Fisher, B., Ravdin, R. G., Ausman, R. K., et al. (1968): Surgical adjuvant chemotherapy in cancer of the breast: Results of a decade of cooperative investigation. *Ann. Surg.*, 168:337–356.
12. Garjn, A. M., Karev, N. I., Bazhenova, A. P., et al. (1973): A summary of the comparative studies of the efficacy of different techniques in treatment of early forms of the mammary gland cancer. *Vopr. Onkol.*, 3:87–93.
13. Månsson, B., Kjellgren, K., and Nissen-Meyer, R. (1974): Cyclophosphamide as adjuvant to the primary surgery for breast cancer, a cooperative controlled clinical study. In: *Proceedings: 11th International Cancer Congress, Florence*, Vol. 3, p. 531 (abstract).
14. Finney, R. (1971): Adjuvant chemotherapy in the radical treatment of carcinoma of the breast. A clinical trial. *Am. J. Roentgenol. Radium Ther. Nucl. Med.*, 111:137–141.
15. Rieche, K., Berndt, H., and Prahl, B. (1972): Continuous postoperative treatment with

cyclophosphamide in breast carcinoma: A randomized clinical study. *Arch. Geschwulstforsch.,* 40:349–354.

16. Yoshida, Y., Miura, S., Murai, H., et al. (1973): Late results in combined chemotherapy for cure of breast cancer (axillary lymph node metastasis and therapeutic effect). In: *10th Annual Meeting of the Japanese Society for Cancer Therapy* (abstract 177).

17. Donegan, W. L. (1974): Extended surgical adjuvant thiotepa for mammary carcinoma. *Arch. Surg.,* 109:187–192.

18. Mrazek, R. G., and McDonald, G. O. (1971): Surgery and adjuvant chemotherapy in the treatment for breast carcinoma. In: *International Cancer Congress, 10th, Houston, 1970,* p. 501 (abstract). Year Book, Chicago.

19. Kholdin, S. A., Deemarsky, L. Y., and Bavly, J. L. (1974): Adjuvant long-term chemotherapy in complex treatment of operable breast cancer. *Cancer,* 33:903–906.

20. Ansfield, F. J. (1974): 5-FU as an adjuvant to mastectomy in high-risk patients. In: *Proceedings: American Association for Cancer Research and ASCO Meetings,* Vol. 15, p. 177 (abstract).

21. Ramirez, G. (1975): Combined chemotherapy-radiotherapy as an adjuvant to mastectomy in patients with positive nodes. In: *Proceedings: American Association for Cancer Research and ASCO Meetings,* Vol. 16, p. 224 (abstract).

22. Zingo, L., Fontanella, U., and Milani, A. (1974): Clinical experience and long-term results of extended mastectomy for breast cancer in 1,578 cases. In: *Proceedings: 11th International Cancer Congress, Florence,* Vol. 3, p. 530 (abstract).

23. Schabel, F. M. (1975): Concepts for systemic treatment of micrometastases. *Cancer,* 35:15–24.

24. Fisher, B., Carbone, P., Economou, S. G., et al. (1975): L-Phenylalanine mustard (L-PAM) in the management of primary breast cancer: A report of early findings. *N. Engl. J. Med.,* 292:117–122.

25. Bonadonna, G., Brusamolino, E., Valagussa, P., et al. (1976): Combination chemotherapy as an adjuvant treatment in operable breast cancer. *N. Engl. J. Med.,* 294:405–410.

26. Canellos, G. P., De Vita, V. T., Lennard Gold, G., et al. (1974): Cyclical combination chemotherapy for advanced breast carcinoma. *Br. Med. J.,* 1:218–220.

27. Taylor, S. G., III, Canellos, G. P., Band, P., et al. (1974): Combination chemotherapy for advanced breast cancer: Randomized comparison with single drug therapy. In: *Proceedings: American Association for Cancer Research and ASCO Meetings,* Vol. 15, p. 175 (abstract).

28. De Lena, M., Brambilla, C., Morabito, A., et al. (1975): Adriamycin plus vincristine compared to and combined with cyclophosphamide, methotrexate, and 5-fluorouracil for advanced breast cancer. *Cancer,* 35:1108–1115.

29. Warne, G. L., Fairley, K. F., Hobbs, J. H., et al. (1973): Cyclophosphamide-induced ovarian failure. *N. Engl. J. Med.,* 289:1159–1162.

30. Canellos, G. P., De Vita, V. T., Arseneau, J. C., et al. (1975): Second malignancies complicating Hodgkin's disease in remission. *Lancet,* 1:947–949.

31. Bonadonna, G., De Lena, M., Banfi, A., et al. (1973): Secondary neoplasms in malignant lymphomas after intensive therapy. *N. Engl. J. Med.,* 288:1242–1243.

32. Sadoff, L., Chan, P., and Tyson, S. (1974): Incidence of second primary cancers in breast patients after prolonged thio-tepa therapy. In: *Proceedings: American Association for Cancer Research and ASCO Meetings,* Vol. 15, p. 145 (abstract).

33. Carbone, P. P. (1975): Chemotherapy in the treatment strategy of breast cancer. *Cancer,* 36:633–637.

34. Tormey, D. C., Waalkes, T. P., Ahmann, D., et al. (1975): Biological markers in breast carcinoma. I. Incidence of abnormalities of CEA, HCG, three polyamines, and three minor nucleosides. *Cancer,* 35:1095–1100.

35. Cuschieri, A. (1975): Urinary hydroxiproline excretion and survival in cancer of the breast. *Clin. Oncol.,* 1:127–130.

Breast Cancer: Trends in Research and Treatment, edited by J. C. Heuson,
W. H. Mattheiem, and M. Rozencweig. Raven Press, New York © 1976.

Current EORTC Study

W. Mattheiem

Institut Jules Bordet, Brussels, Belgium

Protocol 10751 of the EORTC Breast Cancer Group is aimed toward the
evaluation of a postsurgical alternating cyclical hormonal-cytotoxic therapy for
patients with primary breast cancer of poor prognosis.

BACKGROUND AND INTRODUCTION

The most important prognostic factor at the time of the first treatment of
primary breast tumor is the status of the regional lymph nodes. Patients with
tumors of the breast and positive nodes in at least two axillary levels, or patients
with tumors of the central and inner area of the breast with positive internal
mammary nodes, constitute a selected group of patients with a very low prospect
of healing and survival. Only 20–30% of such patients are living after 5 years.
Similarly, approximately 25% of these poor-risk patients are free of apparent
disease after 24 months.

This protocol describes a clinical trial carried out by participating members of
the Breast Cancer Cooperative Group of the EORTC to evaluate the effects of a
regimen of hormonal and cyclic alternating polychemotherapy given for a period
of 1 year following surgery.

OBJECTIVES OF THE STUDY

The primary object of this study is to evaluate postoperative hormonalcytotoxic
therapy for patients with primary breast cancer of poor prognosis with respect to
the following: (a) length of free interval (i.e., time from surgery to local recurrence or metastasis); (b) length of survival; and (c) undesirable effects. Details on
the therapeutic regimen are given in a later section.

SELECTION OF PATIENTS

All female patients with primary breast cancer with no clinical evidence of
distant metastasis are potentially eligible for this study. Specifically, the following
eligibility conditions must be satisfied:

1. Age at time of registration must be less than 65 years.

2. Histologic proof of primary breast carcinoma is required. (Patients with sarcoma of the breast are not eligible.)

3. No distant metastases or additional primaries are allowed. Negative evidence should be based on physical examination, lung X-ray films, skeletal scanning, and hepatic function tests (M0 of TNM classification). In case of a positive skeletal scan, metastasis should be verified by skeletal x-ray films and whenever possible by bone biopsy. A liver scan is desirable but not required.

4. Nodal status must be positive. For outer-quadrant lesions, histologic proof of positive nodes in both the lower and middle axillary level must be available. For central or inner-quadrant lesions, histologic proof of positive nodes in both the lower and middle axillary level *or* in the internal mammary level must be available.

5. No prior anticancer therapy is allowed.

6. The Karnofsky performance index must be at least 80.

7. Kidney function must be intact with creatinine less than 1.2 mg%.

Patients satisfying *all* of the above are eligible for the study and should be registered with the Data Center, *regardless of whether* the patient is actually to be entered on the protocol-specified treatment regimen. (Registration procedures are given in the following section.) All other patients are ineligible and should not be registered.

REGISTRATION PROCEDURES

Registration of a patient on this study is accomplished by completing and sending an on-study form to the EORTC Data Center. This must be done within 4 weeks of surgery.

SURGICAL GUIDELINES

When proof of the malignancy of the breast tumor is obtained for the primary lesion, total mastectomy is performed, removing all breast tissue, nipple, appropriate surface of skin, and the superficial aponeurosis of pectoralis major. For outer-quadrant lesions, axillary nodes external to the outer edge of the pectoralis major are removed and examined by frozen section whenever their involvement is not macroscopically obvious. If negative, the surgical procedure is finished and the patient does not enter the protocol. If nodes from that level (axillary $1 = A_1$) are positive, nodes from behind the pectoralis minor and those situated between the pectoralis minor and between the pectoralis major and minor are also removed (A_2) and examined.

If they are positive, the patient enters the protocol. Nodes internal to the inner edge of the pectoralis minor are then removed (A_3), as are internal mammary nodes in at least the second and third intercostal space. If the internal mammary nodes are clinically small and negative, this could be done by careful ligation of the internal mammary artery and vein at the said interspaces and by removal, for pathologic examination, of that segment of those vessels with the nodes and cellulolymphatic tissue.

If the nodes are enlarged or clinically invaded, removal should be performed, if necessary, down to the fifth interspace and will necessitate section of the costosternal junction for safety and completeness of the procedure. For tumors of the retroareolar (central) area or from the inner quadrants of the breast, the axillary exploration and dissection procedure is the same as described above, but the internal mammary exploration and dissection is done in all cases.

POSTSURGICAL THERAPEUTIC REGIMEN AND DESIGN OF THE STUDY

The postsurgical therapy on this study is indicated in Fig. 1. The 56-day schedule is repeated until the patient has been on treatment for 1 year, after which no further treatment is given unless there is a relapse. In the event of a relapse or metastasis, the patient should be taken off study and a summary and evaluation form completed (see below). Therapy following a relapse or metastasis is not specified in this protocol.

A concurrent ''control'' treatment is not included in this trial since (a) adequate historical information exists on the effects of a potential control treatment such as postsurgical irradiation, and (b) it is desirable to estimate with high precision the effects of the present treatment in as short a time as possible. However, it is intended that the design of this trial be flexible, and the possibility of expanding the trial to include randomization among alternative treatments will be periodically considered. In particular, this possibility will be discussed formally at the end of the first year. This expansion depends partly on the early results from the current therapy and partly on the availability of promising new therapies.

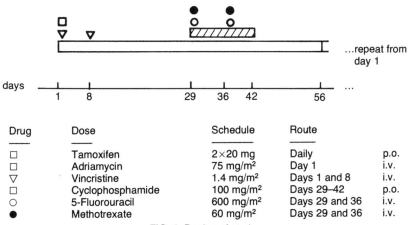

Drug	Dose		Schedule	Route	
□	Tamoxifen	2×20 mg	Daily	p.o.	
□	Adriamycin	75 mg/m²	Day 1	i.v.	
▽	Vincristine	1.4 mg/m²	Days 1 and 8	i.v.	
□	Cyclophosphamide	100 mg/m²	Days 29–42	p.o.	
○	5-Fluorouracil	600 mg/m²	Days 29 and 36	i.v.	
●	Methotrexate	60 mg/m²	Days 29 and 36	i.v.	

FIG. 1. Design of study.

ENDPOINTS OF RESPONSE AND TOXICITY

The primary endpoint on this study is the length of the disease-free interval (see above, *Objectives of the Study*), which is defined as the time from surgery until the first detection of a recurrence or metastasis, regardless of whether the lesion is amenable to surgery and/or irradiation. Survival is measured from the time of surgery.

Toxicity is recorded as either mild, moderate, severe, life-threatening, or lethal. The presence or absence of the following toxicities should be recorded on the flow sheets (see below) at each follow-up examination:

Nausea/vomiting	Blood
Diarrhea	Liver
Infection	Weakness/pain
Bleeding	Cardiac
Skin and mucous membrane	Impairment of shoulder motion
Neurological	Edema of the arm
Respiratory	Weight loss
Genitourinary	

This list represents the minimal requirements. All other toxicities should be noted.

REQUIRED CLINICAL EVALUATIONS AND LABORATORY TESTS

Prior to the start of therapy, a complete patient history should be taken; it must include, but is not necessarily limited to, the following items:

1. Birth date
2. Date of first symptom of cancer
3. Prior cancer therapy information (including dates)
4. Menopausal status and approximate date of menopause, if applicable
5. Other chronic diseases and associated medications (including dates)

In addition, the following clinical evaluations and laboratory tests should be performed prior to starting therapy and at the prescribed intervals throughout the study:

	Procedure	Frequency
1.	Physical examination (includes lesion measurements, if any; Karnofsky index; weight; temperature; blood pressure; and any symptoms of disease)	Monthly
2.	X-ray examination (EPA chest, bone scan)	Every 6 months
3.	Routine blood chemistries (including liver and kidney function tests)	Monthly
4.	Routine hematologic examination (hemoglobin, white cell count and differential, platelets, erythrocyte sedimentation rate)	Monthly

5. Bone marrow examination (spina iliaca anterior   Start of
    superior and spina iliaca posterior superior)   therapy only
6. Urinalysis   Monthly

The above items represent the minimal requirements. Any additional information should also be recorded. All data should be forwarded to the EORTC Data Center on the forms described below.

FORMS AND PROCEDURES FOR COLLECTING DATA

All the data obtained on each registered patient should be mailed to the EORTC Data Center. The required forms for recording the data and the schedule for them are as follows:

Form	Schedule
On-study (form II)	Within 4 weeks of surgery
Flow sheet (form VII)	At least every 3 months
Summary and evaluation (form IX)	When patient is taken off study

For patients who are registered but *not* entered in the protocol treatment, only the on-study form with the reasons for exclusion specified needs to be submitted. However, these patients should be followed and the Data Center notified every 6 months that they are still alive. Immediate notification should be sent of their death.

In addition to the above schedule of sending forms, prior to each meeting of the Group, a special request will be made of each investigator to send in *all* accumulated information on each registered patient. The summary and evaluation form should be sent in only when the patient is removed from the study. Ordinarily, removal from study occurs only if a recurrence or metastasis is observed or if the patient dies. If the patient is taken off study for other reasons, careful documentation of those reasons should be provided with the summary and evaluation form. Regardless of the reasons, all patients taken off study while still alive should continue to be followed, and the EORTC Data Center should be notified of their survival status at least once a year.

STATISTICAL CONSIDERATIONS

It is anticipated that a minimum of 60 patients per year will be entered on this trial. At the end of 1 year, a sufficient number of patients will have been entered to yield a probability of .80 that the estimated median time to recurrence will lie within 20% of the true median time to recurrence. This calculation assumes that the distribution of time to recurrence is roughly exponential in form and that all patients are followed until recurrence. Assuming further that the median time recurrence will be approximately 1 year, sufficient follow-up information will be available on these 60 patients by the end of 2 years (from the opening of the study) to allow a definitive analysis of the results of the trial. Thus there will be a minimum 1-year patient entry period followed by a minimum followup period of 1 year. At the end of the initial year, a decision will be made either to continue the trial without major modification, include a randomization involving a second "promising" therapy, or terminate the trial.

This protocol was prepared by:

W. H. Mattheiem, M.D., Secretary, EORTC Breast Cancer Cooperative Group
S. L. George, Ph.D., Director, EORTC Data Center
J. C. Heuson, M.D., Chairman, EORTC Breast Cancer Cooperative Group

Breast Cancer: Trends in Research and Treatment, edited by J. C. Heuson,
W. H. Mattheiem, and M. Rozencweig. Raven Press, New York © 1976.

Roundtable Discussion: Curative Treatment

Chairman: Y. Kenis

Tubiana: I want to raise two problems that have not yet been discussed. The first is
cosmetic results. It is important to allow a woman to keep her breast if this is possible, and
I think this can be achieved, at least in some types of patients. Remember that in Dr.
Carbone's data, for the patient without lymph node involvement, the proportion of patients
without metastases at long-term follow-up was approximately 75%. If one considers the T1
and T2 tumors without lymph node involvement in the axilla, this proportion rises to 85%,
so it seems that there is a case for conservative treatment. In many centers clinical trials are
comparing radical surgery and more limited surgery, mostly tumorectomy plus radiotherapy
and in some cases axillary lymph node biopsy. The preliminary data suggest that the two
types of treatment are equivalent for small tumors without lymph node involvement, which
is an important point.

The second problem is the importance of psychological factors. It has been noted in this
volume that long-term survival is the same in patients with and without postoperative
radiotherapy; this is true in spite of a higher recurrence rate in patients without postoperative radiotherapy. The long-term survival is about the same because in the control trial in
most cases local recurrence could be cured by local treatment. However, if this is true in
control trials, it may not be true in all cases because under controlled conditions follow-up
is very good and the recurrences are seen at an early stage. This might not be so in routine
practice. Furthermore, one should not overlook the psychological stress linked with recurrence in a patient who hoped for years to have been cured and who now again has the stress
of a new treatment.

A most important problem is that of the role of radiotherapy in the management of
advanced disease. Firstly, to clarify the problem, let me restate the points on which I
disagree and the points on which I agree with Dr. Stjernswärd. The points with which I
disagree concern the higher metastasis rate in patients with postoperative radiotherapy. I am
not convinced of this for two reasons. First, in none of the controlled clinical trials is there
a statistically significant difference between these two groups of patients from the point of
view of metastasis incidence; and second, it is difficult to pool data from different
controlled clinical trials in which the treatment technique and the philosophy were not the
same. So I think we are to keep an eye on this problem, which is a very important one, and
Dr. Stjernswärd was right to raise it. On the other hand, I quite agree with Dr. Stjernswärd
on a few questions, the first being that systematic routine postoperative radiotherapy is not
required. I feel that we have to try to identify that group of patients for whom radiotherapy
is useful, and the group for whom radiotherapy might be not only useless but positively
detrimental. In order to discuss this problem, I want to discuss another one which is linked
purely with surgical treatment, and I do that in order to underline the point that not only
might radiotherapy be detrimental, but also surgery or chemotherapy.

The study I want to discuss is a multicenter trial to compare two types of surgery: radical
mastectomy, and radical mastectomy plus internal mammary chain dissection. A total of
1500 patients were included in the trial, and the 5-year survival rates are 69% for radical
mastectomy and 72% for radical mastectomy plus internal mammary chain dissection; the

difference is not significant, in spite of the large number of patients. On the surface it seems that the two treatments are equivalent, but if one looks more carefully at the data it appears that this absence of difference is due to a balance between two different effects. If one considers the T1 and T2 cases located in the outer half of the breast, without lymph node involvement, the 5-year survival is 87% for radical mastectomy and 77% for radical mastectomy plus internal mammary chain dissection, and the difference is significant. So in these cases the results are better with the less mutilating surgery. On the other hand, if one considers the T1 and T2 located in the internal half of the breast—that is, the patient with a higher probability of involvement of the internal mammary chain—then the results of radical mastectomy are only 52%, and the results of radical mastectomy plus internal mammary chain dissection are much better (71%), a difference that is highly significant. There appeared to be no difference between the two treatments, but there was a balance between the bad results of the overtreatment in the former cases, and the good results of adequate treatment in the latter cases. I think this is by no means specific for surgery or radiotherapy in general—overtreatment is bad, and undertreatment is even worse. The problems are to try to define the groups and choose an adequate treatment.

As a side effect of this trial it has been possible to carry out a control trial, but with nonrandomized patients, in which patients without radiotherapy who were included in the trial were compared with patients who for geographical reasons were not included in the trial but who received radiotherapy. There is no significant difference in the 5-year survival rate for the two types of patients—71% and 63%, respectively. The recurrence rate was higher for patients without radiotherapy, and the metastasis rate was approximately the same for both groups, with no significant difference between them. However, if we again stratify the patients, this apparent lack of difference in survival rate between the two categories of patients is seen to hide much more important data. Considering the patient in whom the internal mammary chain was not involved, the 5-year survival rate for patients with postoperative radiotherapy is 71%, and 82% for patients without postoperative radiotherapy. The difference is not significant, but there is a trend for a better result in patients without radiotherapy. On the other hand, if we now consider the group of patients with involvement of the internal mammary chain who receive postoperative radiotherapy, the survival rate is 65%, compared to 47% for the patients without postoperative radiotherapy; here the difference is highly significant ($p < 0.001$). So again, just to take the routine treatment technique for all patients without trying to distinguish the group for which a more aggressive treatment is required may hide a very important problem.

Moving on to a very different problem, a few months ago we completed a study at Villejuif about the natural history of breast cancer. We measured the doubling time of the tumor on sequential mammography before surgery, or measured the labeling index of the tumor at the time of surgery by *in vitro* incubation with tritiated thymidine. Taking into account the average doubling time of the tumor, one can extrapolate to estimate the time of onset of the disease. I assume for this extrapolation that the tumor has an exponential growth; but, as mentioned by Dr. Carbone, this is not always true, and the growth rate might be faster at the beginning, but this does not make too much difference. Let us say that, on average, when the tumor is detectable, it has already been there for 9 years, with a wide range of from 4 to 20 years, based on our data on both labeling index and doubling time. Now let us consider the problem of metastases, which have a shorter doubling time than the tumor, indicating a faster growth rate. On the average, most of the metastases are detected between the second and third year; considering the second year, this means that the metastases were already there 2 years before the time the tumor was clinically detectable—again with a wide range, a few weeks or months to 5 years.

What conclusion can be drawn from this? It appears that there are two ways to improve the overall results. The first is earlier detection, as this would decrease the number of patients with metastases; on the basis of this model, one can calculate that for every 6 months of earlier detection, the incidence of metastasis would be decreased by 15-20%. This is not negligible but is not very much. The second is early treatment of metastases for patients with a high likelihood of dissemination, and here I completely agree with what has already been said by Drs. Carbone and Bonadonna. I think that if we can identify a group of patients with a high likelihood of metastasis, then it becomes very logical to try to treat them as soon as possible with chemotherapy.

Stjernswärd: Radiotherapy in breast cancer has a limited but well-defined role, and here I think both I and Dr. Tubiana completely agree. There are two questions. Because we have limited resources in oncology, one is the practical aspect, and the second is where does radiotherapy fit within this panel? For instance the pioneer on adjuvant chemotherapy, Dr. Nissenmeyer, has some data showing that adjuvant chemotherapy does not work in those groups when it is given at the time of, or after, radiotherapy. Without doubt there is a proven beneficial effect of local regional radiotherapy in some cases, but there are certain risk groups that worry me, and again I think Dr. Tubiana and I agree completely. If we find a 40% increased mortality by adding postoperative radiotherapy we must be worried. The second point is that few patients have local recurrence without distant metastases, and in Dr. Burn's study from Scotland there were only 4% in this category after 3 years. Therefore if you use routine radiotherapy, you perhaps irradiate 95% in vain. The data show that in uncontrolled disease at death there is no difference between the treated and the observed group who were treated later. Here again people who were not irradiated died without local recurrence, indicating that we irradiate perhaps 70% in vain. Those were the first true data, and now we are down to 95% by "prophylactic irradiation." There is no difference in prognosis after radical mastectomy for lesions medially situated as compared to lateral ones, which makes it very doubtful to argue, as Dr. Tubiana elegantly pointed out, that treating the internal mammary chain node does not necessarily affect the result, whether this is radical mastectomy removing the lymph nodes or irradiation. We also must consider the vascular pulmonary changes which carry a certain morbidity as an argument against radiotherapy.

Perhaps we diminish two things by giving radiotherapy to the tumor locally. There is a local effect. There are vascular changes which prevent the cytotoxic drugs reaching the tissue required. Then there is the systemic effect to the total dose of radiation tolerated by the patient, which is making him lymphopenic for a very long time. Thus we have to examine closely where radiotherapy fits in, if at all, in the adjuvant chemotherapy trials. There are constructive things we can do; we must find and identify the patients at risk because there are clearly those who benefit from postoperative radiotherapy. There may not be as many as we think, but we should try to find them.

Kenis: Dr. Hayward, will you give the advice of a surgeon about adjuvant chemotherapy with cytotoxic agents and hormone therapy?

Hayward: We heard Dr. Carbone, who is a chemotherapist, talking about surgery, so I think I, as a surgeon, can come back and talk about chemotherapy. There are only two points I want to deal with. One is an important factor, which we all have to face when we hear the results of clinical trials: When do we incorporate these results into our own practice? For example, we have heard the very exciting results of Drs. Carbone and Bonadonna's work on adjuvant chemotherapy. Should we then, as surgeons or radiotherapists treating patients with early breast cancer, now use chemotherapy routinely in our practice?

I think one has to bear in mind two things about this. One is that certainly on some of the regimens, and particularly Dr. Bonadonna's, the side effects are formidable, and one ought to remember this. Secondly, we ought to remember that we do not know if any of these regimens is tumorigenic, and indeed there is quite a possibility they may be in the future. So how should we face this? I suggest the following. If you have patients with four or more nodes involved, we know that the recurrence and survival rates of these patients is appalling—50% recur in 18 months, 80% in 5 years. From what we have heard today, and bearing in mind the difficulties, I think this sort of treatment ought to be adopted now, and one can afford to take these risks with this sort of wretched survival experience. However, if you have a patient—and let us suppose it is your wife—with one node marginally involved, do you give her chemotherapy? I feel that, with the information we have at the moment, bearing in mind the side effects and the possible tumorigenic effect, we ought to wait until we have longer follow-up data.

The second thing I want to mention is the question of surgery. As all of you are aware, for the last 30 years, clinical trials have been carried out, slowly and painfully, comparing radical mastectomy with simple mastectomy, simple mastectomy possibly with wide excision, different types of operation for the primary disease—on the whole getting more and more conservative. The results have always been, or look as if they are, that simple mastectomy (in stage I cases anyway) gives results as good as radical mastectomy (that is, with radiotherapy afterwards). Suddenly we are told that unfortunately this is not so any more. The results they give are not as *good* as radical mastectomy but as *bad* as radical mastectomy. So here we are as surgeons, having to read on Dr. Bonadonna's slides the following words: "the primary neoplasm and the regional nodes must be surgically removed." We are back 30 years. Do you know what you have done?

Kenis: This answers the question by Dr. Brennhovd, who asked how effective surgery had been in the curative treatment in breast cancer.

Carbone: The exciting possibility is not that we are competing with each other, but we are beginning to work as a team to treat the patient. I reemphasize that there is a role for all modalities, and the patient is going to benefit if we apply them correctly. The second point, in light of Dr. Bonadonna's presentation, is that there seem to be exciting possibilities. We have been stressing the advanced disease; chemotherapy certainly has been helpful to many patients, but it has not really been curative so people have been discouraged. My feeling is that it is an exciting possibility that we have something like L-PAM, which has a really modest minimal effect against advanced disease, decreasing the recurrence rate by at least 50% up to 2 years. My feeling is that we certainly do not want to make L-PAM in the radical mastectomy mold, where it will take us 40 years to find out if it works. Dr. Fisher and I have already started using two-drug regimen. We now have 300 patients on the second study, and these patients were collected within a matter of 6 months. The exciting possibility is that if the adjuvant situations seem to work in breast cancer, what about colon cancer? There you can almost substitute the same numbers—in other words, stage A is equivalent to stage 1, stage B to stage 2. Our object, therefore, is to find a regimen, not a curative regimen like MOPP, which is very intensive, but possibly a program that has a 20–30% or 40% treatment response in advanced disease, and put this in the adjuvant situation. We should be optimistic, and we should now do this in other tumors. We have a bench mark now of somewhere between 20% and 50% activity—not a highly curative regimen—that should be used in the adjuvant situation. This is the critical issue, the biological point being proved by these clinical trials that we have mentioned today.

Jungi: If adjuvant chemotherapy is effective, why not start it before surgery?

Bonadonna: Surgery is done for two reasons. First, to remove the slow-growing cells in the breast and axillary nodes; and second, to investigate further treatment of the disease on the basis not only of the presence of lymph nodes in the axilla but the number of those nodes, which is crucial in terms of relapse rate and survival. We know that it is very difficult to eradicate a tumor 5, 6, or 7 cm in diameter with chemotherapy because of the slow-growing proliferation of cells. Chemotherapy seems to be much more effective in distant foci of disease where the cells have exponential growth kinetics, at least during the first period of time.

Wybran: Is there a place for immunotherapy and adjuvant therapy, since in this instance we deal with a minimal number of tumor cells? Clinical results in recent leukemia studies are highly suggestive of a positive effect of immunotherapy.

Heuson: Pathological staging requires axillary node dissection and/or internal mammary node dissection, and if found positive and adjuvant chemotherapy is considered, is there a place for radiotherapy in between?

Tubiana: I think that axillary node and intermammary node dissection are not required. We know very well from the pattern of involvement of the axillary lymph node area that a biopsy at the bottom of the region is enough to know whether there is a high or low probability of involvement, so we need only a biopsy; most of the side effects are linked with dissection. Secondly, is internal mammary lymph node dissection required for staging? The study carried out by Dr. Vermès showed that it is possible to estimate the probability of involvement of the internal mammary lymph node just by studying a biopsy of axillary at the bottom. Now we come to the problem—what is the role of radiotherapy in between surgery and chemotherapy? In order to answer this question I think we have to remember that if a lesion is very bulky there is no doubt that surgery is the best way of treating it; if the lesion is small, radiotherapy is very effective; and if the tumor (either primary or metastases) is very, very small (less than 1 mm), chemotherapy seems to be the most efficient treatment. When a tumor is more than 1 mm, chemotherapy is much less efficient, probably because the drug does not reach all the cells of the tumor owing to the oxygen effect. When the tumor is small, there is no oxygen effect because oxygen reaches all the cells of the tumor, and there is a very critical distance between the vessel and the cell. It seems that 1 mm is approximately the critical mass that can be treated efficiently by chemotherapy. To my mind there is no opposition between radiotherapy and chemotherapy, as already pointed out, notably by Drs. Carbone and Stjernswärd. We must use all modalities of treatment possible. Certainly there is room for irradiation of the lymph node area found positive by surgery; here it is less mutilating and probably more efficient than surgery as long as the main mass has been removed by surgery.

Mattheiem: Dr. Heuson wanted to know if adequate radiotherapy will permit chemotherapy afterward, and it seems that this question was not entirely answered.

Tubiana: I do not have enough data to be able to answer that, but again I think you can extrapolate from our knowledge in other diseases. We know from Hodgkin's disease and from nonHodgkin's lymphomas that it is possible to treat efficiently with chemotherapy even after a very extensive course of radiotherapy. In Hodgkin's disease, for instance, it is possible to use MOPP even after total nodular irradiation, which is a very, very wide field of irradiation. I hope there is not much of a problem in giving chemotherapy after a very limited irradiation such as that which is carried out only on the axillary and internal mammary lymph node regions.

Zelen: Could you briefly review the experience of your institute on scientific comparisons of radical surgery with less radical surgery? If there are populations of patients who appear to have the same benefit with less radical surgery, would the medical oncologists recommend this practice plus adjuvant chemotherapy for this group?

Hayward: We compared radical mastectomy plus radiotherapy with wide excision of the lump with conservation of the breast plus radiotherapy in a series now comprised of nearly 800 patients. In the patients who had clinical stage 2 tumors, the patients who had wide excision were demonstrably worse off—they had a higher incidence of distant recurrence and they died earlier. In patients with clinical stage 1 tumors there was a higher incidence of local recurrence, but distant recurrence now at 10 years is identical. As I see it, the problem is that what we are now being told is that even in the stage 1 group (and we know our clinical stage 1 group in fact includes 30% stage 2, because our clinical assessment of the axillary is that inaccurate) we may now be able to do something about the recurrence, but we can only do this effectively by an axillary dissection, and not by axillary node biopsy. There has to be an assessment of the extent of disease, which is all important, and as far as I can see this can be done only by an axillary dissection, which is usually performed nowadays by radical mastectomy. Possibly there might be some future in terms of conservation of the breast with a total axillary dissection in addition. I know of no evidence whatsoever that the sort of regimens that are now being used would be effective in the presence of axillary lymph nodes which are involved with secondary carcinoma, regardless of whether they have been treated by radiotherapy.

Anonymous: What is the meaning of the fourth axillary node?

Carbone: It means that the prognosis is related to the number of nodes involved, but in our experience 1–3 out of 4 is as bad as say 1–3 out of 20. There are some people who feel that it is the percentage, and others (for instance the people at Memorial) feel that it is the level of the nodes. Apparently in their current trial they found that to look at the level of the nodes carefully and scientifically is a very difficult procedure to do on a routine basis, so they are also now looking at 1–3 nodes versus 4 or more. One other point is that right now it is the axillary nodes status that is important to determine prognosis. As I stressed before, one out of four patients with negative lymph nodes is going to recur until we somehow are able to identify those patients. I feel that we need some immunochemical or biochemical marker for this. If the immunologists really want to help us in breast cancer, they should work on giving us a marker so that we can say that a patient postoperatively does or does not have disease left. The therapeutic aspect certainly is helpful and immunology has a tremendous role to play, but a marker is what we really need. If we had something like the HCG assay, we could say with confidence to the patient that the tumors are all gone, and then give chemotherapy based on the marker without the node status. It would simplify the surgical procedure, and it would certainly enable us to answer the question of how long and how intensively to treat. To my way of thinking, this is the most critical area of research in breast cancer.

Stjernswärd: There are very good, clear markers like the CAE, the HCG, and the fetal macroglobulins, but unfortunately these markers work (with a 66% positive rate) only when you have a stage 3 or 4 tumor. We cannot use these markers in stage 1 and 2 disease where we would most like to, but they are very useful, or could be, in the palliative treatment for recurrence.

Burny: Have we thought enough about why the exact number of metastatic axillary nodes is important, or why the size of the primary affects prognosis?

Tubiana: This is a problem we have tried to answer in our model. The probability of dissemination is linked to two parameters. The first one is the number of tumor cells in the tumors; and the second is the probability of migration, which varies very widely from tumor to tumor. For instance, it might be linked to such factors as edema and local congestive reaction; the higher the probability of migration, the greater the number of lymph nodes involved. So lymph node involvement is probably not a prognostic factor *per se,* but it helps to evaluate the probability of migration of a tumor cell.

Spittle: Coming from England, where the National Health Service is stumbling to a halt, may I point out the economic problems associated with this very large group of patients who are going to suddenly flood all radiotherapy or chemotherapy departments needing high doses of chemotherapy, which is extremely expensive? Can we ask those who are organizing prophylactic trials to keep an eye, not only on patient convenience, but also physician convenience, and to make sure that we will not be pouring half an ampule down the drain every time we open one of those expensive things?

Bonadonna: We try to be as precise as possible with dosage. I wish that all the people involved in this trial could be here now so they could explain the efforts in following this large number of patients. We set up a very good system; our research nurses know how to give the drugs, and the patients know how to approach the nurses and be approached in terms of treatment. This is very simple, but it takes a number of years to set up; nevertheless at least in our country, Italy, the drugs are covered by insurance so that patients are not supposed to spend money. I am perfectly aware of the efforts, but if treatment is going to be successful (and probably it will take another year or two to prove it for sure) all these difficulties will be overcome by the fact that the results will force physicians and patients to find a solution from the practical point of view.

Carbone: This is an important point. This is exactly why our philosophy, at least with Dr. Fisher, was to try to do this as simply as possible. The temptation was to use six, seven, or eight drugs. I think our data can tell us how much needs to be done and how much can be avoided and this is very critical.

Breast Cancer: Trends in Research and Treatment, edited by J. C. Heuson,
W. H. Mattheiem, and M. Rozencweig. Raven Press, New York © 1976.

Endocrine Status of Women with an Enhanced Risk of Breast Cancer

R. D. Bulbrook

*Department of Clinical Endocrinology, Imperial Cancer Research Fund Laboratories,
P. O. Box 123, Lincoln's Inn Fields, London, WC2A 3PX, England*

There are three main reasons to search for factors that might identify women with an enhanced risk of breast cancer. The first of these is the acquisition of basic physiological information concerning the mechanisms whereby normal breast cells become malignant and progress to clinical cancer. The second reason is that identification of strong determinants of risk might lead to the possibility of intervention, in the hope that the incidence of the disease might be reduced. A clear analogy is with lung cancer. Cigarette smoking appears to be one of the main causative agents, and measures to reduce tobacco consumption should eventually lead to a reduction in the death rate from this disease. It should be noted that this result could be brought about even if there were no knowledge whatsoever about the biological mechanisms involved. The same argument could be advanced for many industrial carcinogens.

The third reason to search for high-risk groups is that physical methods for the detection of early breast cancer seem to reduce mortality. It is neither practical nor desirable to screen entire populations, however, and any method of identifying women for whom screening would be advantageous would be extremely useful.

The first question to be asked, therefore, is whether sufficient information already exists to enable us to achieve any of the three aims listed above, or if new research is required. If the latter is the case, which areas of exploration might be the most profitable?

RISK FACTORS IN BREAST CANCER

Over the last hundred years a number of factors associated with either an increased or a diminished risk of breast cancer have been described. The chief of these are family history, previous breast disease, age at menarche, age at menopause, age at first baby, premenopausal ovarian status, ethnic group (probably in association with gross national product rather than with genetic susceptibility), religion, social class, height and weight at menopause, excretion of urinary androgen metabolites, and the ratio of urinary estriol to estrone and estradiol.

The majority of these factors are not particularly strong determinants of risk. For example, the increase in risk for women who have a menarche at 11 years of age is only approximately twice as great as that for women with a menarche at 17 years. There are certain categories of women where a given family history is associated with extremely high risk (e.g., 20-fold) but these are rare, and the large majority of women with breast cancer have no familial history of the disease.

Several of these factors are highly correlated and are not additive in their effects on incidence, although satisfactory studies on this aspect of the problem have yet to be carried out. Women with several unfavorable factors do not necessarily run a disproportionate risk when compared with women who have only one high-risk factor present.

The risk factors are not of the same importance in all populations. For example, many retrospective reports indicate that there is an enhanced risk associated with early menarche, but recent work has shown that this correlation is entirely absent in a case-control study carried out in England. More studies from many areas are needed. The correlation between a given factor and risk may not be constant with time: There has been a dramatic increase in the incidence of breast cancer in the large cities of Japan (T. Hirayama, *personal communication*). Under these new circumstances there is no guarantee that correlations between risk levels and age at menarche, etc., still hold. They may be swamped or diminished in importance by new factors. We are not dealing with the immutable laws of physics but with a dynamic situation.

A final complication is that a favorable factor may cancel out the enhanced risk associated with an unfavorable factor. In a prospective study in Guernsey (C. C. Spicer, *personal communication*), it was shown that the increased risk associated with subnormal excretion of androgen metabolites is diminished or abolished by the favorable factor of an early first baby, and vice versa (1).

In our own limited experience with some 50 breast cancers developing in the Guernsey study population of 5,000 women, there was no marked concentration of the classic risk factors (early menarche, late menopause, late first baby, previous breast disease, family history). The strongest predictor of risk was a subnormal excretion of androgen metabolites (2). In summary, it seems improbable that the factors currently known to correlate with risk of breast cancer are sufficiently powerful to be of use in the precise identification of women who are going to develop breast cancer. At best, androgen assays would pick up 80% of the potential cancers, but the risk group would consist of 30% of the population (2).

If these arguments are accepted, it follows that a strong case can be made for searching for new indices of risk. The question is where to look. In view of the vast amount of work on the relation between endocrine function and breast cancer, it appears logical to concentrate on this aspect of the problem.

HORMONE IMBALANCE IN ANIMALS AND MAN

Mammary carcinoma can be induced in many strains of rats and mice by a variety of endocrine manipulations. The underlying concept from the older work with laboratory animals is that "endocrine imbalance" is a key factor in mammary carcinogenesis, and this concept has had a considerable influence on the direction of research in man. Over the last 20 years, a great deal of effort has been expended in attempting to prove that a comparable imbalance exists in women at risk or in patients with breast cancer.

The epidemiological findings noted above have also been interpreted in this light. The inference drawn from the results is that the ovary plays a key role in human breast cancer, and the case has been argued persuasively by MacMahon and colleagues (3). Reduced to the simplest possible terms, it is envisaged that early menarche and late menopause enhance risk by exposing women for a longer period to the carcinogenic action of estrogens. Removal of the ovaries from premenopausal women for reasons other than cancer reduces risk, and the supposition is that the protection is brought about by a diminution in exposure to estrogens. If estrone and estradiol are carcinogenic in women, the beneficial effects of an early first pregnancy are difficult to explain since these hormones are produced in large quantities during pregnancy. Cole and MacMahon (4) suggest that estriol, which is produced in disproportionately large quantities during pregnancy, exerts a protective effect and blocks the action of estrone and estradiol. Among its other merits, this hypothesis preserves intact the original concept of hormone imbalance as an important factor in the genesis of breast cancer in women, a concept for which there is so much support from experimental data in laboratory animals.

ENDOCRINE STATUS IN HIGH-RISK GROUPS

If the inferences drawn from epidemiological work on man and from direct experiments with laboratory animals are correct, it would not be unreasonable to expect that a condition of endocrine imbalance might be detectable in women at high risk or in patients at first diagnosis. Admittedly, the work of MacMahon and his colleagues (5) focused attention on the possibility that very early events might determine life-long risk. Even so, not all risk factors act in this way: Oophorectomy carried out at the age of 40 still diminishes incidence. Weight and height seem to be indices of risk only after menopause. The fall in incidence of breast cancer after menopause in Asian countries is difficult to explain in terms of all-important events occurring at an early age; at least one more factor must surely operate at a later stage. For these reasons, direct measurements of endocrine status in high-risk groups and in patients are certainly worth consideration. The logical choice for such investigations would be the estrogens, progesterone, and prolactin.

While there is still much work to be done, the present results do *not* support the concept that endocrine imbalance is an important factor in the genesis of breast cancer. For example, our own series of women with benign breast disease have plasma estrogens and progesterone levels within the normal range. The majority of women with a family history of breast cancer have normal plasma prolactin values with only a few cases falling outside the normal distribution (7). Kwa and his colleagues (8) showed recently that the circadian rhythm in such women may be abnormal, with a prolongation of the 1900-hr peak. The abnormality, while statistically significant, is small. The normal British population might be considered as a high-risk group when compared with the Japanese. We have been usable to find any significant differences between plasma estrogen, progesterone, and prolactin levels in normal British and Japanese women aged 16–70 years (9; *unpublished observations*). As a broad generalization, therefore, no striking endocrine abnormalities have yet been detected in women with an increased risk of breast cancer.

ENDOCRINE STATUS AT DIAGNOSIS

The bulk of the evidence indicates that patients with breast cancer at diagnosis have normal basal levels of plasma prolactin and a normal response to stimulation by thyrotropin-releasing factor (TRF) (10). We have found plasma estrogen and progesterone levels within the normal range, and differences reported by other workers appear to be small.

DOSE-EFFECT CURVES

While it must be admitted that the endocrine data for high-risk groups or for patients with breast cancer are tenuous, current results support the generalization that estrogen, progesterone, and prolactin levels are within the normal range or that the deviation from normality is minimal. If dose-effect curves for most biological assays are considered, it is usually necessary to increase the dose by a factor of 10 to achieve doubling of a biological effect. In the case of (C57BL $\times$ CBA) F_1 orchidectomized mice bearing pituitary isografts and given estrone in their drinking water for 300 days, estrone concentrations of 1.25, 12.5, 250, and 1,000 μg/liter led to plasma prolactin levels of 0.3, 0.5, 2, and 6 μg/ml: a thousand-fold increase in dose giving a 20-fold increase in effect. In terms of tumor yield, a 200-fold increase in estrone concentration led to an increase in incidence from 33% to 67%. If estrogen brings about its effect via prolactin, then a seven-fold increase in prolactin leads to a doubling of tumor yield (11).

If women are at all comparable, the question must be asked whether the minor endocrine differences so far reported are of such magnitude that they could be expected, in dose-effect terms, to make a substantial difference to incidence, even over very long periods of time. It seems improbable.

POSSIBILITY OF "MAXIMUM ENDOCRINE RISK"

If the proposition so far advanced that the endocrine environment in women at risk and in patients at diagnosis is normal were true, what inferences might be drawn? The first would be that the endocrine system may be already set at a maximum or near-maximum risk level; i.e., the different levels of risk within a population are not now dependent on differences in endocrine function or on hormone imbalance.

This point may be best illustrated by reference to the Anglo-Japanese results already mentioned. Endocrine status appears to be identical in the two populations. Incidence, especially after menopause, is different; and in extreme old age the Japanese incidence is 10- to 20-fold lower than that in Britain. It would follow that the difference in incidence between the two races must depend on factors other than hormones. It is also necessary to consider the incidence of prostatic cancer in Western countries and in Japan. In the latter prostate cancer is rare; whereas in the former it accounts for some 13% of all male cancers. Yet the incidence of latent carcinoma is almost identical in Japan and in Western countries, and rises inexorably in both countries with increasing age. It could be argued that if hormones are involved in the genesis of prostatic cancer and if hormonal status is similar in Japanese and Caucasian men (as it is in their womenfolk), then the difference in clinical expression resides in determinants other than the hormones. The second inference from the suggestion that the endocrine system is "set" at near-maximum risk is that further measurement of endocrine status may not prove to be particularly valuable for identifying women at high risk either for possible schemes of intervention or for selection for physical screening.

ANDROGENS

The androgens are the one class of hormone consistently found to be abnormal in high-risk groups and in patients with breast cancer. Subnormal excretion of urinary androgen metabolites has been found prospectively in precancer cases in Guernsey (1, 2), in women with a family history of breast cancer (12), in nuns (13), in women with benign breast disease (14), and in patients with breast cancer (15). Surely, it could be argued, this is the postulated endocrine abnormality that has been sought for so long.

Unfortunately, the physiological role of the androgens in normal women is not at all clear, especially in terms of the breast. Within the range of androgen titers found in normal women, it remains to be proved that these steroids have any marked effect on breast structure and function. (We should ignore experiments showing destruction of breast tissue in young rodents with pharmacological doses of androgens.) Furthermore, while there appears to be a reasonable correlation between risk and androgen levels in Caucasians, this is totally reversed in Japanese women. Their urinary and plasma androgen levels are significantly lower than those in Western women (16; D. Y. Wang et al., *personal communication*), and rural Japanese women excrete a lesser amount of androgen metabolites than their urban counterparts who have a greater incidence of breast cancer (T. Kodama and M. Kodama, *personal communication*). In the Guernsey prospective study, the curve relating risk to androgen metabolite excretion is suspiciously steep (2). Taken at face value, halving the androgen level leads to a sixfold increase in risk.

Intuitively, this relationship might be better explained, not in terms of a hormonal effect on breast tissue, but on the supposition that the androgens are correlated with other and more fundamental factors concerned with the development of breast cancer.

IMMUNOLOGICAL STATUS AND RISK

The most interesting finding in the Anglo-Japanese study noted above was that the lymph node sinuses in a high proportion of Japanese patients with breast cancer were invaded by histiocytes, whereas this was a rare event in British patients (17). Taken in conjunction with the equivalence of endocrine function in the two races, there is at least the possibility that immunological factors may be important in explaining the differences in incidence, and it may be that the relation between the endocrine and immune systems should be explored in any further searches for high-risk groups.

REFERENCES

1. Spicer, C. C. (1973): Androgens and age at first birth in relation to risk of breast cancer. In: *Host-Environment Interactions in the Etiology of Cancer in Man,* edited by R. Doll and I. Vodopija, pp. 159–162. International Agency for Research, Lyon.
2. Bulbrook, R. D., Hayward, J. L., and Spicer, C. C. (1971): Relation between urinary androgen and corticoid excretion and subsequent breast cancer. *Lancet,* 2:395–398.
3. MacMahon, B., Cole, P., and Brown, J. B. (1973): Etiology of human breast cancer. *J. Natl. Cancer Inst.,* 50:21–38.
4. Cole, P., and MacMahon, B. (1969): Oestrogen fractions during early reproductive life in the aetiology of breast cancer. *Lancet,* 1:604–606.
5. MacMahon, B., Cole, P., Lin, M., Lowe, C. R., Mirra, A. P., Ravnihar, B., Salber, E. J., Valoras, V. G., and Yuasa, S. (1970): Age at first birth and breast cancer risk. *Bull. WHO,* 43:209–221.
6. Swain, M. C., Hayward, J. L., and Bulbrook, R. D. (1973): Plasma oestradiol and progesterone in benign breast disease. *Eur. J. Cancer,* 9:553–556.
7. Wang, D. Y., Bulbrook, R. D., and Hayward, J. L. (1975): Prolactin and risk groups for breast cancer. In: *Workshop Human Prolactin,* edited by H. G. Kwa, J. L. Touber, F. J. Cleton, and C. Robyn. Antoni Van Leeuwenhoek Ziekenhuis, Amsterdam.
8. Kwa, H. G. (1975): Prolactin and breast cancer. *Workshop Human Prolactin,* edited by H. G. Kwa, J. L. Touber, F. J. Cleton, and C. Robyn. Antoni Van Leeuwenhoek Ziekenhuis, Amsterdam.
9. Kumaoka, S., Abe, O., Utsunomiya, J., Bulbrook, R. D., Hayward, J. L., and Swain, M. C. (1973): Plasma oestradiol and urinary oestrogen metabolites in normal Japanese and British women. In: *Host-Environment Interactions in the Etiology of Cancer in Man,* edited by R. Doll and I. Vodopija, pp. 131–135. International Agency for Research, Lyon.
10. Mittra, I., Hayward, J. L., and McNeilly, A. S. (1974): Hypothalamic-pituitary axis in breast cancer. *Lancet,* 1:889–891.
11. Boot, L. M., Kwa, H. G., and Ropcke, G. (1973): Radioimmunoassy of mouse prolactin: Prolactin levels in isograft-bearing orchidectomized mice. *Eur. J. Cancer,* 9:185–193.
12. Wang, D. Y., Bulbrook, R. D., and Hayward, J. L. (1975): Urinary and plasma androgens and their relation to familial risk of breast cancer. *Eur. J. Cancer (in press).*
13. Pitt, P., and Sarfaty, G. (1974): Androgen metabolites in the urine of average women, nuns and women with regional and metastatic breast cancer. *Cancer Forum,* 1:27.
14. Brennan, M. J., Bulbrook, R. D., Deshpande, N., Wang, D. Y., and Hayward, J. L. (1973): Urinary and plasma androgens in benign breast disease: Possible relation to breast cancer. *Lancet,* 1:1076–1079.
15. Bulbrook, R. D., Hayward, J. L., Spicer, C. C., and Thomas, B. S. (1962): Abnormal excretion of urinary steroids by women with early breast cancer. *Lancet* 2:1238–1240.

16. Bulbrook, R. D., Thomas, B. S., Utsunomiya, J., and Hamaguchi, E. (1967): The urinary excretion of 11-deoxy-17-oxosteroids and 17-hydroxycorticosteroids by normal Japanese and British women. *J. Endocrinol.*, 38:401–406.
17. Friedell, G. H., Soto, E. A., Kumaoka, S., Abe, O., Hayward, J. L., and Bulbrook, R. D. (1974): Sinus histiocytosis in British and Japanese patients with breast cancer. *Lancet*, 2:1228–1229.

DISCUSSION

Tagnon: If you take any lymph node, irrespective of whether there is a breast cancer, and compare them for histiocytes in British and Japanese women, do you find the same difference?

Bulbrook: This has not been done. If the general Japanese population, for reasons unknown, have their lymph nodes filled with histiocytes, it would suit us very well—and even better if they do not.

Anonymous: Am I wrong in thinking that an American study found that there was a difference in excretion of one of the estrogen metabolites in Japanese women?

Bulbrook: Yes, McMahon and his colleagues found that the Japanese and most Asian populations excreted more estriol in relation to estrogen and estradiol. This was a urinary measurement, and I think they made a mistake in deducing that it reflected blood levels, because it does not. The plasma levels of the progenitors of these urinary metabolites are identical in our experience. Secondly, Longcope in Worcester has done a beautiful experiment in which he looked at the blood levels of estriol in women with widely different urinary estriol ratios and found them to be identical in all. This looks like a strange liver metabolism, a phenomenon produced by enzymes induced by the diet. However, I think it has nothing whatsoever to do with the etiology of the disease.

Breast Cancer: Trends in Research and Treatment, edited by J. C. Heuson,
W. H. Mattheiem, and M. Rozencweig. Raven Press, New York © 1976.

Critical Appraisal of New Early Detection Techniques

Agnes M. Stark

Women's Cancer Detection Society, Department of Gynaecological Oncology,
Queen Elizabeth Hospital, Gateshead, Tyne & Wear, England

Although the results of treating most cancers have shown considerable improvement in recent years, the survival rates for breast cancer are no better now than 50 years ago (1,2). There is ample evidence (3–6) to show that the smaller the lesion on diagnosis the better the prognosis. It has been estimated (7) that even in an organ as accessible as a breast it is seldom possible to palpate a tumor smaller than 10 mm, and in a fat breast not even one that size.

Eight years ago I set out to attempt the diagnosis of breast cancer in a preclinical phase (i.e., before there is a palpable mass) by screening well women. The basis of this work was the experimental evidence of Lawson (8), who showed that the area of a breast cancer was hotter than that of its surroundings and that this differential could by measured by assessing infrared emission from the skin. During the 1960s sophisticated equipment became available for the pictorial representation and measurement of infrared emission (i.e., thermograms); at about the same time, the technique of mammography greatly improved.

TECHNIQUE

The techniques I used in my screening program are clinical examination, thermography using Aga Thermovision, and film mammography using a Senograph with Kodak Industrial film and more recently vacuum-packed Du Pont Lodose film. I described the details of the technique previously (9,10).

Xerography was considered and rejected on the grounds of the radiation involved. A xerogram gives more information than a film mammogram in the young, highly glandular breast with little fat to give contrast, but screening programs should not include young women.

SCREENING BY CLINICAL EXAMINATION

During the time required to set up this project, screening by clinical examination was offered to a group of self-selected well women aged 40 years and older.

Seven hundred such women were examined, and 85% were considered to be clinically normal.

Of the other 107, 104 had knotty fibrocystic breasts and were later thermogramed and mammogramed, confirming the diagnosis. One woman had a palpable mass considered to be an adenoma. She refused biopsy and 12 months later was found to have a breast cancer. There was one patient with a 60-mm carcinoma with palpable axillary glands, and the final patient had skin dimpling but no palpable mass. Mammography suggested a carcinoma, and biopsy confirmed a 5-mm intraductal cancer.

Pick-Up Rate

By means of clinical examination, with mammography in selected women, this is a pick-up rate of two cancers in 700, only one of which was confined to the breast; i.e., the detection rate of early breast cancer was 1.4 per 1,000, which is considered to be quite inadequate.

INTERPRETATION OF FINDINGS ON THERMOGRAPHY AND MAMMOGRAPHY

A thermograph is a pictorial representation of infrared emission, and there are three basic patterns in the breast: 30% are of an avascular type, 60% show a linear vascular pattern, and 10% a mottled type of vascularity. Each woman has a characteristic thermal pattern that remains stable during her reproductive life unless she is pregnant. This fact is most useful when reviewing women, as any variation from the baseline pattern is an indication of abnormality.

The thermographic features which I consider abnormal are: (a) a localized area of increased heat emission, or hot spot (a differential of 1.5°C or more is significant); (b) localized increased vascularity; (c) increased heat of the areolar area, particularly if the breast is fatty; and (d) generalized increased temperature of the breast. The essential element is comparison of symmetrically opposite areas, as well as an overall impression of the heat pattern, using one breast as a control for the other. For some years only relative temperatures were employed in breast thermography, but with increasing interest in the possibility of computerization absolute temperatures are assessed now.

The mammographic features of an early malignancy are (a) an opacity which may be circumscribed or stellate in outline and have a clear halo due to edema; (b) microcalcification in or adjacent to an opacity, or in a localized group without an opacity; and (c) localized increased vascularity. A generalized increased density of the breast and edema or thickening of the skin are late signs.

RESULTS OF FOUR-YEAR PROJECT

These are the results of a 4-year project during which two groups of well women were screened.

Screening by Clinical Examination and Thermography

The first group of 4,621 self-selected well women, aged 21–75, were screened by clinical examination and thermography, and with mammography when either of the first two examinations was abnormal. Six of the women had asymptomatic clinical cancers; the thermogram had been negative in one and abnormal in the other five.

There were 628 women (13.6%) with abnormal thermograms, and they were investigated further by mammography. Forty-two of the mammograms were positive for malignancy, and biopsy was recommended. Biopsy confirmed 27 cancers, 22 of which were preclinical; the other 15 were negative for malignancy, i.e., epitheliosis, adenosis, fat necrosis, etc.

Sixty-two mammograms were considered to be suspicious for malignancy and for early follow-up; 326 were abnormal but negative for malignancy (i.e., showed dysplasia, cysts, or fibroadenomas); and 198 were negative. Among the suspicious group of 62, 9 were found at repeat mammography after 6 months to have a progressive lesion that proved on biopsy to be cancer; thus thermography may indicate malignant change at a time when the lesion is too small to be demonstrated on X-ray films.

As these figures show, thermography plays no part in the differential diagnosis of breast conditions; the temperature difference can be as great with a fibroadenoma as with a very invasive carcinoma. Because of the relatively high incidence of abnormal thermograms, this alone has not been considered an indication for biopsy but is used purely as an index of suspicion. It does call for further investigation by mammography, with early follow-up should the latter be negative.

Pick-up Rate

Using clinical examination with thermography as an initial screening, with subsequent mammography when the thermogram is abnormal, there was a detection rate among 4,621 well women of 27 asymptomatic cancers, 22 of which were preclinical—i.e., an overall pick-up rate of 5.8 per thousand, and for preclinical breast cancer 4.8 per thousand. If women under the age of 35 are excluded from this group, there was a pick-up rate among 3,543 well women of 7.6 per thousand, 6.2 per thousand being preclinical.

For some years now I have not accepted women under the age of 35 for screening. With my limited resources, I consider that I must concentrate my efforts on the older women since only 3% of all breast cancers occur in women under 35 (3,11); also, it is unwise to submit young women to annual radiation exposure. On the other hand, I consider that a lower age limit of 50 years, as in some screening projects (12), is too high: In my clinic 6.4% of the cancers found have been in the age group 35–39 years and 55% in the age group 40–49 years, so that 61.4% would have been missed if my lower age limit had been 50.

False-Negative Rate

Breast cancer is such a complex clinical problem that criteria for false-negative screening are debatable. I consider the result to be a false-negative if a clinical lesion develops within 12 months of a negative screening test. Seven women in this group developed a clinical lesion within 1 year. Including the patient with a clinical lesion who had a negative thermogram, this gives a false-negative rate for thermography of 1.7 per thousand women screened.

Screening by Clinical Examination, Thermography, and Mammography

A second group of women, considered to be at higher than average risk of breast cancer, have been screened by clinical examination, thermography, and mammography. Women were assigned to this group when they had:

1. A previous abnormal thermogram and/or doubtful mammogram.
2. A family history of breast cancer, especially in their mother or a sister.
3. No children or low parity. Women who had had their first child after age 35, irrespective of subsequent parity, were also included.
4. A past history of a benign breast lesion or knotty fibrocystic breasts.
5. A late menopause.
6. A history of endometrial cancer.

(Now any woman who has been treated with one of the reserpine group of drugs is included in this high-risk category.)

Up to May 1972, 2,684 women, aged 33–70, in one or more of these categories, had been screened by clinical examination, thermography, and mammography. Thirty-nine of these women had biopsies because of clinical findings, revealing 14 cancers. Eighty-three biopsies were done on clinically normal breasts that had an abnormal thermogram and/or mammogram. Of these 83, there were 52 cancers, 3 adenomas, 3 cases of fat necrosis, 1 with normal tissue containing much fine calcification, and 24 cases of papillomatosis, epitheliosis, etc., 10 of which were very severe with many active cells—a histological picture which some people consider to be premalignant (13–16).

Pick-up Rate

This gives an overall pick-up rate of 24.5 asymptomatic cancers per thousand, of which 19.3 per thousand were preclinical cancers. It should be emphasized that these women were selected as being "at risk.'

False-Negative Rate

In this highly selected group, the false-negative rate for thermography was 6.3 per thousand, while the false-negative rate for the overall screening by clinical examination, thermography, and mammography was 1.49 per thousand.

TABLE 1. *Pick-up rates on annual review of high-risk well women*

Year[a]	Rate per 1,000 women
1970	11.4
1971	4.5
1972	13.2
1973	5.4
1974	8.0
1975 (first 6 months)	7.0

[a] Project commenced in 1968.

Since the completion of this 4-year project, I have continued to screen women by this routine, concentrating on the high-risk group. The pick-up rates have been maintained, and the false-negative rate for those screened at least 12 months ago is 1.9 per thousand women screened.

ANNUAL REVIEW

At the same time, an active attempt has been made to review all the women in the high-risk group at annual intervals. The follow-up rate is 82.9%. The pick-up rates in these rescreened women are as shown in Tables 1 and 2. I consider that rates of 4.5 to 13.2 per thousand (Table 1) justify annual rescreening of high-risk women.

The rates for the fifth and sixth reviews in Table 2 are low because a smaller number of women have been attending the clinic for 5–6 years. Also, in 1941 Muir (15) postulated that *in situ* breast lesions may be present for several years before becoming invasive. It may be that most of these *in situ* lesions are found during the first 5 years of screening. If this trend continues, however, the routine of annual rescreening after the fifth year may have to be reconsidered.

ACCURACY OF SCREENING

It was found that the accuracy of screening was greater in the case of preclinical cancer when both the thermogram and the mammogram were abnormal than when biopsy was performed on the grounds of an abnormal mammogram alone (Table 3).

Of 40 women submitted to biopsy on the grounds of only an abnormal mammogram, 40% were found to have cancer and 2.5% to have a possibly premalignant lesion (e.g., gross epitheliosis, papillomatosis); but in 108 women with both an abnormal thermogram and mammogram, 64.8% had histologically proved cancer and 27.8% lesions of a premalignant nature.

For a screening program to be successful, there must be a coordinated team involved, with a surgeon and a pathologist interested in such work. It is essential that the biopsy specimen is X-rayed to ensure that a nonpalpable lesion is included

TABLE 2. *Annual review at which cancer was diagnosed in high-risk well women*

No. of annual reviews	% of total pick-ups in rescreened women
1	46.5
2	16.6
3	14.3
4	17.7
5	2.4
6	2.4

in the biopsy. The frozen section technique is not applicable to this type of biopsy in which there is seldom a macroscopic lesion. I have found it worthwhile to do a scrape smear of the surface of the area of the lesion as located by X-ray films of the biopsy. Similarly, needle or drill biopsy is applicable only when there is a palpable lesion.

CONCLUSION

There is no doubt that it is possible to diagnose breast cancer in a preclinical phase, but it has yet to be shown that this will materially improve the long-term results, as it takes no account of tumor type or host response. At least 10-year results are required to allow for the lead time. After 8 years of screening, I am feeling cautiously optimistic because none of the women who had a preclinical lesion have yet shown any evidence of spread.

ACKNOWLEDGMENTS

This work is financed by the Women's Cancer Detection Society of the North-East of England. I wish to acknowledge the cooperation of my technical staff and the invaluable help of Mrs. Carole Lawson in preparing the manuscript.

TABLE 3. *Influence of thermogram on final diagnosis in women submitted to biopsy in the absence of clinical indications*

Thermogram	Total No.	Histologically proved cancer		Premalignant lesion		Benign lesion		Negative biopsy	
		No.	%	No.	%	No.	%	No.	%
Thermogram positive Mammogram positive	108	70	64.8	30	27.8	7	6.9	1	0.5
Thermogram negative Mammogram positive	40	16	40	1	2.5	21	52.5	2	5

REFERENCES

1. Gershon-Cohen, J. (1967): Diagnosing breast cancer earlier. *Lancet*, 1:1389.
2. Fisher, B., Nelson, H. S., Bross, I. D. J. (1969): Cancer of the breast: Size of neoplasm and prognosis. *Cancer*, 24:1072.
3. Dunn, J. E. (1969): Epidemiology and possible identification of high risk groups that could develop cancer of the breast. *Cancer*, 23:775.
4. Forrest, A. (1970): Cancer of the breast—early diagnosis. *Br. Med. J.*, 2:465.
5. Gershon-Cohen, J. (1969): *Postgraduate Med.*, 45:84.
6. Strax, P., Shapiro, S., and Venet, L. (1968): In: *Prognostic Factors in Breast Cancer*, edited by A. P. M. Forrest and P. B. Kunkler, p. 242. Livingstone, Edinburgh.
7. Lawson, R. (1957): Thermography—a new tool in the investigation of breast lesions. *Can. Serv. Med. J.*, September: 517.
8. Lawson, R. (1956): Implications of the surface temperatures in the diagnosis of breast cancer. *Can. Med. Assoc. J.*, 75:309.
9. Stark, A. M., and Way, S. (1974): The screening of well women for the early detection of breast cancer using clinical examination with thermography and mammography. *Cancer*, 33:1671.
10. Stark, A. M., and Way, S. (1974): The use of thermovision in the detection of early breast cancer. *Cancer*, 33:1664.
11. Haagenson, C. D. (1956): *Diseases of the Breast*. Saunders, London.
12. Sellwood, R. A. (1975): Feasibility of clinical and radiological screening for breast neoplasm. *Proc. R. Soc. Med.*, 68:434.
13. Muir, R. (1934): Pathogenesis of Paget's disease of the nipple and associated lesions. *Br. J. Surg.*, 22:728.
14. Muir, R. (1939): Carcinoma of the breast. *J. Pathol.*, 49:289.
15. Muir, R. (1941): The evolution of carcinoma of the mamma. *J. Pathol.*, 52:155.
16. McLaughlin, C. W., Schinken, J. R., and Tamisica, J. X. (1961): A study of pre-cancerous epithelial hyperplasia and non-invasive papillary carcinoma of the breast. *Ann. Surg.*, 153:735.

Breast Cancer: Trends in Research and Treatment, edited by J. C. Heuson, W. H. Mattheiem, and M. Rozencweig. Raven Press, New York © 1976.

Theory of Early Detection of Breast Cancer in the General Population

Marvin Zelen

State University of New York at Buffalo, Buffalo, New York 14226

During the past 10 years there has been an accelerated interest in the early detection of breast cancer utilizing special screening programs. Much of this interest has been motivated by the pioneering study carried out by the Health Insurance Plan of Greater New York (HIP) (1,25). This study utilized both a clinical examination and X-ray mammography in a program of periodic screening. The reported results of this program indicated a one-third decrease in mortality due to breast cancer. These encouraging conclusions prompted the initiation in 1973 of a National Breast Cancer Demonstration Project in the United States in which 26–30 institutions would periodically screen 10,000 women annually over a 5-year period.

The interpretation of the HIP results in reference to nationwide public health programs requires careful consideration of the available data. It has not been generally recognized that data obtained from screening examinations generate significant biases that are subtle and not immediately recognizable. The objectives of this paper are to: (a) discuss the general background of screening programs; (b) review the HIP study; and (c) discuss the cost implications for large public health programs modeled on the early detection procedures associated with X-ray mammography and clinical examinations.

GENERAL THEORY OF SCREENING PROGRAMS

Background

The two principal questions which arise in evaluating the efficacy of early detection screening programs are:

1. How much earlier is the disease detected by the early detection program as compared to the time when the disease would have been detected under routine medical care?

2. What is the relation between earlier detection of the disease and increased benefit from therapy? Are there more cures? Do people live longer?

These questions are related to one another and depend on the natural history of the disease. The latter is defined as the biological events which would occur if the course of the disease had not been interrupted by treatment, as well as those biological events which happened from the inception of the disease until treatment.

Consider the detection of breast cancer. It is a widely held belief that the smallest tumor that can be detected by palpation is that which has a 1 cm diameter. If we make the idealized assumptions that the tumor started with a single cell, 10 μm in diameter, and experienced exponential growth with a doubling time of 100 days, then it would take approximately 8 years for the tumor diameter to reach 1 cm. (The estimate of a 100-day doubling time is not out of line with current experimental evidence.) Figure 1 describes this situation. The time from inception of disease to the visible tumor state may be called the *preclinical phase* and the time after that, when the tumor is "visible," is called the *clinical phase*. During the clinical phase it appears as if the tumor is growing very rapidly, but this is only the result of its exponential growth.

Had the disease been surgically removed when it was still localized, the treatment would have resulted in a cure and the patient would lose no years of life because of the disease. On the other hand, if the disease is diagnosed and treated after it has spread, treatment of the primary tumor does not result in a cure. The patient eventually dies with metastatic disease and a shortened life (Fig. 2). Therefore even if the disease is found early, it does not result in increased benefit if the disease has already metastasized.

Now consider a population of women having breast cancer. There may be a period during which all the women have localized disease. If diagnosed and treated, all are cured, resulting in no years of life lost because of the disease. As time goes on and the disease is not diagnosed, some women enter the metastatic

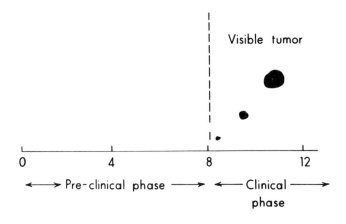

FIG. 1. Relation of early detection of disease to natural history. (Assumption is that tumor doubling time is 100 days and a tumor in the clinical phase is palpable.)

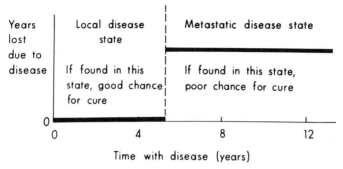

FIG. 2. Years of life lost due to having disease versus time with disease for an individual patient.

disease state and the population consists of a mixture of localized and metastatic disease. The average years of life lost for this population then becomes positive and continues to increase with time as more individuals in the population enter the metastatic disease state. Eventually almost all women in the population destined to go into the metastatic disease state will be there. The years of life lost due to having disease then no longer increase with time and approach an asymptote. Figure 3 shows this situation; the time scale can be divided into three parts: a *local phase,* a *local-metastatic phase,* and a *metastatic phase.*

It is clear that the value of an early detection program depends on: (a) the phase in which standard methods of detection find the disease; and (b) whether earlier detection of the disease results in a larger proportion of cases having treatment during the local or local-metastatic phase.

An early detection program is of small value if it succeeds in detecting disease significantly earlier but the bulk of the cases are in the metastatic phase. Alternatively, if the curve depicting time at detection versus years lost because of disease

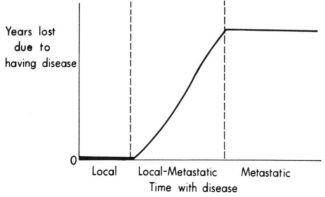

FIG. 3. Years of life lost due to having disease versus time with disease for a population of patients.

has a sharp slope in the local-metastatic phase, a relatively short earlier detection time may result in substantial therapeutic enhancement for the population.

Lead Time and Lead Time Biasing

It is convenient to have an "abstract" model for the natural history of the disease. Let us assume that an individual is in one of three disease states at any point in time:

Apparent disease-free state (S_o)
Preclinical state (S_p)
Clinical state ($S_{\hat{c}}$)

The state S_o signifies the state where individuals are disease-free or have a form of the disease that cannot be detected by the early disease detection program. The preclinical state S_p refers to the situation where the individual has the disease but is unaware of it. The early detection program is capable of identifying individuals in S_p. The clinical state Sc is defined as one where the disease has become clinical and is diagnosed. Throughout we shall assume that the idealized natural history of breast cancer is progressive, i.e., the individual goes from the apparently disease-free state, to the preclinical state, to the clinical state.

Consider a woman's individual natural history of breast cancer. The time history is depicted in Fig. 4. If the woman was fortunate enough to have participated in an early detection program, then she would have been diagnosed early. The cross-hatched portion of the line in Fig. 4 represents the time gained by early diagnosis. This is called the *lead time*. One of the important problems in evaluating a screening program is to estimate the mean lead time for a population

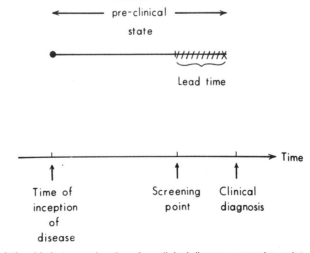

FIG. 4. Relationship between duration of preclinical disease, screening point, and lead time.

or a group participating in a screening program.

The problem of estimating the mean lead time does not lend itself to an obvious solution. If the disease is treated at the time of detection (in a screening program), then the disease is interrupted and it cannot be observed how long the individual would have gone until diagnosed under routine medical care. This problem was solved, however, by Zelen and Feinleib (3) using a stochastic model to represent the early detection process (4).

The value of an early detection program depends on whether women whose cancers are found early live significantly longer than those not participating in such a program. In judging if a woman actually lives longer, one must take into account the bias of finding the disease earlier. The origin for women found in an early detection program is at the point of earlier detection and treatment, whereas if the same women had been found by routine medical care the origin for measuring survival would have been advanced to the time at which the clinical disease had been detected. Thus even if the earlier detection does not result in increased therapeutic benefit, it would appear as if women found in an early detection program would live longer. This is called the *lead time biasing*.

Table 1 summarizes the history of a tumor that progressed to the preclinical state when the patient was 50 years old, metastasized when she was 55, and would cause her to die at age 62 if diagnosed and treated after the time of metastasis. Note that under routine medical care she would have lived 2 years after treatment, but if she was found by an early detection procedure after metastatic spread she would have had a 4-year survival. Of course she received no benefit from the earlier detection. Early detection simply resulted in longer observed time with disease.

Length-Biased Sampling

There is still another kind of bias which arises in early detection programs. It is due to the fact that the people found with disease by an early detection program

TABLE 1. *Hypothetical time history*

Event	Age (years)	Observed survival
Entered preclinical state	50	
Disease metastasized	55	
Early detection	58	4
Detection under routine medical care	60	2
Death	62	

cannot be considered as a representative or random sample of the general diseased population. Actually they have biologically different disease. Consider a population of women having breast cancer. The duration of preclinical disease varies from woman to woman according to some probability law. At a particular point in time this population is examined in an early detection program and those in S_p identified. Figure 5 summarizes this situation. The probability of detecting a case is equivalent to "throwing" a vertical line at random on the figure. The event of identifying an individual as being in the preclinical state corresponds to the vertical line intersecting a horizontal line. Clearly, longer horizontal lines are more likely to intersect the vertical line than shorter horizontal lines. In other words, individuals with a long preclinical duration of disease are more likely to be found. People with short preclinical durations tend to be diagnosed more quickly and present in smaller numbers in a screening program. Thus women with longer preclinical duration of disease tend to be picked up more often by a screening program. Undoubtedly women with longer preclinical durations have more slowly advancing disease and tend to live longer even if the early detection did not result in any therapeutic enhancement.

This phenomenon is called *length-biased sampling*. Thus people who are diagnosed by an early detection program do not constitute a random sample of preclinical cases. In other words, cases found by a screening examination tend to be less advanced.

Table 2 summarizes the HIP experience with patients having negative nodes at treatment. Note that the cases found at the screening examination have 63% negative axillary nodes compared to the reduced figure of 52% for those who were diagnosed between screening examinations. It is interesting that the (weighted) average of individuals not detected by screening and those who refused screening is 47%, which is close to the figure of 46% for the control group. This table merely confirms the results of length-biased sampling and *should not be interpreted as scientific evidence of an advantage for a screening program*. The detection program always selects cases with slower-growing disease, which in the case of breast cancer refers to women having less of a tendency for the disease to spread.

One way to confirm the existence of length-biased sampling is to examine the age at detection in an early detection program compared to the age at detection when individuals would be diagnosed under their usual routine medical care. One

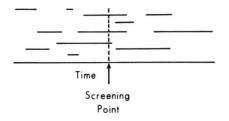

Time ↑

Screening
Point

FIG. 5. Population of individuals with varying duration of preclinical disease. Length of horizontal line represents duration of preclinical disease for an individual. (Observe that the vertical dashed line has a higher probability of intersecting a longer horizontal line.)

TABLE 2. *Proportion of breast cancer cases by histologic evidence of negative axillary node involvement*

Group	No. of cases	Proportion having negative nodes	Extent of disease unknown
Total screened group	296	0.57	0.04
Detected by screening	132	0.63	0.04
Not detected by screening	91	0.52	0.01
Refused screening	73	0.40	0.06
Control group (not screened)	284	0.46	0.05

Adapted from Shapiro et al., ref. 5.

would expect that if there existed two comparable populations—one of which was screened and the other observed (control group)—that the individuals detected in an early detection program would tend to be younger than those who become incident in the control group. The HIP program simulated this situation. Shapiro et al. (5) reported that the average age of diagnosis for women detected in the screening program was 54.9 years compared to 54.5 years for women incident in the control group. Thus the women found earlier tend to be slightly older than the average age of incidence. The difference is not statistically significant and for all practical purposes is the same.

How could women found earlier with asymptomatic disease have the same average age as women who are found when the disease is symptomatic? It appears to be a paradox. The explanation is that women who are found earlier in a detection program tend to be asymptomatic longer, i.e., have slower-growing disease. As a result, we have two compensating factors. Although the women are found earlier (and thus should be younger), they are selected by the length-biased sampling procedure and tend to be in the preclinical state longer and thus are older. When the average age at case finding is the same as that of incidence, then the duration of the preclinical disease follows an exponential probability law (3).

Periodic Screening

The discussion in the preceding sections has been mainly concerned with problems associated with an initial screen or a so-called "one-shot" screening program. Most programs involve a protocol in which individuals are screened periodically. The lead-time biasing and the length-biased sampling may be different for the first screen compared to subsequent screens. Theoretical results for periodic screening programs can be found in Hutchison and Shapiro (6), Zelen (7), and Prorok (8), the latter of whom discusses the problem extensively.

When the probability law for duration of preclinical disease follows an exponential distribution, the mean lead time for the initial screen and all subsequent periodic screens are the same. The estimate for the mean lead time under this assumption takes the simple form:

Mean lead time = prevalence of disease/incidence of disease

Zelen and Feinleib (3) discuss the above formula and prove that the necessary and sufficient condition for the duration of preclinical disease to follow an exponential distribution is that the average age at prevalence (detection) is the same as that of incidence.

The mean lead time for the HIP breast cancer screening program can be estimated from the first year's results. The investigators reported for the first year:

Prevalence $(P) = 55/20,166 = 2.73$ cases per 1,000 women

Incidence $(I) = 1.94$ cases per 1,000 women per year

Therefore an estimate of the mean lead time (L) is

$L = P/I = 2.73/1.94 = 1.41$ years $= 16.9$ months

Shapiro and colleagues (9) discussed the problem of lead time determination and estimated the lead time for the initial screen to be 7–8.4 months. This calculation is based on the questionable assumption that everyone detected by screening has exactly the same lead time. Their estimate for the mean lead time for the subsequent periodic screenings ranges from 11 to 13 months. The model on which these latter estimates are given requires further clarification.

Multimodality of Case Finding

The HIP screening program consisted of examining women utilizing both a clinical examination and X-ray mammography. Some cancers were detected by both modalities, whereas others could be found with only one. Shapiro et al. (5) reported that of the 132 cases detected by screening 33.3% were detected by mammography alone, 44.7% by clinical examination alone, and 22.0% by both modalities. Thus two-thirds of the cases could be detected if the screening program consisted of only a clinical examination.

In order to plan public health programs for breast cancer screening, one must attempt to evaluate the potential therapeutic enhancement for each case-finding modality. This is especially important when the different modalities vary greatly in cost.

The lead-time biasing and length-biased sampling depend on modality of case detection. One can envision that the disease in the preclinical state can be in one of three states corresponding to the means of case finding, i.e., clinical examination, mammography, or both. Although it may be conceptually possible to adjust for lead-time biasing by modality of case detection, there is no way at this time in which the length-biased sampling can be adjusted for modality of screening when both modalities were used simultaneously. This is an open problem in mathematical modeling. Screening programs especially designed to investigate the benefits of different screening modalities could supply answers.

HIP BREAST CANCER SCREENING PROJECT

Experimental Plan

In December 1973 HIP started a long-term randomized trial to determine whether periodic breast cancer screening with X-ray mammography and a clinical examination results in a reduction in breast cancer mortality (5). Briefly, approximately 62,000 women aged 40–64 years were randomly assigned to two groups, each of equal size. One group (called the study group) received an invitation to participate in the breast screening program; the other was simply observed and served as a control group. The women in the study group were offered an initial screening examination. Those who accepted were invited to three more screening examinations at annual intervals. Approximately 65% of the women assigned to the study group agreed to the initial screening examination. From this initial group 79% had a first annual re-examination, 73% a second annual re-examination, and 69% had all annual re-examinations. A total of 64,810 mammographic and clinical examinations were given to 20,166 women. The study is now in follow-up. This investigation represents one of the most interesting and certainly the best study ever carried out for the purpose of evaluating the benefits of a screening examination.

Mortality Results

The real test of the early detection program is if the screened group as a whole exhibited a reduced number of deaths from breast cancer. At the end of 5 years there were 40 breast cancer deaths in the study group compared to 63 among the controls. At the end of 7 years the cumulative figures were 70 deaths in the study group and 108 in the control group—highly significant results. This is a valid comparison of beneficial effect due to screening, and it is not biased by the lead time or length-biased sampling considerations discussed earlier.

Table 3 summarizes the death rates associated with breast cancer, as well as the total death rates from all causes by age at death. There is no therapeutic advantage to the younger age group induced by screening. The demonstrated significant reduction in mortality from breast cancer is confined to the women aged 50–59 years. It appears that there is an apparent advantage to the older group 60–69 years of age, but it is not statistically significant. One possible explanation is that there is a substantially elevated risk of dying from other causes in this age group. Hence any potential beneficial effects of breast screening would be "obscured" by the large number of deaths from other causes.

It is noteworthy that in the age group in which the screening program has

TABLE 3. *Death rates per 10,000 person-years by age of death*

Cause	Control group, by age at death			Study group, by age at death		
	40–49	50–59	60–69	40–49	50–59	60–69
Breast cancer death rates	2.4	5.0	5.0	2.5	2.3	3.4
Total death rates	23.6	52.5	103.8	25.3	53.0	100.4
Ratio	0.092	0.087	0.046	0.099	0.042	0.033

These data are based on first 5 years of follow-up after study.
Data from Shapiro et al., ref. 5.

proved to be effective (50–59), it only succeeded in reducing the deaths by 2.7 per 10,000 person-years—or over a 5-year period this figure results in an average *reduction* of 13.5 deaths per 10,000 women. Over the entire screened group the death rate (all ages) was 3.4 deaths per 10,000 person-years compared to 5.0 deaths per 10,000 person-years for the control group. Thus the net overall gain due to screening is 1.6 deaths per 10,000 person-years, which implies over a 5-year period an average reduction of 8.0 deaths per 10,000 women.

Benefit by Detection Modality

The benefits from early detection of breast cancer can result in: (a) a larger number of cures, or (b) prolonged survival even if the cancer is not detected in a curable state. In order to plan large-scale public health programs, it is important to evaluate the benefits of each detection modality. In this section we attempt to investigate the relative advantages of a screening program utilizing a clinical examination only, compared to both clinical and mammographic examinations.

Cancers in women in the HIP program could be detected by a clinical examination alone, mammography alone, or by both kinds of examinations. Table

TABLE 4. *Summary of breast cases detected according to initial or subsequent screen, detection modality, and age*

Detection modality	Age < 50	Age ≥ 50	Totals
Initial screen			
Clinical only	10 (63)[a]	14 (36)	24 (44)
Mammography only	3 (19)	18 (46)	21 (38)
Both modalities	3 (19)	7 (18)	10 (18)
Total	16	39	55
Subsequent screens			
Clinical only	9 (60)	26 (42)	35 (45)
Mammography only	3 (20)	20 (32)	23 (30)
Both modalities	3 (20)	16 (26)	19 (25)
Total	15	62	77

[a]Numbers in parentheses denote column percentages.

TABLE 5. *Case-finding rates if mammography omitted*

Age	Initial	Subsequent	Totals
< 50	13/16 = 0.81	12/15 = 0.80	25/31 = 0.81
≥ 50	21/39 = 0.54	42/62 = 0.68	63/101 = 0.62
Total	34/55 = 0.62	54/77 = 0.70	88/132 = 0.67

4 summarizes the HIP experience by modality of detection, age at detection, and whether the case was found during the initial examination or one of the subsequent screening examinations. (This table has been culled from various publications by the HIP investigators.) It is clear that the proportion of cases found by the different modalities is the same for the initial and subsequent screenings by age group.

Table 5 shows the case-finding rates had the mammographic examination been omitted. Overall, two-thirds of the cases would have been detected by the clinical examination. Furthermore, cases in older women would not be detected at the same rate as in younger women.

Another characteristic, which may reflect a beneficial aspect of the screening modalities, is the proportion of women detected who have negative axillary nodes. Table 6 presents this information by screening modality. (This table was culled from several HIP published papers.) As was pointed out above, cases found during a screening examination tend to have longer preclinical durations. Hence one would expect a higher proportion of negative-node patients compared to the control group. However, this information could be analyzed by modality of detection, as a comparable proportion of negative nodes would indicate comparable lead times.

Note that the proportion of negative nodes for either the clinical or mammographic examination groups alone is nearly the same and does not change depend-

TABLE 6. *State of axillary nodal involvement at time of treatment as a function of detection modality*

Detection modality	Negative	Positive	Total
Initial screen			
Clinical examination only	17 (71)[a]	7	24
Mammography only	17 (81)	4	21
Both	2 (20)	8	10
Totals	36 (65)	19	55
Subsequent screen			
Clinical examination only	28 (80)	7	35
Mammography only	17 (74)	6	23
Both	12 (63)	7	19
Totals	57 (74)	20	77

[a] Numbers in parentheses refer to row percentages.

ing on whether the case was found during the initial or subsequent periodic examinations. It is only those cases that could be found by both screening modalities where the proportion of negative-node cases depend on whether the case was found by the initial or a subsequent screen ($p = 0.03$). This observation implies that the duration of preclinical disease for cases found only by a single modality is the same and does not depend on whether the screen is the initial or a subsequent periodic examination. Hence the biases due to lead times and length-biasing sampling would be the same for each modality. However, those cases found by both modalities may have lead times that depend on whether the case was detected at the initial or a subsequent screen.

The HIP investigators reported that the control group over the 5-year period of observed incidence had 46% negative axillary nodes. This allows one to obtain an *upper bound* to the increased proportion of negative-node patients discovered solely by mammography. The proportion of negative-node patients discovered by mammography is $34/44 = 0.77$. It might be expected that if this group of women had received their usual routine medical care they would exhibit the same proportion of negative nodes as the control group. Hence the increase in proportion of negative-node patients solely due to mammography is $0.77 - 0.46 = 0.31$. This figure is an upper bound, as the 0.77 figure is "inflated" owing to the length-biased sampling; i.e., we estimate from available information that the increase in discovery of negative-node patients from mammography was 31% at most. Since 44 cases were found solely from a mammographic examination, it would be expected that (on the average) $(0.31)(44) = 13.6$ cases were detected in women with negative nodes because of the mammographic examination; these women would have had positive nodes at the time of detection if left to routine medical care. This is an upper bound due to the length-biased sampling problem.

Another way to attempt to judge the therapeutic enhancement associated with mammography is to regard the procedure as having the same therapeutic benefit as a clinical examination. This is not unreasonable owing to the comparable figures on nodal involvement associated with both detection modalities. Among the 132 cases found by a screening modality, $44/132 = 0.33$ were detected only by mammography. Since at the end of 7 years there were 38 fewer deaths in the screened group, one could attribute $(0.33)(38) = 12.67$ of this reduction to the use of mammography. It is interesting that this figure is approximately the same as the upper bound of the number of additional negative-node patients detected by mammography. Thus the estimated contribution of mammography to raising the cure rate is $12.67/20,166 = 6.3$ per 10,000 women screened.

Costs of Mammography Screening

The cost of a single mammographic examination is approximately $40. Table 7 summarizes the case-finding rate and costs of detecting a cancer using mammography. The overall cost per case found by mammography is nearly $59,000. Similarly one could also calculate the costs on the basis of a gain of 13.6

TABLE 7. *Case-finding rate and costs per case found for mammography ($40/examination)*

Mammography	No. of mammograms	Cases found only by mammography	Case-finding rate (per thousand exams)	Cost per case
Initial	20,166	21	1.04	$38,411
Subsequent	44,644	23	0.515	$77,642
Total	64,810	44	0.679	$58,918

additional negative-node patients (who may be positive if detected at a later time and 12.67 "cures" induced by mammography. The costs are $185,000 per "cure" or per negative-node patient.

Clearly the costs shown above and in Table 7 nullify the use of mammography as a general public health measure to detect breast cancer early in an asymptomatic population. The use of mammography should be confined to high-risk populations.

On the other hand, if one wants a public health program for early detection that uses only a clinical examination, then only two-thirds of the cases found by using both mammography and a clinical examination would be detected. Assuming that the cost of a clinical examination is $5, then an early detection program which uses only a clinical examination will result in 5.4 times more cases detected compared to a combined mammography program having equal costs.

Radiation Hazard

A recent investigation by Bailar (10) concluded that there is a serious possibility of radiation hazard to women undergoing mammographic examinations. Bailar estimated that the HIP early detection program may generate up to eight additional cases of breast cancer among the 20,166 screened women for each 10 years of follow-up. This induced breast cancer would require an approximate 10-year latency period. He points out that the evidence for this radiation hazard is not conclusive and requires additional information and study. Nevertheless, although the hazard is undoubtedly small for each woman, when multiplied by the total number of mammographic examinations in the HIP study, Bailar concludes that there "seems to be a possibility that routine use of mammography in the screening of asymptomatic women may eventually take almost as many lives as it saves."

SUMMARY

This chapter reviews the general theory of screening for early disease. The concepts of lead time and length-biased sampling are discussed in relation to the interpretation of data from early detection programs. The HIP breast cancer screening program is reviewed and the value of both initial and subsequent periodic screens discussed. Among the conclusions are that: (a) the cure rate associated solely with mammography is estimated to be 6.3 "cures" per 10,000 women screened (on the average, 3.2 mammograms per woman); and (b) for equal costs an early detection program utilizing a clinical examination will find 5.4 more cases than are found using both clinical and mammographic examinations.

ACKNOWLEDGMENT

This research was supported by Public Health Service Grant CA-10810 from the National Cancer Institute.

REFERENCES

1. Shapiro, S., Strax, P., and Venet, L. (1971): Periodic breast cancer screening in reducing mortality from breast cancer. *J.A.M.A.,* 215:1777–1785.
2. Strax, P., Venet, L., Shapiro, S., Gross, S., and Venet, W. (1970): Breast cancer found on repetitive examination in mass screening. *Arch. Environ. Health,* 20:758–763.
3. Zelen, M., and Feinleib, M. (1969): On the theory of screening for chronic diseases. *Biometrika,* 56:601–614.
4. Zelen, M. (1974): Problems in cell kinetics and the early detection of disease. In: *Reliability and Biometry,* pp. 701–726. Society of Industrial and Applied Mathematics, Philadelphia.
5. Shapiro, S., Strax, P., Venet, L., and Venet. W. (1973): Changes in 5-year breast cancer mortality in a breast cancer screening program. In: *Proceedings: Seventh National Cancer Conference,* pp. 663—678. American Cancer Society and National Cancer Institute.
6. Hutchison, G. B., and Shapiro, S. (1968): Lead time gained by diagnostic screening for breast cancer. *J. Natl. Cancer Inst.,* 41:655–681.
7. Zelen, M. (1971): Problems in the early detection of disease and the finding of faults. *Bulletin of the International Statistics Institute,* Proc. 38, Session I, pp. 649–661.
8. Prorok, P. (1973): The Theory of Periodic Screening for the Early Detection of Disease. Ph.D. dissertation, State University of New York at Buffalo.
9. Shapiro, S., Goldberg, J. D., and Hutchison, G. B. (1974): Lead time in breast cancer detection and implications for periodicity of screening. *Am. J. Epidemiol.,* 100:357–366.
10. Bailar, J. C. III (1976): Mammography—a contrary view. *Ann. Intern. Med.,* 84:77–84.

Roundtable Discussion: Epidemiology and Screening

Chairman: H. J. Tagnon

Tagnon: Dr. Tubiana, do you agree with the very sobering view that we may kill as many patients as we save by giving them mammography, a view proposed by Dr. Zelen? Additionally you quote a study by Dr. Bailar. What evidence does he present on the hazards of radiation diagnosis?

Zelen: This is a study which will be published shortly and is based on figures from a study by the U.S. National Academy of Sciences on the hazards of low-level radiation. Dr. Bailar hedged his conclusion, and he does not say that these are facts, he just says that there seems to be a possibility. I do not know if the women who were involved in the screening program were advised that there was a radiation hazard, or if the 250,000 women who are currently involved in the demonstration project in the United States have been advised that there is a radiation hazard. However, if there is a possibility, and this is a view held by several people, it seems to me the women should have been informed that there is that potential risk.

Van Putten: A crude estimate was made in Holland based on some data on mammography equipment still widely available, giving a radiation dose at 1 cm depth, which if used would induce as many tumors as are detected. Of course, if you keep on detecting them the prognosis of those tumors will be relatively better, which implies that you will gain from the operation. Nevertheless, there is great urgency for improving the quality and the type of mammography and in using a low dose.

Tubiana: I agree that there is a possibility of reducing the doses given in mammography by a factor of 10 if we use modern equipment.

Zelen: It is a scientific fact that you can reduce the depth dose to about 0.2 of a rad with these newer systems, but let me remind you that the gain from mammography over 20,000 women screened on the average 3.2 times each is approximately 13 or 14 per 10,000. With regard to cure rate, this is a very small number indeed for the costs involved.

Powles: By choosing the high-risk patients for screening, may these not theoretically be the patients that are most likely to have radiation-induced tumors?

Van Putten: We must make an educated guess about extrapolation, and this is a situation where we just do not have enough data. It is unlikely that from the human material we will ever have enough, because to make this statistically significant we need data on several hundreds of thousands of patients.

Tagnon: Perhaps we could discuss the cost, because although human life is worth anything in terms of money we must consider priorities. Any money spent on detection cannot be spent on any other potentially more useful undertaking. The price quoted for detection was very high, and one wonders what could be done if this money were used for other purposes. I am very surprised that no one here has noted the possibility of biochemical detection of tumors. A start has been made in this area for certain tumors. Franchimont in Liege, for example, just published a very interesting study in which he showed that he can detect small amounts of casein in the blood of patients with breast cancer. Of course this is just the beginning, and there are some false-negatives and some false-positives; but one can imagine that with refinement such tests, combined with the already existing ones, could provide a very inexpensive way to detect the presence of a breast tumor—although this is still far away. Someone else, I think, has detected blood lactose levels in patients with cancer, but I am not sure if this has been confirmed.

Bulbrook: These biochemical markers must be regarded with enormous suspicion because what Barts Hospital or Franchimont in Liege calls a healthy population of normal controls are probably nice, healthy nurses. If you take people in off the street, these are walking sacks of drugs and disease. The moment you start looking at cancer in this population, and we have published this recently (or it may be just coming out), they look like nothing in the literature at all. We can find no differences between cancer in our controls—that is, in random women—and cancer cases except in very advanced disease. We have to take all these tests with enormous pinches of salt, although I agree with you that they ought to be done, because the calculation is that if you use a rather weak predictor such as the androgen assay you could probably knock the cost of finding tumor down in Britain from £ 8000 per tumor found to £ 2000. The experiment has yet to be done, however, and it would cost an enormous amount of money, whether the result was positive or not.

Anonymous: Dr. Stark, have you had any experience with liquid crystals in thermography?

Stark: Yes, but from what I have seen in other centers I would say it is very messy. Patients do not like it, and there is very much less definition.

Anonymous: Could you give us some more specific data on the danger of xerography compared to thermography and mammography?

Stark: With xerography you have to use a rigid casette, which means that in order to project the whole breast you need to take more than two views, which increases the radiation involved. I now use a plastic vacuum pack with a back screen so that you need to take only two views, which cuts down the radiation.

Clarysse: The reason we talk of early detection is because we believe that early detection leads to early treatment with resultant reduced morbidity and mortality. However, while we are awaiting effective means for early detection of cancers, we should at least make sure that those patients who do have tumors get proper treatment. A lot needs to be done in this area.

For example, I had a patient who in 1969 when she was 50 years old had a small localized tumor in the left breast, confirmed by mammography to be very suspicious. Clinical examination at that time showed no detectable axillary nodes. Unfortunately this woman was never referred by her general practitioner to a surgeon, radiotherapist, or medical oncologist. The GP treated her for 6 years with steroids, she developed cushinoid features, and eventually when she had massive infiltration of the axilla with edema of the left arm, the edema was treated with insertion of needles to drain out the fluid. The point is that while we spend a great effort in early detection we should not forget to ensure that those who do have signs and symptoms of cancer receive proper treatment. I am surprised every day in my daily practice, about how little physicians in general practice know of the current world-wide treatments and how often they are surprised to hear that cancer can be treated and that it is worth treating. So a lot needs to be done in the area of educating the primary physicians. We also need more cancer centers in Europe where we can ensure adequate treatment.

Tagnon: Can the virologists propose hypothetical methods of detection of cancer of the breast at the viral stage?

Schlom: This is not strictly a viral situation, but more one of tumor-specific antigens, which may be related to viral-specific antigens. An area in great need of pursuit and clarification is the identification and/or detection of breast tumor-specific antigens. One of the very recent studies, published a couple of months ago at the National Cancer Institute, used chromatography and chromo-gel electrophoresis to isolate specific fractions from membranes of human malignant breast tumor cells and other carcinomas compared to benign tumors. I believe that they have a breast tumor-specific antigen via skin testing, but this has not been followed up yet and work is continuing. This is a very important area of pursuit that may very well be related to viruses.

Bentvelzen: I do not see how we can delineate high-risk groups, which is what we are after, by looking for viral proteins. Looking at the family history does not make too much sense to me either, because many of us belong to a family in which breast cancer is common. There are a few high-risk cancer families, but these are exceptional; there is also some scanty evidence for the release of viral proteins or proteins related to known viral proteins. At the moment we have the technology available to trace them in the human population; and although some problems are still to be resolved, that might make sense in the near future. An epidemiological prospective study of a confined population, without much social mobility, might yield some kind of correlation between the release of viral proteins and the genesis of breast cancer in man. Once more I would emphasize that I do not think it will ever be useful as a tool; but in case such a correlation could be established in a few studies, we might think about antiviral methods.

Tagnon: Dr. Burny has been working on such a study in relation to leukemia.

Burny: Two or three years ago when I was in New York, we tried to correlate the presence of viral-reversed transcriptase in the blood of leukemic patients with the onset or diagnosis of the disease. Out of approximately 100 patients screened, we found transcriptase in three. In one of them with acute leukemia there was as much reverse transcriptase as free enzyme as in the blood of a leukemic mouse. We stopped that study because of the cost of the effort and the very poor results we finally got. Looking at these results now that 2 or 3 years have elapsed, maybe we could have expected that because the release of virus particles is probably exceptionally bad during the course of the disease. We are encountering the same type of problem and arriving at the same sort of conclusions in the bovine system, where there really is a strict correlation between the detection of viral protein and the presence of the disease. The viral protein is not reversed transcriptase, however, and does not look like it is bound to the presence of virus particles. Probably 2–3 years ago when we started that study we were too optimistic and made the wrong choice, but it does not mean that it is not worth going after viral markers or viral proteins now that we begin to know them better, at least in some animal systems.

Heuson: What is your interpretation, Dr. Stark, of the remarkable decrease in pick-up rate over the 5-year follow-up in high-risk women?

Stark: I think the reason for the remarkable drop in pick-up after 5–6 years is perhaps because during the first 4 years of screening the slow-growing lesions were already found. I think we must accept that breast cancer is like an iceberg, and that the clinical bit is only the one-eighth which is visible; and the other seven-eighths have been obscured for a long time.

Tagnon: Dr. Juret, what about those low-risk patients with cancer of the breast, i.e., women who have had a child early in life?

Juret: Let me draw your attention to two facts concerning the high-risk problem in mammary cancer—age at menarche and age at first pregnancy. Most of the studies on the relationship between age at menarche and breast cancer have concluded that the earlier the onset of menstruation the earlier the risk of breast cancer. In our center we have figures for the follow-up of more than 800 patients who were operated on by radical mastectomy, 500 of whom have been followed for 5 years. It is obvious that having had an early menarche is a factor for poor prognosis and is very significant at 1, 3, and 5 years. The 3-year follow-up on patients and the survival in relation to the age at menarche shows that patients who menstruated at 11 years or earlier have a poorer prognosis than the others, and if one compares this group with the others who menstruated later, the difference is significant ($p > 0.01$–0.001). At 5 years one finds exactly the same figures, but we have not enough patients and it is not significant. It seems that at 3 years, as at 5 years, the most favorable situation is to have been menstruating at 15 years.

We also studied the relation between the number of children and the risk of breast cancer. You will remember that the earlier the first birth the smaller the risk of having a breast cancer, and from these data we had thought that there was also a prognostic value in parity. We found exactly the opposite of what we expected; that is, women with no children had a very good survival rate of 80%. The rate falls with parity, and with more than 12 children the survival rate is only 55%. It therefore appears that what was previously thought to be a factor of high risk concerning breast cancer is a favorable factor. In conclusion, the notion of high risk is one that has to be interpreted with caution when considered in terms of the obstetrical history, since what appears to be a favorable factor as far as morbidity is concerned is unfavorable as regards mortality. Do we have the right to say that nulliparity is a high-risk factor even if it does increase the chances of disease, while it also improves the prognosis?

Concluding Remarks

P. P. Carbone

I want to add my congratulations to the organizers of the committee and thanks to Professor Heuson and Professor Tagnon for their kind hospitality on behalf of the Americans and others who have come from abroad. This has certainly been an interesting meeting.

I have been asked to say a few words about the concept of the Breast Cancer Task Force. Since the mid-1960s there has been in the United States an effort to form the Breast Cancer Task Force. By definition, a task force is an organization composed of some existing operational divisions; in other words, people are taken from various aspects of different programs, put together, and called a task force. A very important part of the task force concept is that it should not be perpetuated indefinitely. Although our task force had been formed in the 1960s, it became active only in 1970–71, under Dr. Berlin, who was then the chairman. It is interesting that Dr. Berlin's experiences are as a hemotologist; he has had practically no experience of breast cancer work but was given the responsibility by the NCI to organize the breast cancer program. It is my feeling that, as an administrator, he has done a tremendous job in getting the proper people together and finding out what had to be done. For a year or so we met and tried to develop the programs and then what we felt were high-priority items along various lines.

The Task Force is organized under the chairmanship of Dr. Berlin and is composed of consultants in the NCI, people from the internal organization, and others. It meets annually, and the steering committee, which is composed primarily of NCI individuals, representing all the disciplines, including virology, epidemiology, pathology, surgery, radiotherapy, chemotherapy, and endocrinology meets regularly. Part of this organization requires four separate committees on diagnosis, epidemiology, biology, and treatment. The chairman of the steering committee was once an individual from the NCI, but currently this is an outside person supported by an executive secretary who develops the activities of the committee. In each of the committees there is a consultant, usually representing outside people, people who are known in the field, people who are interested, plus those from the intramural program. This is a very large organization but in fact has developed into a very effective one. We have been interested in the Iceland study and have supported its activities in looking at epidemiological factors. The interesting point is that between 1840 and 1940 there has been a tremendous increase in the incidence of breast cancer along with, surprisingly enough, prolongation of the first menses; in other words, the age at first pregnancy has also correspondingly increased, and the reasons behind this are being investigated by the epidemiology committee. In terms of risk factors, I think there are groups working in Holland with the Cancer Institute looking at the question of height and weight. There are also groups, as mentioned by Dr. Zelen, looking at the detection of breast cancer and at the relative role of physical examination in terms of thermography and mammography. The breast screening projects are not under the Task Force directly, it is a conjoint program of what we call "cancer control" and the American Cancer Society. I think they estimate now that there are more than 100,000 women who have been screened at least once.

An important function of the Task Force is education. For example, there was a lot of scattered information on the estrogen receptors, so Dr. McGuire organized a meeting in Bethesda last summer in which all the people working on this got together. It was a very interesting meeting, and one that not only had the biochemists who were doing the methodology but also the clinicians and Dr. McGuire presenting data.

Our own committee is the Treatment Committee, and this has been working primarily in the area of clinical trials. We have also been developing projects in cell kinetics, in particular trying for very rapid methods, because, as you know, the long-term radiolabeled technique is somewhat tedious. One of our contractors feels that he can develop growth fractions and proliferation rates in a matter of hours. We also heard Dr. Bogden give a presentation earlier involving animal models, trying to determine what aspects of breast cancer could be predicted or determined from *in vitro* studies. We consider this to be very important. We have already heard a bit about markers, a very important aspect to breast cancer work. We certainly do not have the answer, and I have often said that if the biologists, virologists, or immunologists want to contribute something in this area, the marker deserves the highest priority.

We have described clinical trials, particularly the ones in adjuvant therapy and it has been estimated in the United States that there are approximately 80,000 breast cancer patients included in trials in 16 cooperative groups, five or six of which have research activities in breast cancer work. There are also contractors related to one of the programs of the Cancer Institute, but surprisingly enough until 1971 or 1972 none of these programs had fostered or developed a combined modality approach; it was done through Dr. Fisher. In addition to sponsoring activities, it is important to know what is going on, and there are many people who are willing to work together under different funding mechanisms to get the activities of the Task Force working. It is not necessary to control or direct, nor is it meant to do the only research, as far as I am concerned, in breast cancer treatment in the United States. However, it certainly is important for this group to identify the gaps, to find out what is going on and to stimulate and develop new projects, and this is basically what we did. We sponsored very little work in the area of advanced breast cancer, which is all done through the cooperative groups and others.

I agree with Dr. Bulbrook completely—we certainly are looking for a marker. There is no single marker, for example; there are elevated levels of CEA, HCG, and fetal macroglobulins in advanced disease patients, and roughly 97% of these patients do have evidence of one of these markers. There is no evidence to indicate that one marker is sufficient, and I think that what we are looking for particularly is some indication that there is a more sensitive marker that could relate to clinical course. In advanced disease, patients who fail to respond have a progressive decrease particularly in CEA, but we do not have a sensitive marker for the patients with N-positive disease who have no evidence of liver involvement. This is the critical area of research.

It is important not to get bogged down in repeating work that has been done elsewhere, and that the Task Force not be used as a political mechanism to get things done that only you want to do. It should be a mechanism to facilitate work that you think is important scientifically. One final point: what we are interested in is not to develop a single remedy or a single treatment—the proverbial chicken soup that cures all, that can be administered to all patients with breast cancer—but rather to develop a specific treatment for individual patients, to apply the right amount of surgery, the right amount of endocrine therapy, the right amount of immunotherapy or chemotherapy. This is a very important area of research that certainly will not only benefit the patients but will answer some important biological questions that might be helpful elsewhere.

As to cost, the Task Force started off with less than $1 million. It now has much more because as you get results you tend to get more support; many of the programs can be interrelated, and what you really want to do is not to support all the research but find out what has to be done and support those aspects. The Task Force, I suspect, supports less than 30% of all the breast cancer treatment research in the United States.

THE NEED FOR AN EORTC BREAST CANCER TASK FORCE

J. C. Heuson

I had the privilege of attending some of the task force meetings in the United States, and I was impressed by the success of its multidisciplinary work. This symposium has also been a success, and has demonstrated that the various disciplines working in a given field of cancer can communicate and successfully inform each other of the meaning of their respective researches. What really seems to be lacking in Europe is the mechanism by which these individual efforts can be coordinated to increase efficiency and to avoid duplication.

A year ago the EORTC Breast Cancer Co-operative Group decided to organize this symposium, and it also decided to make an attempt to create such a mechanism. We proposed that a small group be formed comprising clinicians, fundamentalists, and epidemiologists; the group would define its own operational rules and report to both the Breast Cancer Co-operative Group and the EORTC. Dr. Mattheiem and I were given the responsibility of selecting the core of this group. The first meeting took place last June in Geneva and was attended by some 10 people. All participants agreed on the principle of the task force and most agreed to be members of it. Additional members to be invited at the next meeting were proposed, and a steering committee was nominated. Objectives were discussed and were defined broadly as follows: first, to support research for a better understanding and treatment of breast cancer; second, to select key questions and formulate relevant research projects; third, to assess current and new approaches in research of treatment of breast cancer; fourth, to improve coordination between fundamental research and clinical investigation, implement this program, and finally critically appraise activities and make periodical progress reports.

In practice, an immediate objective should be to evaluate the socioeconomic impact of breast cancer in Western Europe, and if possible to assess the cost of treatment and of loss of lives. Such estimates would be instrumental in the justification of the task force activities and provide firm grounds in discussion with European, governmental, and other agencies. A second initial objective would be to make a catalogue of resources and activities in breast cancer research in Europe. Dr. Carbone is currently visiting cancer centers and laboratories and has offered to evaluate the potentialities in the field of clinical investigation. The various specialists of the task force might do the same in their own specialties. After this has been accomplished, the task force should carry out the specific and important objective of selecting key questions and formulate relevant research projects. In practical terms, it was proposed that the task force should hold meetings with four or five invited specialists in a given field; the corresponding specialists on the task force would select these experts and serve as their interpreters for the benefit of the other members. These discussions would result in the formulation of key questions and well-defined research projects. The latter would then be fostered and implemented according to feasibility either stepwise or at the end of a limited period of enquiry, say 1 year.

Financial support should be sought, especially when the projects have direct clinical implications in prevention, diagnosis, or treatment. At this stage no definitive decision was taken as to how the task force should be financially supported, especially to help in implementing specific research projects. It was expected and hoped that the EORTC will soon be successful in raising funds for such purposes. The task force will meet for a second time tomorrow, its agenda comprising several points, among which are: (1) consideration of additional membership; (2) definition of research projects and evaluation of socioeconomic impact of breast cancer in Europe; (3) constitution of working parties for a

European inventory of fundamental and clinical research activities and resources in the breast cancer field; (4) working plans and schedule of meetings for 1975/1976. The members of the task force at the present time comprise four medical oncologists, one clinical chemotherapist, two surgeons, one epidemiologist, one specialist in screening and diagnosis, one radiotherapist and immunologist, one virologist, one specialist in experimental tumor therapy, and one of molecular endocrinology. From the nationality standpoint, two members are from France, two from Germany, two from Belgium, two from the Netherlands, two from Britain, and one each from Italy, Sweden, and Switzerland. Dr. Carbone has agreed to work as consultant. The composition will be reconsidered in 1 year.

EORTC: Definition and Function

H. J. Tagnon

Service de Médecine et d' Investigation Clinque, Institut Jules Bordet, Brussels, Belgium

The European Organization for Research on Treatment of Cancer (EORTC) was created to stimulate and coordinate therapeutic research on cancer in Western Europe. It has an administration board, coordinating office, data center, and cooperative research groups active in laboratory and clinical research. It is a nongovernmental, multinational body that is supported by private donations and receives additional financial support from the Euratom to some of its laboratories. It has also been given a grant by the National Cancer Institute, Bethesda, Maryland (United States), which covers administrative and coordinating activities and has been an indispensable factor in the success achieved so far.

While it is true that each country of Western Europe has adequate research talents as well as good hospital and laboratory facilities, one important factor for success in many research areas is lacking: the continental, as opposed to the national, dimension of cancer research as exemplified, for instance, in the United States. National responsibility for research may be quite enough for certain programs, but by and large training in clinical medicine and research is more successful when carried out in a broader environment. The occasional exchanges of personnel and techniques as they take place among our small European nations are useful but insufficient. At the other extreme, worldwide organizations have their special usefulness, which is not primarily the training of research personnel or the production of original data and new concepts. In contrast, the rapid circulation of people and exchange of ideas with the resulting cross fertilization of minds and elimination of "parochial" types of planning and working is characteristic of the continental dimension as is well illustrated by medical science in the United States.

As the situation is now, much of the research potential of Europe is badly underused. For instance, the limited resources of a small or medium-sized nation may not be sufficient for the acquisition of certain types of equipment. Furthermore, despite meetings and symposia, there remains a basic deficiency of communications among scientists, leading to needless duplication of identical research in adjoining countries supported by distinct national foundations. Pharmacological and clinical research requires large financial investments, access to several well-equipped hospitals, extensive experimental support, and early availability of results to achieve speedy progress. The continental dimension of medical performance and training for research has lasting educational value and improves the general level of medical care throughout the continent, thereby making available everywhere the highest quality of medical care.

These factors have been invoked to explain the spectacular progress of medical research and especially clinical medical research in the United States, which contributes over 75% of the medical publications of the world. Another factor is the integration and continuous confrontation of multiple disciplines.

This is why the EORTC is committed to the promotion of "biomedical research," understood as a synthetic approach to laboratory and clinical science. Despite many declarations to the contrary, the distinction between basic and applied research appears to be entirely artifical. Progress in medicine results from clinical observation and experimentation, as well as laboratory work. The history of medicine demonstrates that new important data and concepts originate as often in the clinic as in the laboratory. While it is true that the majority of clinicians are not scientists, there is nevertheless a class of clinicians who have developed a scientific approach to clinical medicine and have acquired an experimental turn of mind. They are as scientific and basic in their approach to disease as the laboratory scientist. This type of clinician should be distinguished from the ordinary practitioner and be identified as a "clinical scientist." It is quite useless for laboratory and clinical scientists to oppose one another, as is too often done. The truth is that they should work together in biomedical research for better and more rapid results. This is why the EORTC promotes the association of laboratory and clinical scientists in definite programs and research projects.

The ultimate aim in cancer research is to find a treatment for the disease. This will come about more rapidly by constant communication among the workers at all levels than by exclusive reliance on one type of research. Ultimately, advances in biology and medicine are utilized for the treatment of patients, and this should be carried out in a strictly scientific manner, with a specific and sophisticated methodology, and considerable mathematical and statistical support. The *clinical trial,* a major and difficult undertaking, represents the culmination of the research effort and mobilizes all biological sciences. Results of significance flow from the clinical trial back to the laboratory worker, bringing him new ideas and orientation.

This free flow of communications needs developing in Europe, where laboratory workers as well as clinical scientists do not always have the modesty to realize that little can be achieved by proud isolation and dogmatic pronouncements on who will discover the cure of cancer and how it will come about. Actually, the cure of cancer is being discovered every day, and the most important contributions so far have come from workers who ignored the distinction between "basic" and "applied" research.

The EORTC is fulfilling a third function: By promoting therapeutic clinical research as a scientific discipline, it responds to the ethical obligation to advance knowledge and improve patient care. This obligation is binding on the whole medical profession and especially on clinical scientists working in institutions and hospitals supported by public funds since these make available to them the tools of research.

Subject Index